Laparoscopic Hepatectomy

Xiujun Cai

Laparoscopic Hepatectomy

Atlas and Techniques

ZHEJIANG UNIVERSITY PRESS
浙江大学出版社
Springer

Xiujun Cai
Department of General Surgery
Sir Run Run Shaw Hospital
Zhejiang University
Hangzhou
China

ISBN 978-94-017-9839-6 ISBN 978-94-017-9840-2 (eBook)
DOI 10.1007/978-94-017-9840-2

Jointly published with Zhejiang University Press, Hangzhou
ISBN: 978-7-308-14361-5 Zhejiang University Press, Hangzhou

Library of Congress Control Number: 2015939600

Springer Dordrecht Heidelberg New York London

Printed on acid-free paper

Springer Science+Business Media B.V. Dordrecht is part of Springer Science+Business Media (www.springer.com)

Foreword I

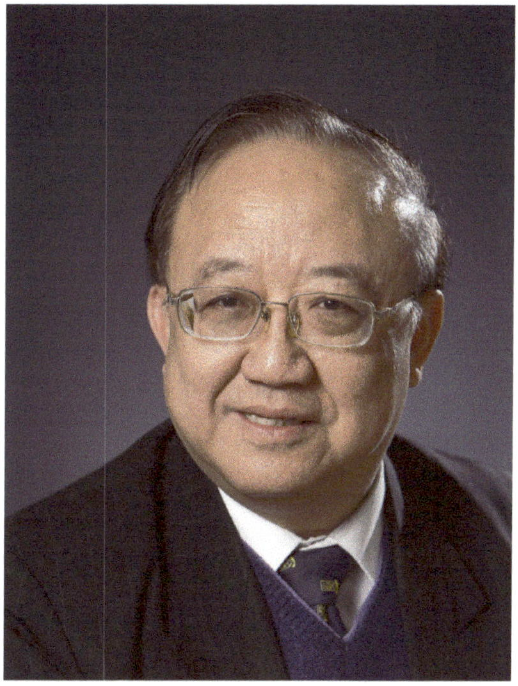

Surgery, which is as old as mankind, is an art of working with hands. The introduction of laparoscopic surgery has drastically changed the way in which surgeons operate. In the past two decades, laparoscopic surgery has invaded and conquered all bastions of open surgery. It is the first time in the history of surgery that such drastic and sweeping changes have occurred within such a short period of time. Even complex liver resectional surgery, which has always been considered as one of the most difficult operations in open surgery, can be carried out laparoscopically now.

This metamorphosis of surgical techniques has promoted how a change in a surgical atlas could be documented. Instead of the simple description of techniques by written words or by drawings, the use of a lot of high-definition digital operative photographs enabled by modern laparoscopic instruments has created a good instructional format to illustrate how a complex liver resectional surgery is carried out.

This book, *Laparoscopic Hepatectomy: Atlas and Techniques,* is written by Prof. Xiujun Cai. His operative techniques have been based on the procedures in open surgery, which he developed during his surgical training under Prof. Shuyou Peng. However, the translation of open techniques to the laparoscopic arena is entirely through Prof. Cai's own efforts, and these techniques are beautifully displayed in this book. Prof. Cai has also adopted the use of Peng's multifunctional operative dissector (PMOD), which was invented by Prof. Peng for safe liver parenchymal transection in open surgery, to laparoscopic surgery by extending the length of the stalk and modifying the aspiration system of the instrument to fit laparoscopic use. This instrument (the laparoscopic Peng's multifunctional operative dissector, LPMOD) can execute all the functions necessary for liver parenchymal transection including blunt dissection, cutting, coagulation, and aspiration. Thus, it decreases transection time by avoiding frequent changes of instruments. LPMOD is cheap, and with experience, it can be used to safely dissect out large vessels and bile ducts within the liver parenchyma for subsequent ligation, thus avoiding major bleeding or postoperative bile leak.

Another innovative operation which has been beautifully illustrated in this book is the completely laparoscopic ALPPS (associating liver partition with portal vein ligation for staged hepatectomy) using round-the-liver ligation to replace liver splitting in the stage I operation. Both the stage I and II operations have been shown clearly with digital operative photographs in this book.

I highly recommend this book to surgeons who have some experience in liver surgery, especially those who would like to extend their surgical techniques into laparoscopic liver resectional surgery. Even for surgeons who are experienced in laparoscopic liver surgery, there is a lot to learn by reading this book.

Lau Wan Yee Joseph, MD, DSc, FRCS, FACS, FRACS (Hon)
Academician, The Chinese Academy of Sciences
Hongkong, China
October 17, 2014

Foreword II

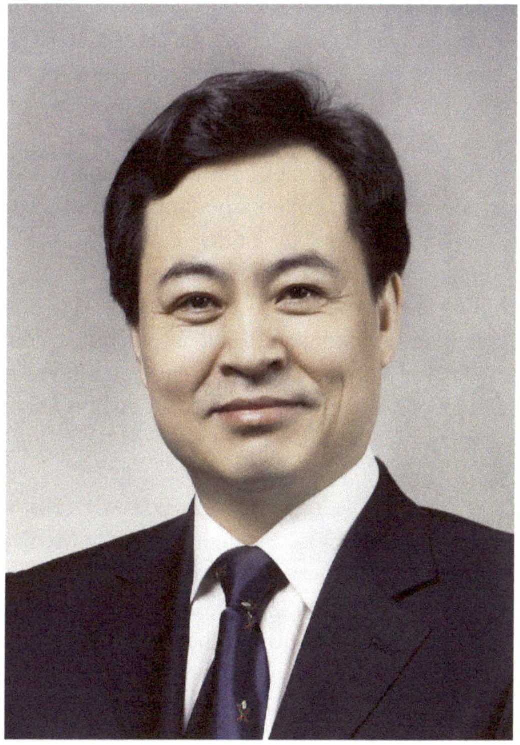

Laparoscopic hepatectomy first appeared in the 1990s and has been developing ever since. It is regarded as one of the most difficult procedures in abdominal surgeries because of the high risk of massive bleeding and performed as a routine procedure only in a few hepatobiliary centers in the world. Prof. Xiujun Cai developed an effective technique for laparoscopic hepatectomy by using the innovative instrument called the laparoscopic Peng's multifunctional operative dissector (LPMOD). He has completed a great number of cases of laparoscopic hepatectomy by curettage and aspiration, and all the cases make up the largest case resource pool in the world. Massive bleeding is the major complication of laparoscopic liver resection, which hinders the development of this procedure. In 1998, Prof. Cai started the research for laparoscopic liver resection, and procedures extended to hemihepatectomy, isolated resection of caudate lobe, and ALPPS, with technique innovations in decreasing or avoiding intraoperative bleeding.

Patients with malignant liver tumors require radical resections. Anatomical resection is usually performed on these patients but mostly with the open approach. Prof. Cai developed the technique of laparoscopic selective inflow occlusion, in which branches of the hepatic artery and the portal vein were occluded before the liver transection. This technique would facilitate the anatomical liver by decreasing the intraoperative blood loss. Laparoscopic hepatectomy by curettage and aspiration is an effective technique for the laparoscopic liver transection. Differing from other available instruments for liver resections, LPMOD could preserve and dissect vessels in liver transection. It is an instrument for meticulous dissection combining the function of cutting, coagulation, and aspiration, which makes it a satisfying instrument for transecting the liver parenchyma. These techniques and the instrument developed by Prof. Cai have solved the major problem in laparoscopic hepatectomy.

This book introduces the instrument, techniques, and procedures of laparoscopic hepatectomy by curettage and aspiration space with figures and videos including the introduction of initial cases of ALPPS using the round-the-liver ligation. All the figures and videos were collected from Prof. Cai's video recording and were carefully selected. This is a high-quality book about laparoscopic liver resection, and I am sure that this book would draw the attention of many hepatobiliary surgeons and could serve as a good textbook for young surgeons who are interested in hepatobiliary surgeries and laparoscopic surgeries.

Yupei Zhao, MD, FACS (Hon), FRCS (Hon)
Vice President, Chinese Medical Association
Chairman, The Surgery Branch of Chinese Medical Association
President, Peking Union Medical College Hospital
Academician, The Chinese Academy of Sciences
Beijing, China
December 24, 2014

Foreword III

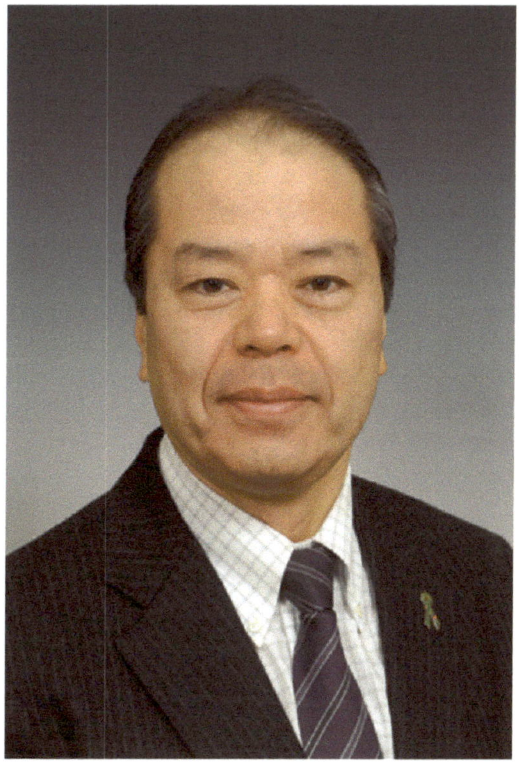

First of all, I would like to congratulate Prof. Xiujun Cai for his remarkable accomplishment of completing this book, entitled *Laparoscopic Hepatectomy: Atlas and Techniques*. I met him for the first time during my visit to his hospital in Hangzhou from August 2 to 4, 2009. He kindly welcomed us and showed his warmest hospitality during our stay. Prof. Cai hosted an international symposium on laparoscopic liver resection, so we had a meaningful time to observe his live surgeries and to discuss vividly regarding techniques and essentials in laparoscopic major hepatectomy. What amazed us most was his parenchymal transection technique. It is very speedy and simple. He knows the basic skills and essentials of laparoscopic parenchymal transection, i.e., meticulous dissection, direct visualization, and sealing of the vascular structures. This book is about his techniques regarding laparoscopic hepatectomy.

When I hosted the 2nd International Consensus Conference on Laparoscopic Liver Resection in Morioka, IWATE, from October 4 to 6, 2014, I invited Prof. Cai to serve as a member of the expert panel. He was assigned in a working group on a clinical question regarding "*What is the best technique for parenchymal transection?*" I believe he is one of the best laparoscopic liver surgeons in China and can represent this huge country in terms of both patient number and potentially largest market in the world. He has published numerous important articles on laparoscopic liver resection and knows how to perform laparoscopic parenchymal transcction speedily and efficiently as I observed from his live surgeries. Prof. Cai contributed a lot to create statements and recommendations on laparoscopic parenchymal transection. I have to mention one thing about the process of creating these recommendations. Although Prof. Cai insisted to include the laparoscopic Peng's multifunctional operative dissector (LPMOD) in these recommendations, it was not accepted by the writing committee because unfortunately, LPMOD is not used worldwide at this time.

I know LPOMD is a very useful device, and it is important to know the basic skills and essentials of laparoscopic parenchymal transection to perform this surgery safely and efficiently. I strongly recommend this book to be widely circulated and read by many liver surgeons who are involved or interested in laparoscopic liver resection. If LPOMD becomes widely used in the world with the help of this book, it will be mentioned with its name at the next consensus conference on laparoscopic liver resection for sure.

Go Wakabayashi, MD, PhD, FACS
Chairperson of the 2nd International Consensus
Conference on Laparoscopic Liver Resection
Tokyo, Japan
December 15, 2014

Foreword IV

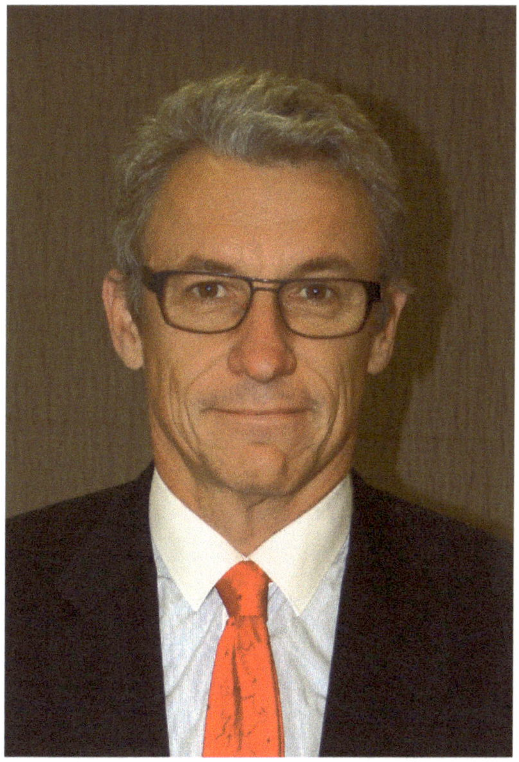

It gives me great pleasure to introduce this wonderful atlas of laparoscopic liver resection (LLR).

Since the first reports in the mid-1990s, LLR has been slowly accepted worldwide as an improvement on open liver surgery in many cases. Pioneers like Prof. Xiujun Cai have been very important in demonstrating the safety of LLR. Thanks to enthusiasts like Prof. Cai, LLR is much more widely practiced, as was shown at the recent 2nd International Consensus Conference.

Laparoscopic surgery of the liver can be more expensive, with many surgeons using disposable energy devices and multiple firings of linear staplers. I have had the privilege of visiting Prof. Cai and his team at Sir Run Run Shaw Hospital in Hangzhou. The skills of the surgeons were very advanced, and a complicated left hepatectomy and bile duct clearance was completed in

90 min! Not only was the surgery beautifully performed, but it was done with minimal expense and minimal blood loss using Peng's dissector and a few clips.

This book serves as a wonderful guide to both simple and advanced LLR. As such, it is of benefit to students and experts. Most importantly, patients will be the lucky ones as they can be offered safe, cost-effective liver surgery with much less pain.

Nicholas O'Rourke FRACS
President of the Australian New Zealand's Hepato
Pancreatico Biliary Association (ANZHPBA)
Brisbane, Australia
December 11, 2014

Foreword V

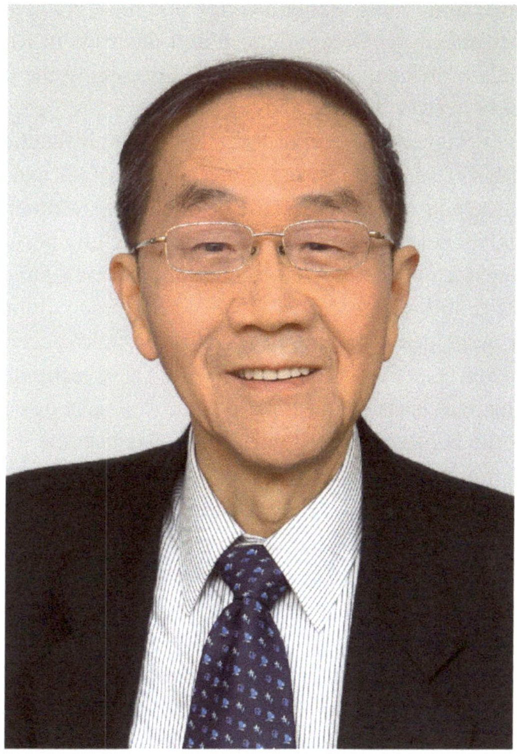

Xiujun Cai is my best student. In the 1990s, when he was a postgraduate, we worked together trying to develop a practical scalpel for liver resection as there were so many HCC patients waiting to undergo operation. We were anxious to have an instrument that is supposed to be simple but efficient, safe, and cheap, as we have been abiding by the maxim: The patient is the center of medical universe, around which all our works revolve and towards which all our efforts trend (Benjamin Murphy). Day in and day out, finally we designed a multifunctional dissector, which is known as Peng's multifunctional operative dissector (PMOD). This instrument can execute all the functions necessary for liver parenchymal transection, including blunt dissection, cutting, coagulation, and aspiration.

Usually, in the process of liver transection, we pursue the three-"I" principle, which is "Identification," "Isolation," and "Individually" dealing with.

That is to say, vessels and bile ducts in the parenchyma should be identified and isolated before being either divided or preserved. This is especially true when the transection is being carried out at a very risky area where some important vessels or ducts must be protected and preserved. The beauty of PMOD is its simplicity and versatility; using it, quite a variety of difficult HCCs, which were previously thought to be unresectable, are successfully resected. Up to now, the instrument is widely used in liver surgeries in China and some other countries even after the emergence of some expensive instruments for liver transection, such as harmonic scapel, CUSA, LigaSure, and so on.

Laparoscopic liver resection arose in the beginning of the 1990s, but it encountered huge difficulties. Being a young and most creative surgeon, Cai at that time was already very experienced and dextrous in using PMOD to perform all kinds of difficult liver resections. Foreseeing the developmental tendency of modern liver surgery and problems in laparoscopic liver resection as well, he designed the laparoscopic Peng's multifunctional operative dissector (LPMOD) as an improved version of PMOD and preliminarily established the technique of laparoscopic hepatectomy by curettage and aspiration on animal models. In August 1998, he successfully performed the first laparoscopic hepatectomy by curettage and aspiration on a patient with HCC, and this patient is still well and alive, free of recurrence. Subsequently, Cai established the technique of laparoscopic selective inflow occlusion for anatomical major liver resection in the early 2000s. These techniques effectively solved the problem of massive bleeding in laparoscopic hepatectomies. Since then, laparoscopic hepatectomy using LPMOD has become the most widely used procedure for laparoscopic liver resection in China.

In the past 16 years, Cai developed and established all kinds of laparoscopic procedures for different liver diseases and lesions using LPMOD and achieved very good clinical outcomes. "To study the phenomenon of disease without books is to sail an uncharted sea while to study books without patients is not to go to sea at all "(Sir William Osler). It is really necessary to write this book to introduce these original techniques and procedures to liver surgeons all over the world. With the anticipation that this book will represent a springboard for knowledge exchange that will not only benefit the clinicians but also the patients that they serve, I highly recommend this book to liver surgeons and residents who are interested in liver surgeries.

Shuyou Peng, MD
FACS (Hon), FRCSG (Ad eundem), ESA (Hon)
Professor of Surgery, Zhejiang University
February 11, 2015

Preface

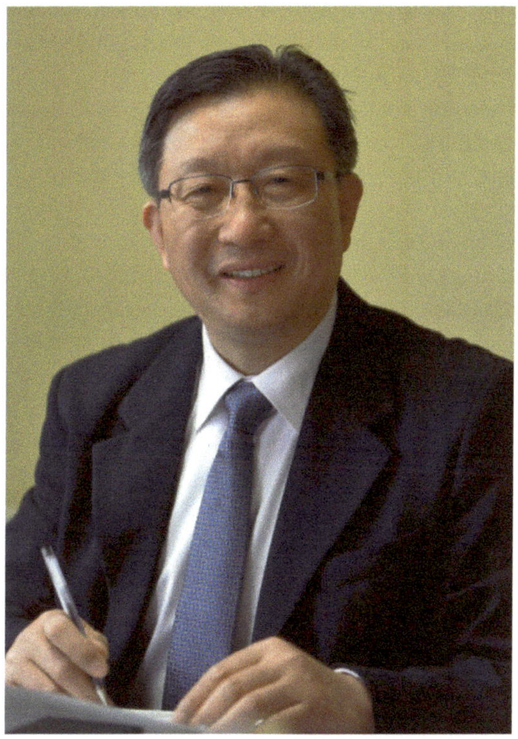

The laparoscopic approach, which has been adopted worldwide, allows patients a rapid return to daily activity with less postoperative pain. Even though the advantage of laparoscopic surgery is widely recognized by surgeons, laparoscopic hepatectomy is still a rarely performed procedure, as open liver resection is still the most widely used procedure for liver lesions in most hospitals worldwide. The main reasons include the difficulty of dissecting the intrahepatic vessels, the risk of intraoperative massive bleeding, and the inefficiency of mobilizing liver lobe in the laparoscopic situation.

We began to perform laparoscopic hepatectomy in August 1998. The technique of laparoscopic hepatectomy by curettage and aspiration was developed, and a special instrument, the laparoscopic Peng's multifunctional operative dissector (LPMOD), was designed. Local resection of liver tumors was the major procedure in the initial stage, and then, laparoscopic left lateral segmentectomy became the first anatomical liver resection in our institute, Sir Run Run Shaw Hospital, School of Medicine, Zhejiang University, and also became the major procedure performed in our institute before 2005. In 2005, laparoscopic left hemihepatectomy was performed as a routine procedure, and the technique of laparoscopic selective inflow occlusion was developed for controlling intraoperative bleeding. After that, anatomical major liver resections with selective inflow occlusion were performed routinely in our institute.

For the purpose of safe transection of liver parenchyma and of dissecting small vessels in the transection plane, a special surgical instrument was designed and was named LPMOD. This instrument could be used for blunt dissection, cutting, electric coagulation, and aspiration. It can execute all the functions at the same time, which facilitates the manipulation and decreases the operating time by avoiding frequently changing instruments. LPMOD was designed based on Peng's multifunctional operative dissector (PMOD), which was invented by Prof. Shuyou Peng and was used in open surgery. We extended the length of the stalk and modified the aspiration system to fit the laparoscopic purpose.

Blunt dissection is the major point of the technique of laparoscopic hepatectomy by curettage and aspiration. By using LPMOD, liver parenchyma can be crashed and aspirated immediately, the intrahepatic ducts and small vessels can be preserved and safely dissected for ligation, and massive bleeding can be avoided by the meticulous dissection. Laparoscopic selective inflow occlusion is routinely performed in anatomical major hepatectomies, including left hemihepatectomy and right hemihepatectomy. It is more technically difficult than total vascular occlusion, but it can avoid complications of ischemia–reperfusion injury and gastrointestinal congestion. Furthermore, the selective inflow occlusion does not require fast liver transection to decrease the occlusion time, which allows surgeons to have sufficient time for meticulous dissection. Total vascular occlusion is the conventional procedure for controlling intraoperative bleeding in open major liver resections and is used in some laparoscopic liver resections. It is easier to perform laparoscopically compared with the selective inflow occlusion. In our opinion, in local resections, especially in patients with severe liver cirrhosis, the occlusion tape could be placed before liver resection and total vascular occlusion executed only if encountering unmanageable massive bleeding.

Recently, a new two-stage surgery named ALPPS (associating liver partition with portal vein ligation for staged hepatectomy) is drawing the attention of surgeons. This procedure enables the rapid growth of the future liver remnant (FLR) and extends surgical indication to patients with "insufficient" FLR. The first-stage operation includes the in situ splitting of the liver, which could lead to the high occurrence of postoperative biliary leakage. In 2014, we performed the completely laparoscopic ALPPS using round-the-liver ligation, which replaced liver splitting and got good results. The surgical technique is also presented in this book. We hope this procedure could give patients who are waiting for liver transplantation another alternative to fight liver diseases.

This book introduces the surgical technique of laparoscopic hepatectomy by curettage and aspiration and different procedures for laparoscopic hepatectomy with LPMOD, which were explored and established by our group in 16 years of practice. We want to share our experience with hepatobiliary–pancreatic surgeons and deliver an understanding of laparoscopic liver resection by writing this book. Finally, I would like to express my deepest gratitude to my teacher Prof. Shuyou Peng, who taught me the technique of open liver resection hand by hand when I was a resident student, leading me into the field of hepatobiliary–pancreatic surgery. He also gave me much valuable advice in the exploration of laparoscopic hepatectomy by curettage and aspiration.

Hangzhou, China Xiujun Cai
September 2, 2014

Acknowledgments

I would like to express my thanks to these persons, as follows, for their work in assisting operations, collecting pictures and videos, drawing figures, and helping me edit the book.

Hong Yu, MD, PhD (Sir Run Run Shaw Hospital, Zhejiang University, Hangzhou, China)

Xiao Liang, MD, PhD (Sir Run Run Shaw Hospital, Zhejiang University, Hangzhou, China)

Yifan Wang, MD, PhD (Sir Run Run Shaw Hospital, Zhejiang University, Hangzhou, China)

Zhiyi Zhu, MD, PhD (Sir Run Run Shaw Hospital, Zhejiang University, Hangzhou, China)

Yuelong Liang, MD, PhD (Sir Run Run Shaw Hospital, Zhejiang University, Hangzhou, China)

Ren'an Jin, MD (College of Medicine, Zhejiang University, Hangzhou, China)

Tu'nan Yu, MD, PhD (Sir Run Run Shaw Hospital, Zhejiang University, Hangzhou, China)

Jie Zhao, MD (School of Medicine, Zhejiang University, Hangzhou, China)

Han Yan, MD (School of Medicine, Zhejiang University, Hangzhou, China)

Zheyong Li, MD, PhD (Sir Run Run Shaw Hospital, Zhejiang University, Hangzhou, China)

Lian Duan, MD (School of Medicine, Zhejiang University, Hangzhou, China)

Xianfa Wang, MD (Sir Run Run Shaw Hospital, Zhejiang University, Hangzhou, China)

Libo Li, MD (Sir Run Run Shaw Hospital, Zhejiang University, Hangzhou, China)

Xiaodong Sun, MD (Sir Run Run Shaw Hospital, Zhejiang University, Hangzhou, China)

Linghua Zhu, MD (Sir Run Run Shaw Hospital, Zhejiang University, Hangzhou, China)

Bin Xu, MD (Sir Run Run Shaw Hospital, Zhejiang University, Hangzhou, China)

Diyu Huang, MD (Sir Run Run Shaw Hospital, Zhejiang University, Hangzhou, China)
Jin Yang, MD (Sir Run Run Shaw Hospital, Zhejiang University, Hangzhou, China)
Xueyong Zheng, MD (Sir Run Run Shaw Hospital, Zhejiang University, Hangzhou, China)
Yucai Hong, MD (The Second Affiliated Hospital, Zhejiang University, Hangzhou, China)
Yuanqiang Lu, MD (The First Affiliated Hospital, Zhejiang University, Hangzhou, China)
Yong Wang, MD (Sir Run Run Shaw Hospital, Zhejiang University, Hangzhou, China)
Liuxin Cai, MD (Sir Run Run Shaw Hospital, Zhejiang University, Hangzhou, China)
Zhengxu Zhou, MD (The First Affiliated Hospital of Wenzhou Medical University, Wenzhou, China)
Xiaoping Yang, MD (Hangzhou First People's Hospital, Hangzhou, China)
Hai Huang, MD, PhD (Affiliated Guangxing Hospital of Zhejiang Chinese Medical University, Hangzhou, China)
Jida Chen, MD, PhD (Sir Run Run Shaw Hospital, Zhejiang University, Hangzhou, China)
Heming Zheng, MD (Sir Run Run Shaw Hospital, Zhejiang University, Hangzhou, China)
Jinhua Mei, MD, PhD (Sir Run Run Shaw Hospital, Zhejiang University, Hangzhou, China)
Xiaoyan Cai, MD, PhD (Sir Run Run Shaw Hospital, Zhejiang University, Hangzhou, China)
Yin Xin, MD, PhD (Zhejiang Provincial People's Hospital, Hangzhou, China)
Lizhong Lin, MD (Taizhou Central Hospital, Taizhou, China)
Qiken Li, MD (Zhejiang Cancer Hospital, Hangzhou, China)
Tie Fang, MD (Ningbo No. 2 Hospital, Ningbo, China)
Bo Shen, MD, PhD (Sir Run Run Shaw Hospital, Zhejiang University, Hangzhou, China)
Hui Lin, MD, PhD (Sir Run Run Shaw Hospital, Zhejiang University, Hangzhou, China)
Zhifei Wang, MD (Zhejiang Provincial People's Hospital, Hangzhou, China)
Bingjie Zhang, MD (Taizhou Hospital of Zhejiang Province, Taizhou, China)
Yi Dai, MD, PhD (Sir Run Run Shaw Hospital, Zhejiang University, Hangzhou, China)
Jin Yang, MD (Zhejiang Provincial People's Hospital, Hangzhou, China)
Yuhua Zhang, MD, PhD (Zhejiang Provincial People's Hospital, Hangzhou, China)
Jianfeng Li, MD (The Affiliated Wenling Hospital of Wenzhou Medical University, Wenling, China)

Hong Fu, MD (Shaoxing People's Hospital, Shaoxing, China)
Hai Hu, MD (The Second People's Hospital of Sichuan, Chengdu, China)
Xin Zhu, MD (Shaoxing People's Hospital, Shaoxing, China)
Yiming Zhao, MD (Sir Run Run Shaw Hospital, Zhejiang University, Hangzhou, China)
Yichen Yu, MD, PhD (Sir Run Run Shaw Hospital, Zhejiang University, Hangzhou, China)
Hang Yuan, MD (Zhejiang Provincial People's Hospital, Hangzhou, China)
Kun Liu, MD, PhD (Fuwai Hospital, Peking Union Medical College, Beijing, China)
Huajie Cai, MD (The First Affiliated Hospital of Wenzhou Medical University, Wenzhou, China)
Zhengfeng Wang, MD (Peking University Health Science Center, Beijing, China)
Liang Hu, MD (The First Affiliated Hospital, Zhejiang University, Hangzhou, China)
Jikai He, MD (Affiliated Zhoushan Hospital of Wenzhou Medical University, Zhoushan, China)
Lei Zhu, MD (Lishui Central Hospital, Lishui, China)
Rui Ma, MD (Zhejiang University, Hangzhou, China)
Xu Feng, MD, PhD (Sir Run Run Shaw Hospital, Zhejiang University, Hangzhou, China)
Shihui Zhen, MD (Hangzhou First People's Hospital, Hangzhou, China)
Ning Meng, MD (The Affiliated Hospital of Hangzhou Normal University, Hangzhou, China)
Yale Zhang, MD (Hangzhou First People's Hospital, Hangzhou, China)
Xinye Hu, MD (Zhejiang Provincial People's Hospital, Hangzhou, China)
Weijia Wang, MD (Tufts Medical Center, Boston, United States)
Jiangbo Ying, MD (Institute of Mental Health, Singapore)
Hua Jin, MD (Zhejiang Hospital, Hangzhou, China)
Jiemin Lv, MD (Sir Run Run Shaw Hospital, Zhejiang University, Hangzhou, China)
Xiang Li, MD (Ningbo No. 2 Hospital, Ningbo, China)
Hanglin Wu, MD (Hangzhou First People's Hospital, Hangzhou, China)
Shilin He, MD (Hangzhou Xiasha Hospital, Hangzhou, China)
Shouzhang Yang, MD (The First Affiliated Hospital of Wenzhou Medical University, Wenzhou, China)
Junru Dai, MD (Sir Run Run Shaw Hospital, Zhejiang University, Hangzhou, China)
Chong Lai, MD (The First Affiliated Hospital, Zhejiang University, Hangzhou, China)
Xuan Yang, MD (Sir Run Run Shaw Hospital, Zhejiang University, Hangzhou, China)
Chuyan Yan, MD, PhD (Sir Run Run Shaw Hospital, Zhejiang University, Hangzhou, China)
Feng Lou, MD, PhD (Sir Run Run Shaw Hospital, Zhejiang University, Hangzhou, China)

Xin Zheng, MD (Sir Run Run Shaw Hospital, Zhejiang University, Hangzhou, China)

Jing Xu, MD (Sir Run Run Shaw Hospital, Zhejiang University, Hangzhou, China)

Contents

Abbreviations

ALPPS	Associating liver partition with portal vein ligation for staged hepatectomy
BPV	Bifurcation of portal vein
CA	Cystic artery
CBD	Common bile duct
CD	Cystic duct
CHD	Common hepatic duct
CL	Caudate lobe (of the liver)
CP	Caudate process
CPT	Caudate portal triad
CUSA	Cavitron ultrasonic surgical aspirator
FL	Falciform ligament
FLR	Future liver remnant
FLT	Fissure for ligamentum teres
GB	Gallbladder
HCL	Hepatocolic ligament
HD	Hepatic duct
HDL	Hepatoduodenal ligament
HP	Hilar plate
HRL	Hepatorenal ligament
IIVC	Infrahepatic inferior vena cava
IVC	Inferior vena cava
LCL	Left coronary ligament
LHA	Left hepatic artery
LHCA	Technique of laparoscopic hepatectomy by curettage and aspiration
LHCA	Laparoscopic hepatectomy by curettage and aspiration
LHD	Left hepatic duct
LHV	Left hepatic vein
LIFV	Left inferior phrenic vein
LL	Left lobe (of the liver)
LLR	Laparoscopic liver resection
LLS	Left lateral segment
LO	Lesser omentum
LPMOD	Laparoscopic Peng's multifunctional operative dissector
LPV	Left branch of portal vein

LTL	Left triangle ligament
LV	Ligamentum venosum
MHV	Middle hepatic vein
OF	Omental foramen
PH	Porta hepatis
PHA	Proper hepatic artery
PMOD	Peng's multifunctional operative dissector
PP	Paracaval portion
PV	Portal vein
RAPV	Right anterior branch of portal vein
RCL	Right coronary ligament
RHA	Right hepatic artery
RHD	Right hepatic duct
RHV	Right hepatic vein
RL	Round ligament
RLL	Right lobe of the liver
RPPV	Right posterior branch of portal vein
RPV	Right branch of portal vein
RTL	Right triangle ligament
SHV	Short hepatic vein
SIVC	Suprahepatic inferior vena cava
SP	Spiegel process

1 Anatomy of the Liver in the Laparoscopic Situation

Knowledge of the anatomy of the liver is most important for surgeons to perform liver resection. It includes perihepatic ligaments, the biliary system, the portal vein system, the hepatic vein system, and the hepatic artery system (Fig. 1.1). Due to the different viewing angles in open liver resection and laparoscopic liver resection, the laparoscopic view of the liver's anatomy might be a little different from the open condition.

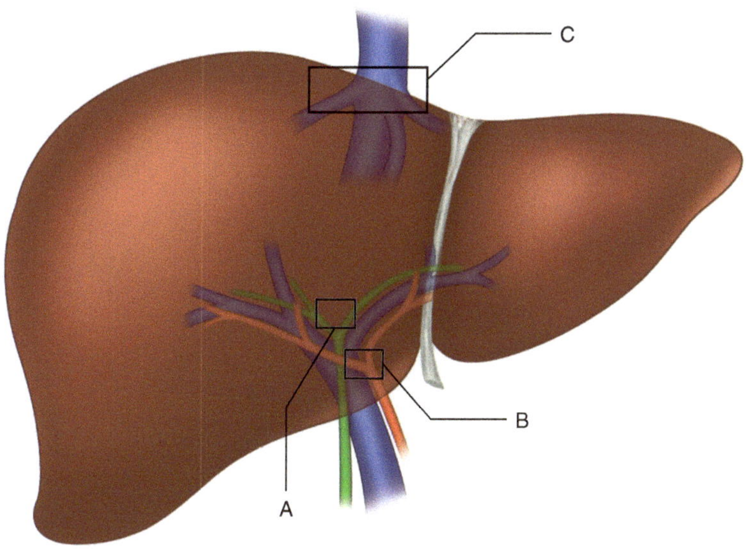

Fig. 1.1 Major structures which should be properly managed in anatomical hepatectomies. (*A*) Biliary system; (*B*) Portal vein system and hepatic artery system; (*C*) Hepatic vein system

X. Cai, *Laparoscopic Hepatectomy: Atlas and Techniques*,
DOI 10.1007/978-94-017-9840-2_1,

1.1 Perihepatic Ligaments

The observation port is usually located infraumbilically or supraumbilically, and the liver is observed and manipulated from the middle abdomen (Fig. 1.2). The hepatoduodenal ligament (HDL) can be exposed by mobilizing the liver upward by the traction of the round ligament (RL) or/and the gallbladder (GB) (Figs. 1.3 and 1.4). The RL (Fig. 1.5), the falciform ligament (FL) (Fig. 1.6), and the hepatocolic ligament (HCL) (Fig. 1.7) can be visualized and be divided firstly in laparoscope. The lesser omentum (LO) could be exposed by elevating the left lobe (LL) of the liver (Fig. 1.8). The left triangle ligament (LTL) can be exposed by pulling the left lobe to the right with a forceps (Fig. 1.9). The left coronary ligament (LCL) can be fully exposed after dividing the LTL (Fig. 1.10). It also can be exposed by pressing LL downward after dividing the FL (Fig. 1.11). The hepatorenal ligament (HRL) should be divided in right hemihepatectomy. It could be exposed by elevating the right lobe of the liver (RLL) or by pulling the right lobe to the left (Fig. 1.12). The right triangle ligament (RTL) and the right coronary ligament (RCL) might be the most difficult to expose in laparoscope for the limited space in the right upper quadrant. Before exposing them, RLL should be fully freed; the RL, FL, HCL, HRL, and even some short hepatic veins (SHVs) in the right wall of the inferior vena cava (IVC) should be divided; and RLL should be pushed to the left with forceps or a retractor to expose RTL (Fig. 1.13) or be pressed downward to expose RCL (Fig. 1.14). Additionally, in the division of LCL or RCL, inferior phrenic veins should be taken care of to avoid bleeding (Fig. 1.15).

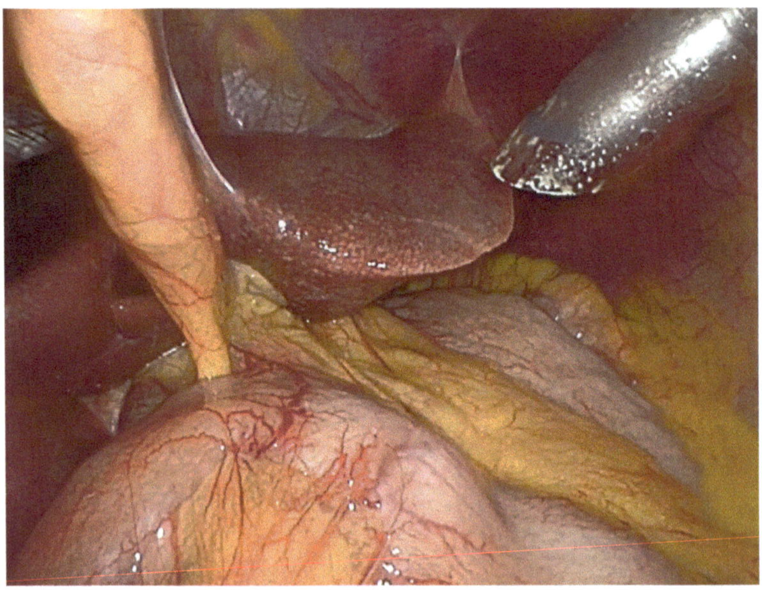

Fig. 1.2 The view of the liver observed from the middle abdomen

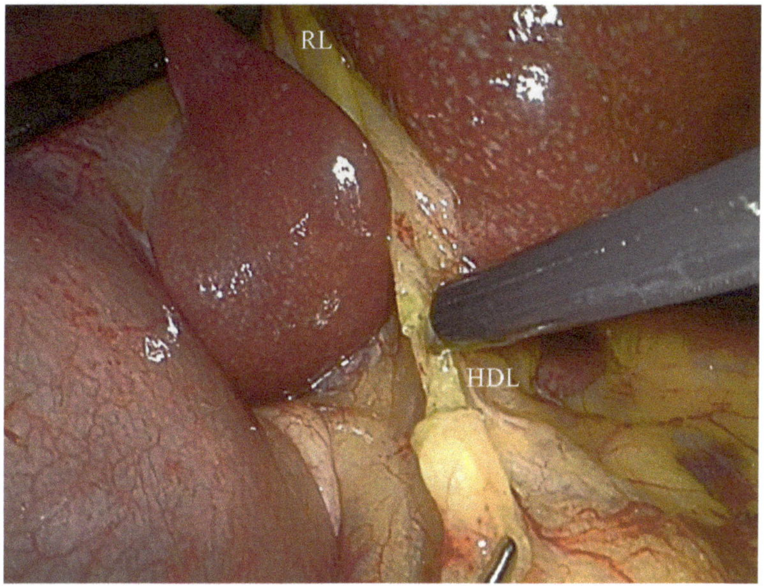

Fig. 1.3 The HDL is exposed by the traction of RL with a forceps

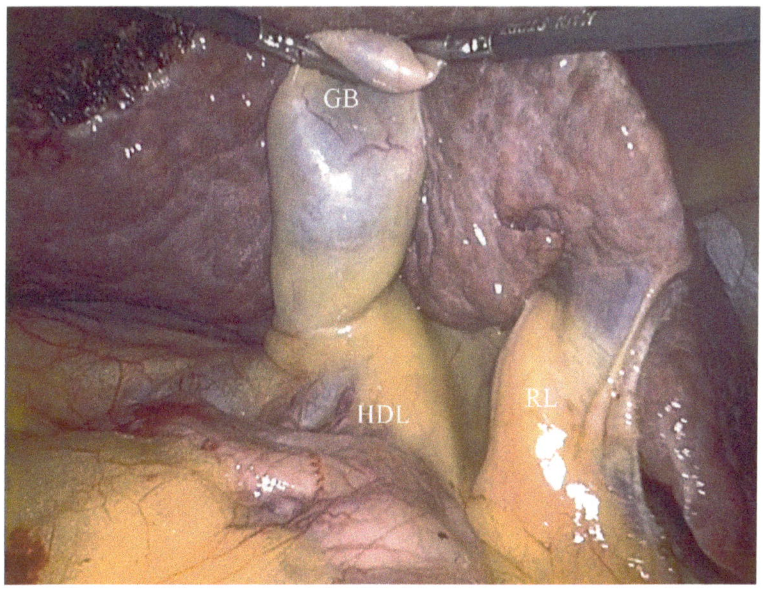

Fig. 1.4 HDL is exposed by the traction of GB with a forceps

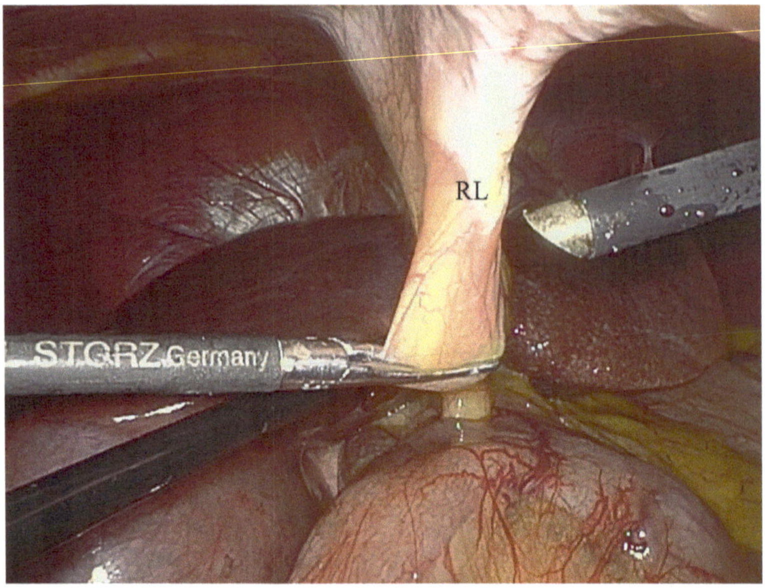

Fig. 1.5 RL is visualized laparoscopically. It is being drawn by a curved dissecting forceps and is to be transected by LPMOD

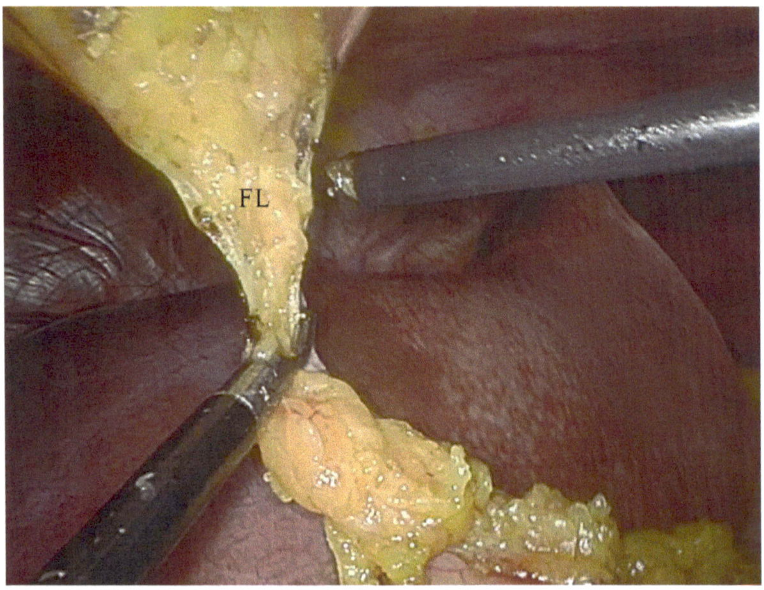

Fig. 1.6 FL is visualized laparoscopically after RL was divided

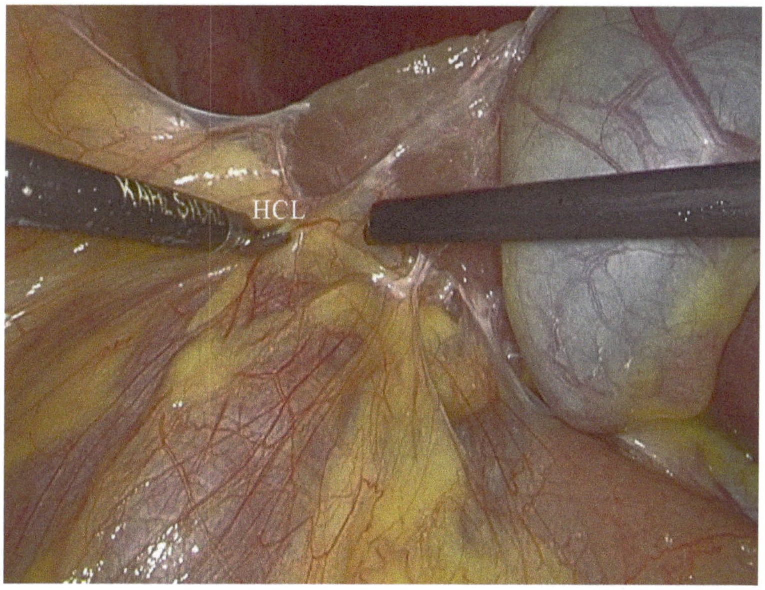

Fig. 1.7 HCL is visualized laparoscopically

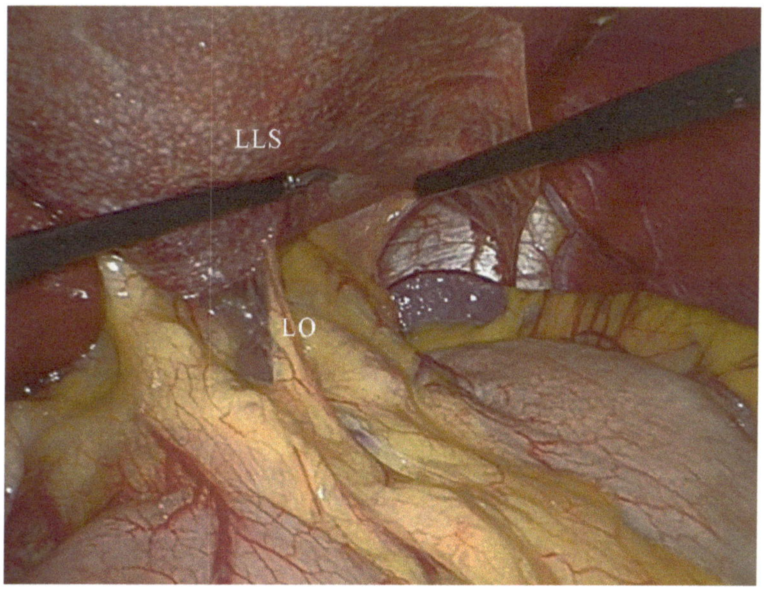

Fig. 1.8 The left lateral segment (*LLS*) is elevated with a curved dissecting forceps, and LO is exposed

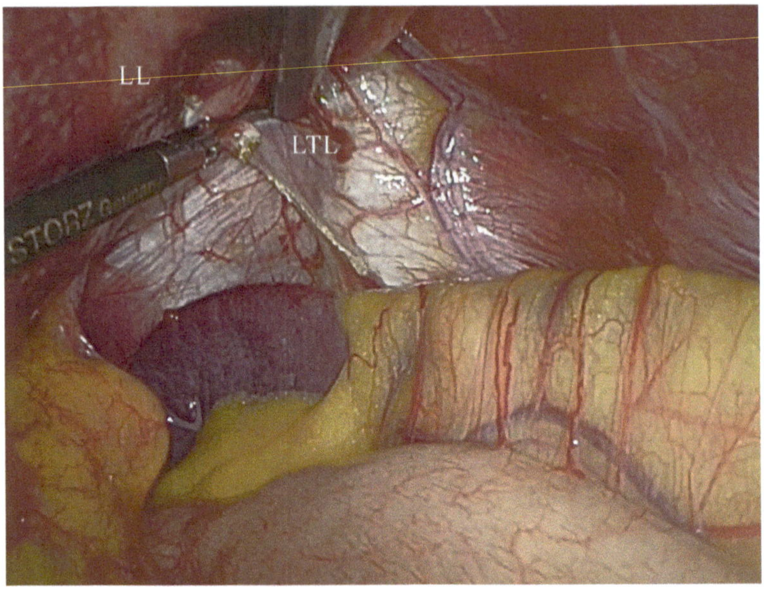

Fig. 1.9 The left lobe (*LL*) of the liver is mobilized to the right and LTL is visualized

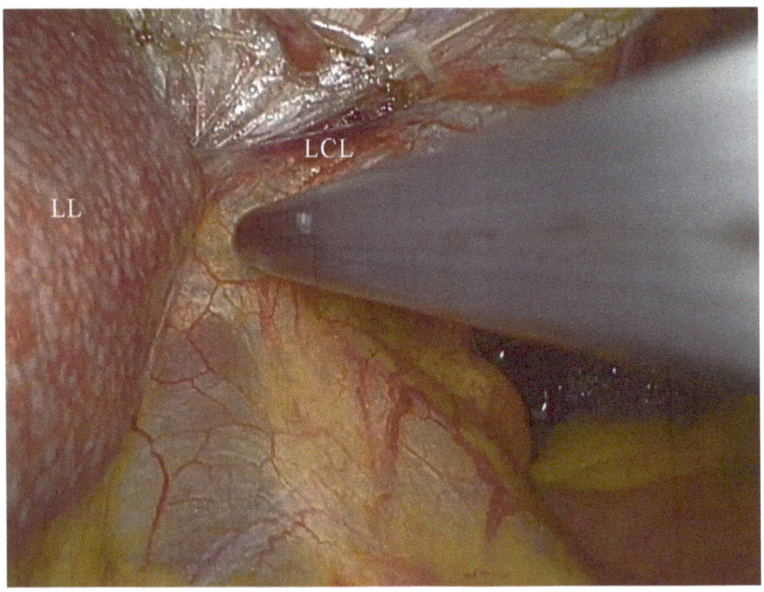

Fig. 1.10 The LL is mobilized to the right after LTL was divided and LCL is well exposed

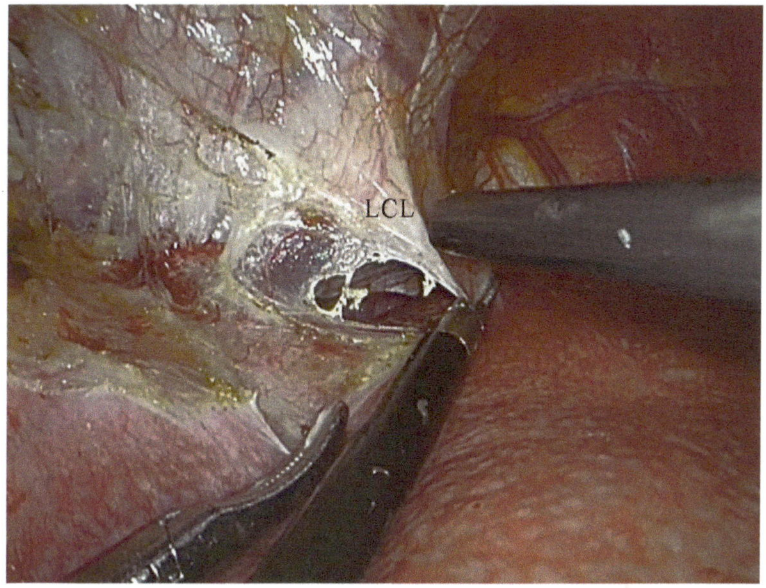

Fig. 1.11 After FL was divided, the left lobe of the liver is pressed downward with two pairs of forceps, and LCL is exposed for the division

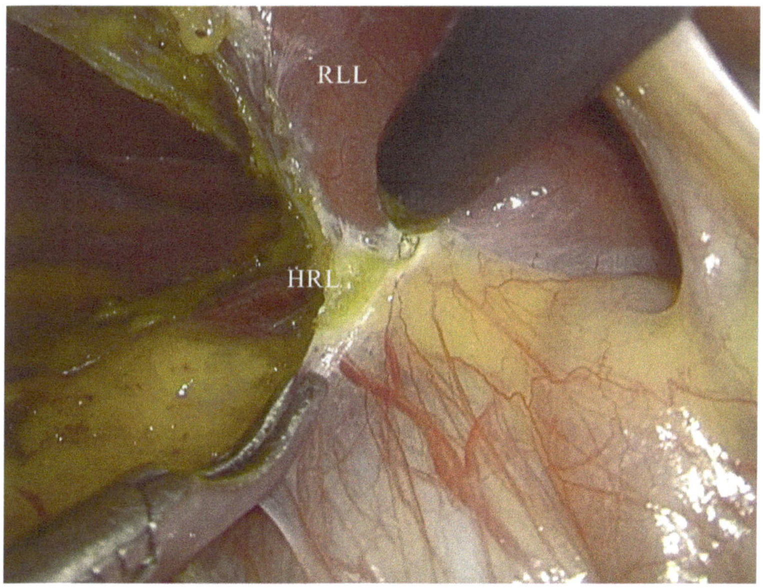

Fig. 1.12 The RLL is elevated and HRL is exposed, and then HRL should be divided

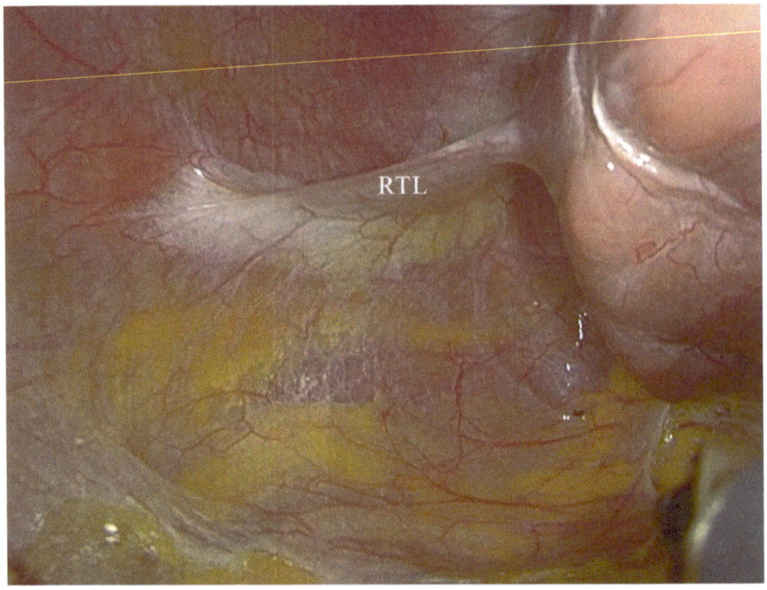

Fig. 1.13 RLL is mobilized to the left after HCL and HRL was divided. RTL is exposed

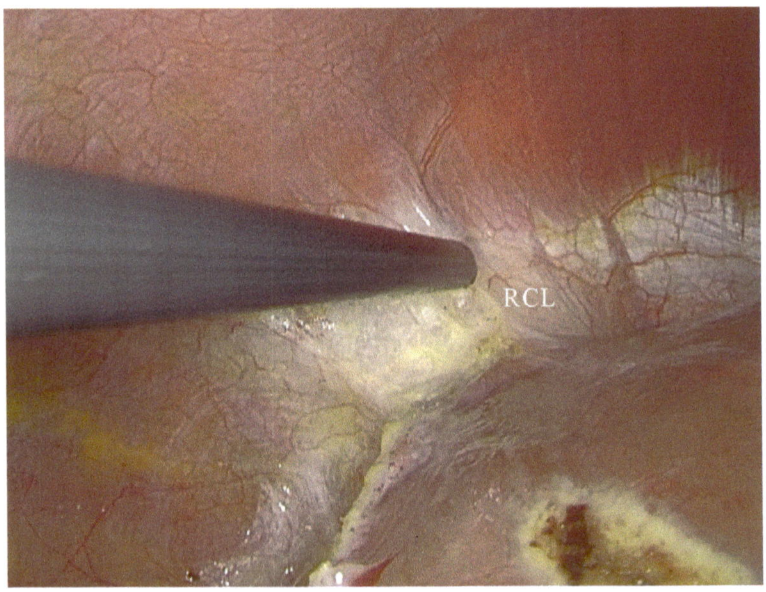

Fig. 1.14 RCL is exposed for the division, after RLL was pressed downward

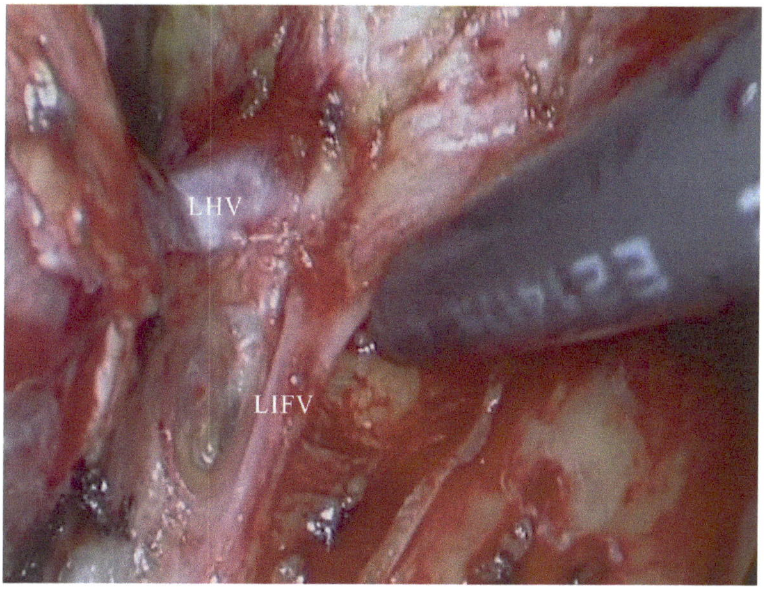

Fig. 1.15 The left inferior phrenic veins (*LIFV*) and the left hepatic vein (*LHV*) are visualized when dividing LCL

1.2 The Porta Hepatis

The porta hepatis (PH) can be exposed by mobilizing the liver upward by pulling the round ligament and/or the gallbladder with laparoscopic grasping forceps. It can be further exposed by pulling the hilar plate (HP) with curved dissecting forceps after preliminarily dissection (Fig. 1.16). The hepatic artery and its branches can be dissected firstly (Fig. 1.17). The branches of the portal vein (PV) usually can be visualized after the left hepatic artery (LHA) or the right hepatic artery (RHA) has been divided (Fig. 1.18). In most cases, the branch of PV is difficult to distinguish from the trunk of PV, and the bifurcation of the portal vein (BPV) should be visualized for identifying the branch of PV (Fig. 1.19). The bifurcation of the common hepatic duct (CHD) is usually higher than the bifurcation of the hepatic artery and PV and is difficult to dissect laparoscopically, especially in left hemihepatectomies.

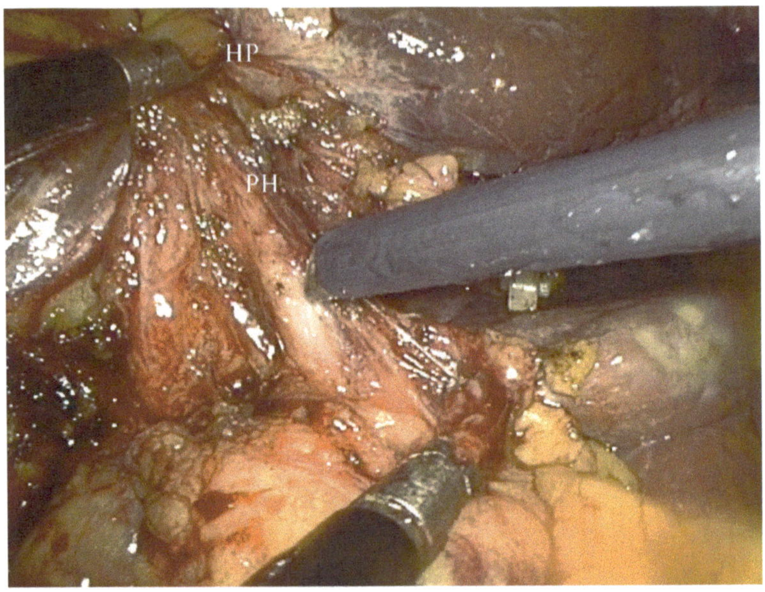

Fig. 1.16 The PH is well exposed by the traction of the HP with a curved dissecting forceps

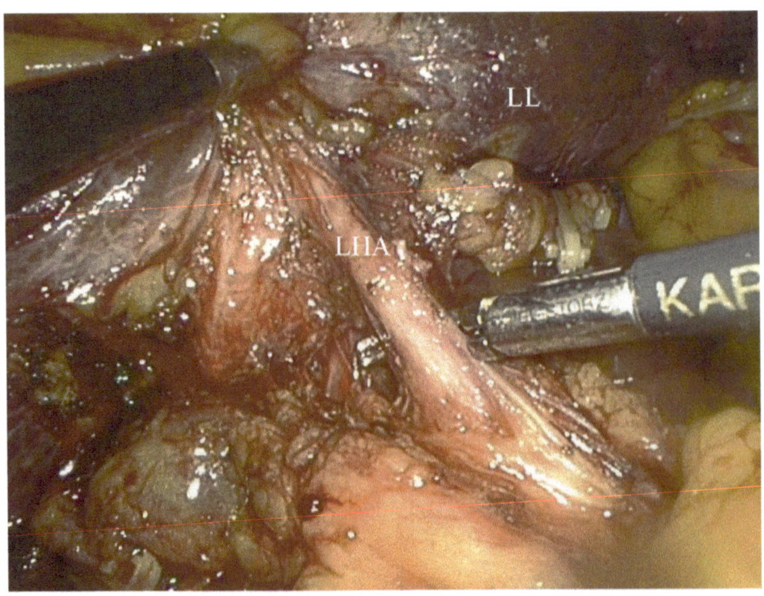

Fig. 1.17 LHA is firstly visualized and is freed with a curved dissecting forceps

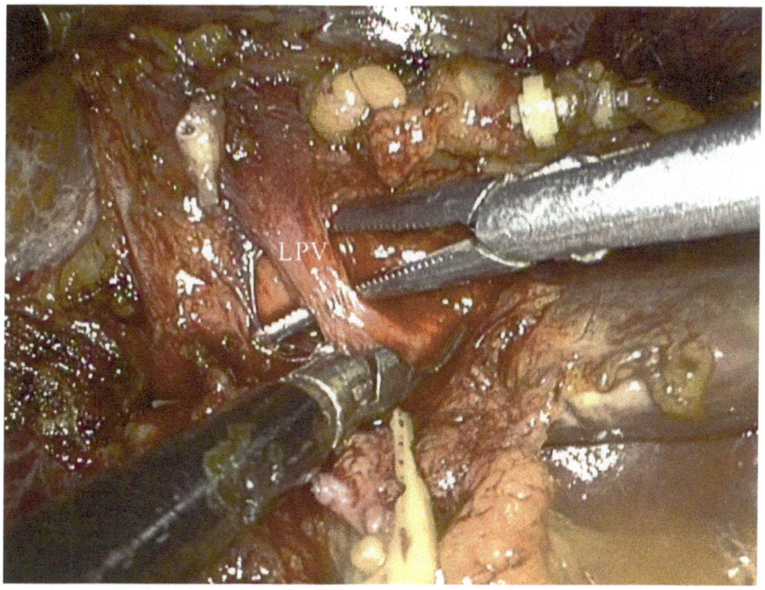

Fig. 1.18 The left branch of the portal vein (*LPV*) is visualized after LHA was divided

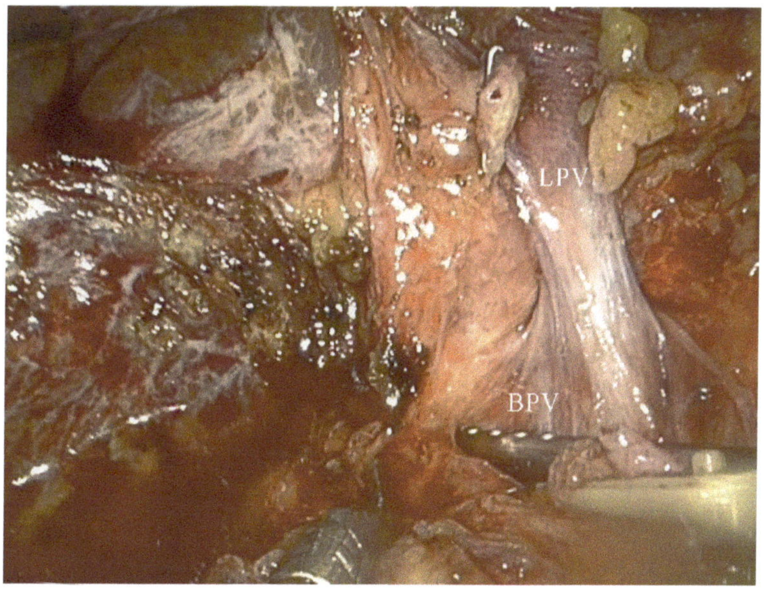

Fig. 1.19 LPV is identified by the vision of BPV

1.3 Hepatic Veins

Laparoscopic dissection of hepatic veins before liver transection is a highly skilled and riskful procedure due to the limited manipulation space and the poor vision field, which may lead to unmanageable bleeding and emergent conversion. In hemihepatectomy, it is performed on selected patients whose hepatic veins can be exposed sufficiently and dissected safely.

1.4 Short Hepatic Veins

Short hepatic veins (SHVs) can be exposed by elevating RLL or the caudate lobe (CL) of the liver after perihepatic ligaments are properly divided (Figs. 1.20 and 1.21). The dissection of SHVs is not a difficult procedure as long as they are well exposed.

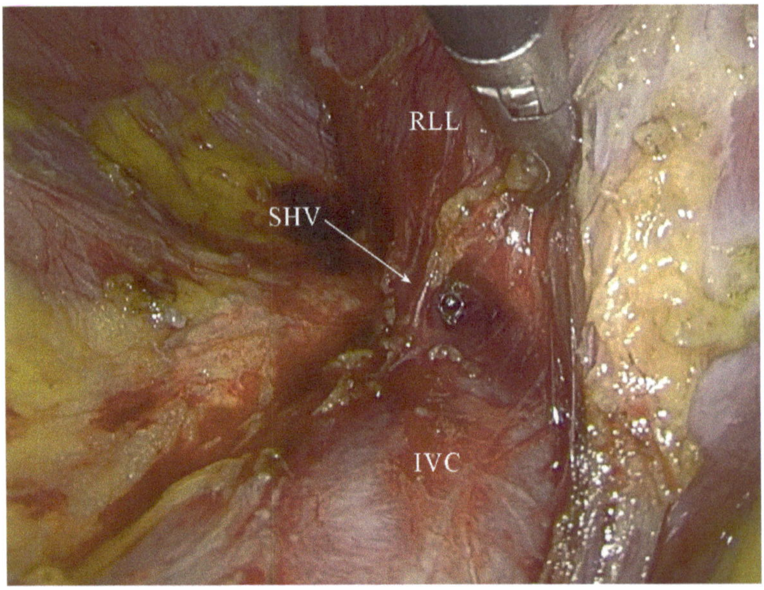

Fig. 1.20 RLL is mobilized to the left, and the IVC and a SHV are visualized

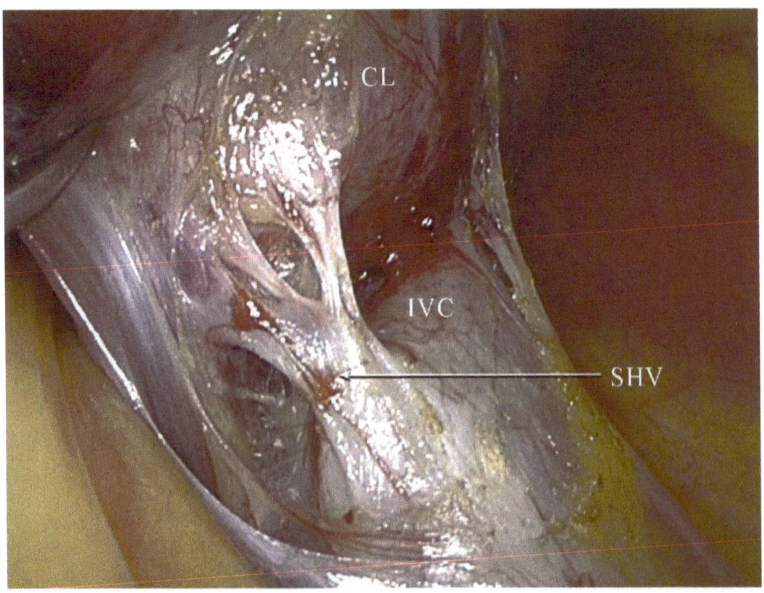

Fig. 1.21 CL of the liver is elevated, and the IVC and a SHV vein are visualized

2 Instruments for Laparoscopic Hepatectomy by Curettage and Aspiration

Laparoscopic cholecystectomy is a mature laparoscopic surgery and is supposed to be the basic laparoscopic hepato-biliary-pancreatic procedure. Laparoscopic hepatectomy by curettage and aspiration was developed on the basis of the laparoscopic cholecystectomy. Equipments, instruments, trocars' position, and even the laparoscopic surgical technique for laparoscopic cholecystectomy were applied to the laparoscopic hepatectomy in the early stage and were modified or developed in practice.

X. Cai, *Laparoscopic Hepatectomy: Atlas and Techniques*,
DOI 10.1007/978-94-017-9840-2_2,

2.1 Basic Equipments

Equipments for laparoscopic hepatectomy by curettage and aspiration are the same as the basic laparoscopic equipments used in laparoscopic cholecystectomy including the insufflators, the light system, and the image system (Fig. 2.1).

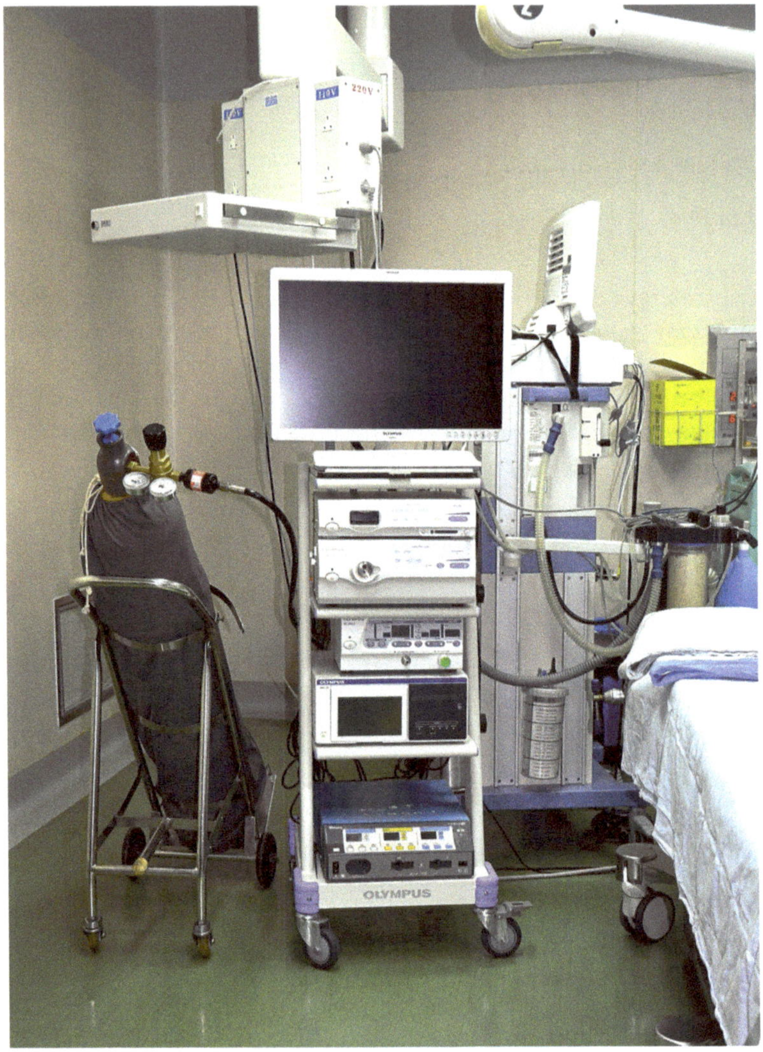

Fig. 2.1 Basic equipments for laparoscopic hepatectomy including the monitor, the image system, the light system, the insufflators, the video recording system, and the electric cutting and coagulation system (*up to down*)

2.2 Trocars

A 10-mm trocar is used for observation port and two 5-mm trocars are used for assistant ports. A 12-mm bladeless trocar is used for the manipulation port. The 12-mm bladeless trocar allows 5–12 mm laparoscopic instruments to pass without gas leakage. No accessories need to be changed or adjusted when changing among different instruments that could facilitate the manipulation and decrease the operating time.

2.3 Instruments for Liver Transection

The special instrument for liver transection is the laparoscopic Peng's multifunctional operative dissector (LPMOD) (Cai et al. 2006) (Figs. 2.2 and 2.3). It was developed on the basis of the Peng's multifunctional operative dissector (PMOD) which was invented by Prof. Shuyou Peng and is used for open surgery (Peng et al. 2003). We extended the length of the stalk of PMOD and modified the aspiration system to fit the laparoscopic purpose. It can be used for blunt dissection, electric coagulation, cutting, and aspiration and can bluntly dissect intrahepatic ducts and vessels. It can execute all the functions at the same time that facilitates the manipulation of liver transection and can decrease the operating time by avoiding frequently changing instruments. By using this instrument, the liver parenchyma can be crashed and be aspirated immediately, and intrahepatic ducts and small vessels can be preserved and be safely dissected for ligation, and massive bleeding could be avoided by the meticulous dissection.

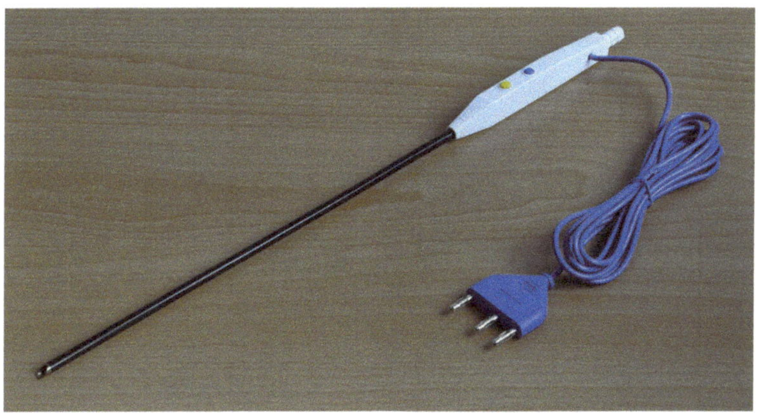

Fig. 2.2 LPMOD

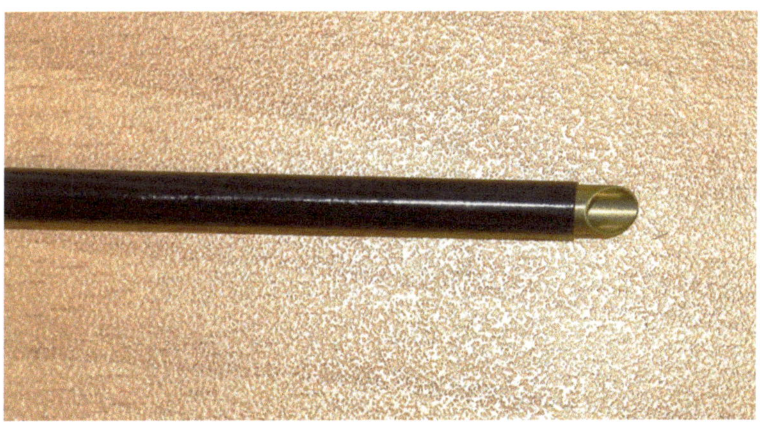

Fig. 2.3 The tip of LPMOD

2.4 Instruments for Liver Mobilization

For the mobilization of liver lobe in left hemihepatectomies, right hemihepatectomies and left lateral segmentectomies, the laparoscopic fan retractor or the laparoscopic liver retractor is used. The laparoscopic grasping forceps are also used for liver mobilization by drawing the liver capsule, perihepatic ligaments, or the gallbladder. In some cases, the stalks of grasping forceps can be used for the elevation of liver lobe as well.

2.5 Instruments for Dissection

LPMOD is an ideal instrument for the bluntly meticulous dissection. The majority of vessels and hepatic ducts can be dissected with it. Some other instruments are used to assist LPMOD in meticulous dissection. Curved dissecting forceps are usually used to dissect the back wall of vessels and hepatic ducts, and are sometimes used to grasp vessels or hepatic ducts to assist the dissection. In addition to normal types of curved dissecting forceps which is used in laparoscopic cholecystectomy, a special 10-mm and 90° curved dissecting forceps (Figs. 2.4 and 2.5) was manufactured and is used in our institute, the Sir Run Run Shaw Hospital, School of Medicine, Zhejiang University, for dissecting large vessels, dilated hepatic ducts, or the common hepatic duct. In addition, a laparoscopic liver retractor, Goldfinger, is used in freeing branches of portal veins and hepatic veins in some cases. It can be fixed in different curves, and its smooth tip could safely pass through the back space of major vessels.

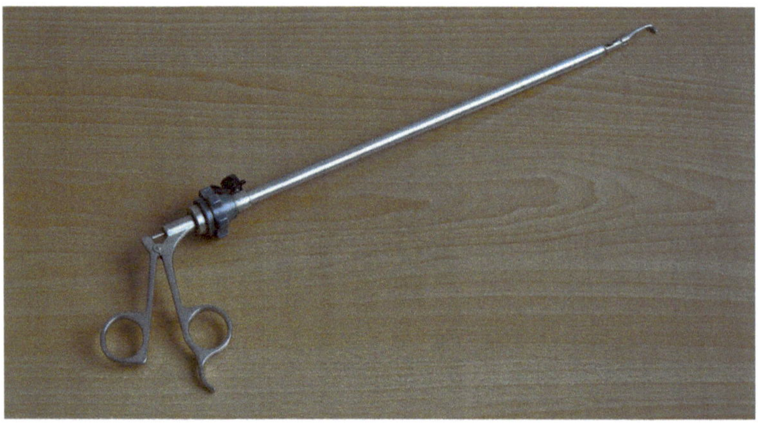

Fig. 2.4 The laparoscopic 10-mm 90°-curved dissecting forceps

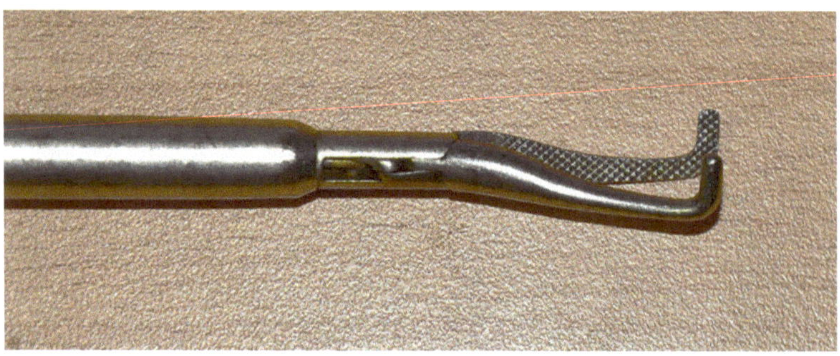

Fig. 2.5 The tip of the laparoscopic 10-mm 90°-curved forceps

2.6 Instruments for Ligation

Normally, the titanic clip is usually used to clamp the distal portion of vessels and hepatic ducts or small vessels less than 1 mm. The major vessels and hepatic ducts are usually managed with absorbable clips or nonabsorbable polymer clips. A laparoscopic linear staple is usually used in the transection of the right hepatic vein and, sometimes, is used in the transection of the left pedicle or the left hepatic vein. Needle holding forceps is needed in some cases of intrahepatic hepatolithiasis for suturing the stump of dilated hepatic ducts.

2.7 Instruments for Tissue Division

LPMOD is the main instrument for tissue cutting such as in the division of perihepatic ligaments, liver capsule, and hepatic ducts. Laparoscopic bipolar hook electrode and laparoscopic curved scissors were are also used for cutting in some cases.

2.8 Other Instruments Used in Laparoscopic Hepatectomy

In open liver resection, tumors and intrahepatic stones can be located by the feeling of hands, but in laparoscopic surgeries, intra-abdominal organs cannot be touched. It becomes a major problem for laparoscopic surgeons to locate tumors or intrahepatic stones in laparoscopic hepatectomies, especially in non-anatomical liver resections. Laparoscopic ultrasound is used in place of hands. Furthermore, it is more accurate than the hand's feeling and can be used to calculate size and depth of tumors. In non-anatomical liver resection, it should be repeated in the parenchyma transection to secure enough free margin for malignancy or to make a proper transection line to remove intrahepatic stones completely. For removing liver specimens, an Endobag is used by which the specimens could pass through small abdominal incisions without incision tumor implantation or incision contamination.

References

Cai XJ, Yu H, Liang X, et al. Laparoscopic hepatectomy by curettage and aspiration: experiences of 62 cases. Surg Endosc. 2006;20:1531–5.

Peng SY, Li JT, Mou YP, et al. Different approaches to caudate lobectomy with "curettage and aspiration" technique using a special instrument PMOD: a report of 76 cases. World J Gastroenterol. 2003;9:2169–73.

3 Laparoscopic Left Lateral Segmentectomy

In 1996, laparoscopic left lateral segmentectomy was reported by Azagra et al. (1996). For now, this procedure can be performed in most institutes of hepato-biliary-pancreatic surgery worldwide. Furthermore, laparoscopic left lateral segmentectomy was supposed to be a standard practice according to "The Louisville Statement" (Buell et al. 2009). Management of the hepatic pedicle is the point of this laparoscopic procedure. In some cases, the branches of the hepatic artery could be dissected outside the liver parenchyma before liver transection. The falciform ligament (FL) and the fissure for ligamentum teres (FLT) are the anatomical lines for liver transection along which the secondary branches of the portal vein and the hepatic artery can be well managed by meticulous dissection and the left lateral segment can be anatomically resected.

3.1 Indications and Contraindications

The indications include liver tumors in lateral segment or left intrahepatic bile duct stones with irreversible diseases (biliary stricture, severe parenchymal fibrosis or atrophy) requiring left lateral segmentectomy and liver function of Child A to B classification. The contraindications include history of biliary surgeries such as exploration of common bile duct or cholangiojejunostomy (cholecystectomy is not regarded as a contraindication), extrahepatic bile duct stricture, or acute suppurative cholangitis.

Electronic supplementary material The online version of this chapter at (doi: 10.1007/978-94-017-9840-2_3) contains supplementary material, which is available to authorized users.

X. Cai, *Laparoscopic Hepatectomy: Atlas and Techniques*,
DOI 10.1007/978-94-017-9840-2_3,

3.2 Patient Position and Trocars' Position

Patients are placed in the supine position under general anesthesia. Three surgeons are needed in the operation. As shown in Fig. 3.1, the senior surgeon stands on the left side of the patient, one assistant surgeon stands on the right side of the senior surgeon manipulating the aspiration device, and the other assistant surgeon stands on the right side of the patient. Four entries are made. A supra-umbilical 10-mm trocar is inserted as the observation port. A 12-mm trocar below the left costal margin is inserted as the main manipulation port. And two 5-mm trocars are inserted at the right flank area as assistant manipulation ports.

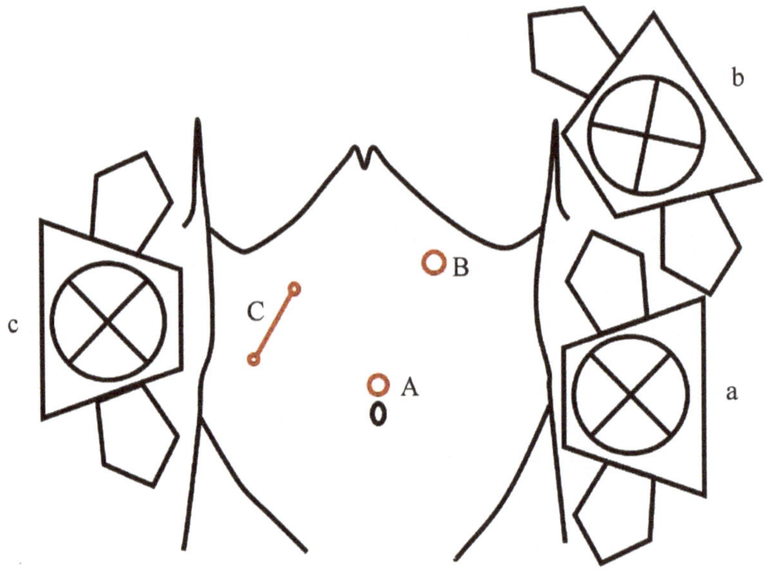

Fig. 3.1 The trocars' position and surgeons' position. (*A*) Observation port; (*B*) Main manipulation port; (*C*) Two assistant ports and the incision for removing specimen; (**a**) The senior surgeon stands on the *left side* of the patient; (**b**) One assistant on the *right side* of the surgeon controlling the aspiration device; (**c**) The other assistant stands on the *right side* of the patient

3.3 Laparoscopic Left Lateral Segmentectomy

See Figs. 3.2, 3.3, 3.4, 3.5, 3.6, 3.7, 3.8, 3.9, 3.10, 3.11, 3.12, 3.13, 3.14, 3.15, 3.16, 3.17, 3.18, 3.19, 3.20, 3.21, 3.22, 3.23, 3.24, 3.25, 3.26, 3.27, 3.28, 3.29, 3.30, 3.31, and Video 3.1.

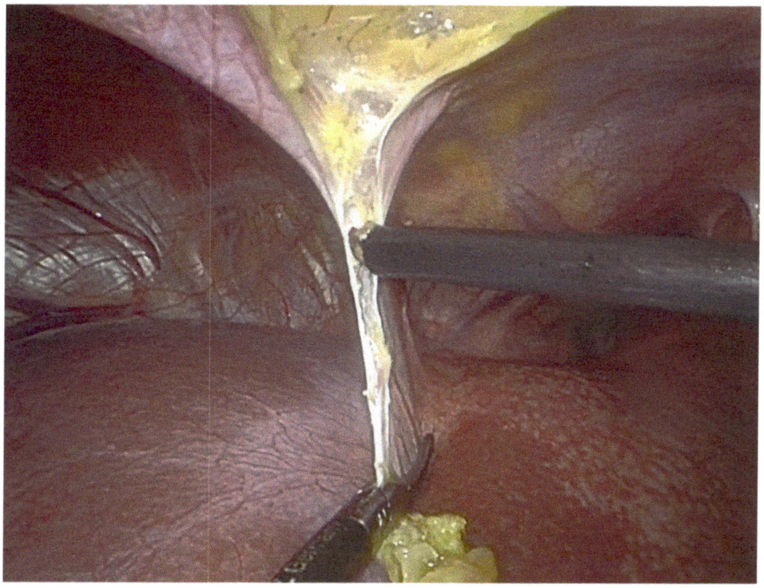

Fig. 3.2 The round ligament (RL) and the falciform ligament are divided with LPMOD

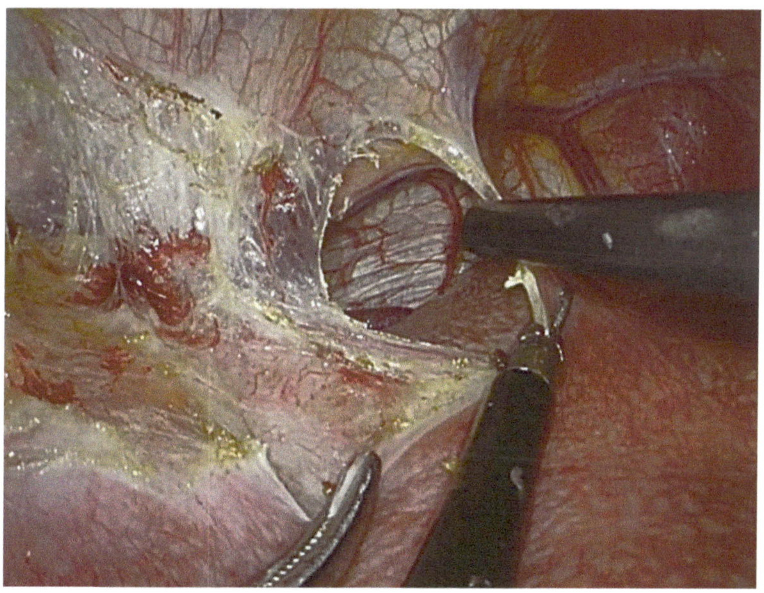

Fig. 3.3 The left coronary ligament (LCL) is divided with LPMOD

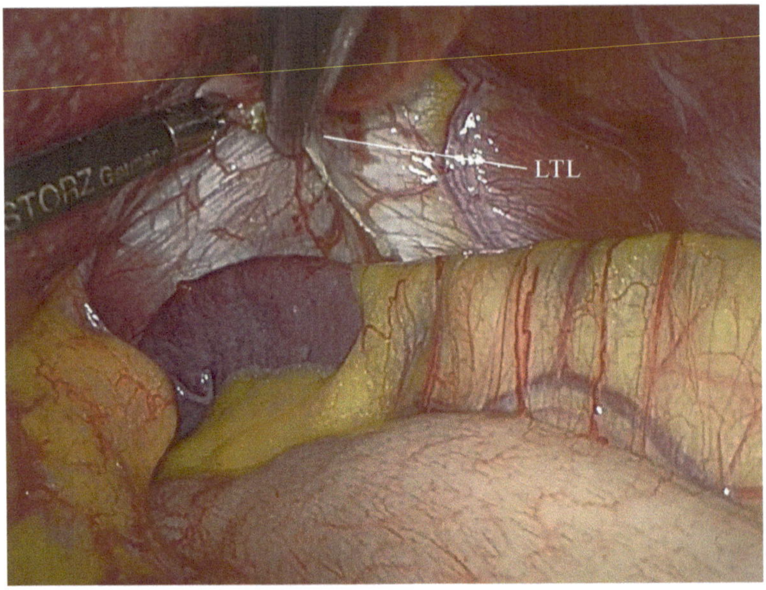

Fig. 3.4 The left lobe (LL) of the liver is elevated and the left triangle ligament (*LTL*) is divided with LPMOD

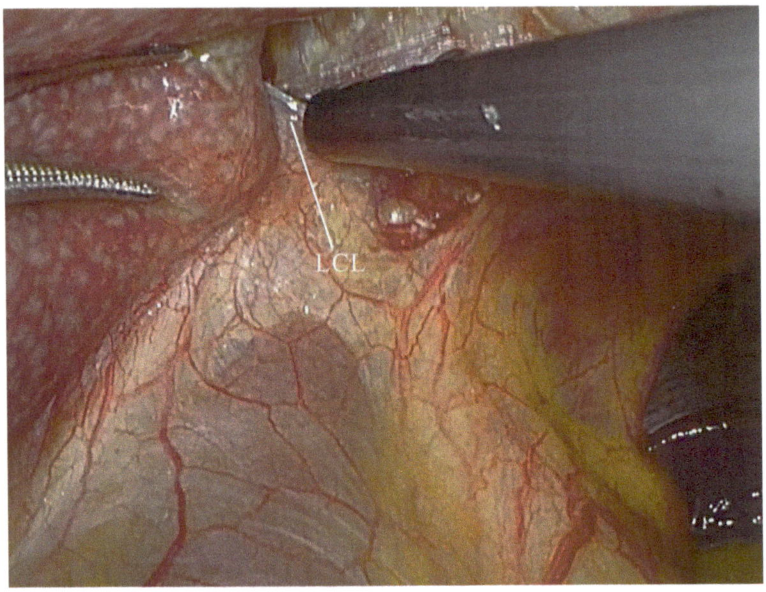

Fig. 3.5 The left lobe of the liver is elevated and LCL is further divided with LPMOD

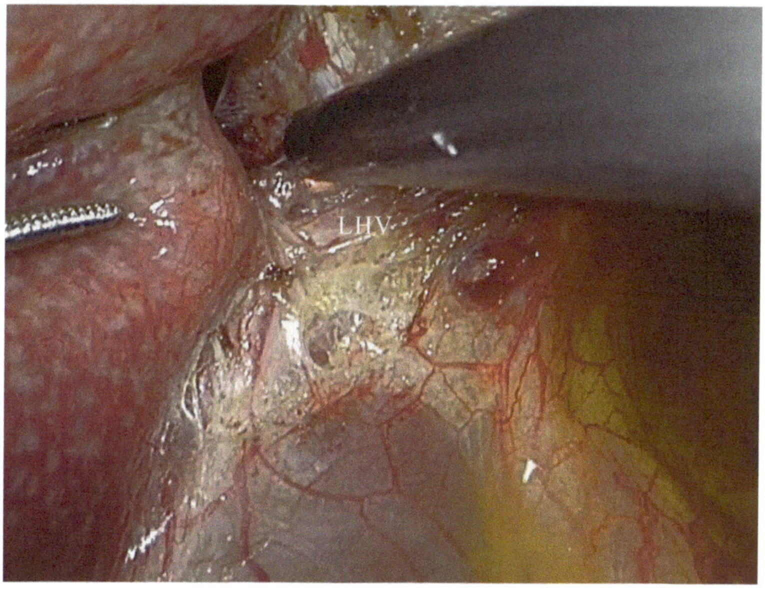

Fig. 3.6 The left hepatic vein (*LHV*) is visualized after the left coronary ligament was divided

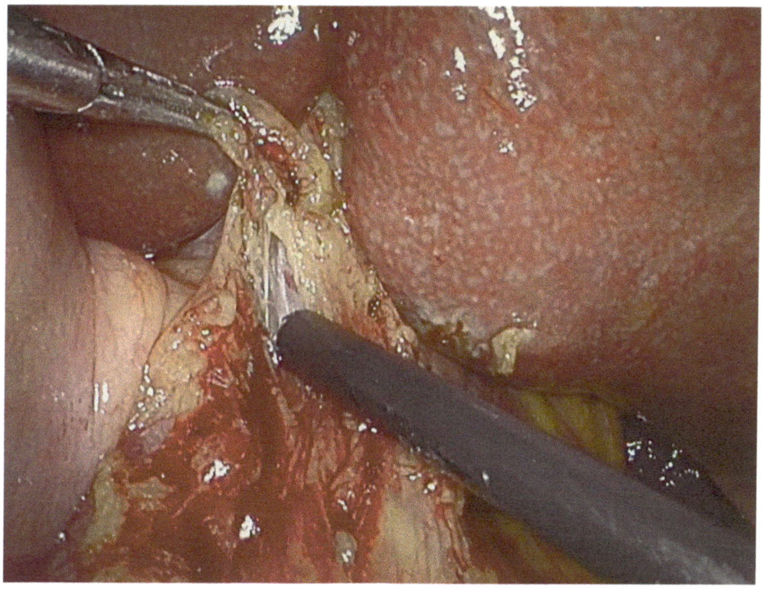

Fig. 3.7 The liver is mobilized upward by the traction of the round ligament, and the hepatoduodenal ligament (HDL) is dissected with LPMOD

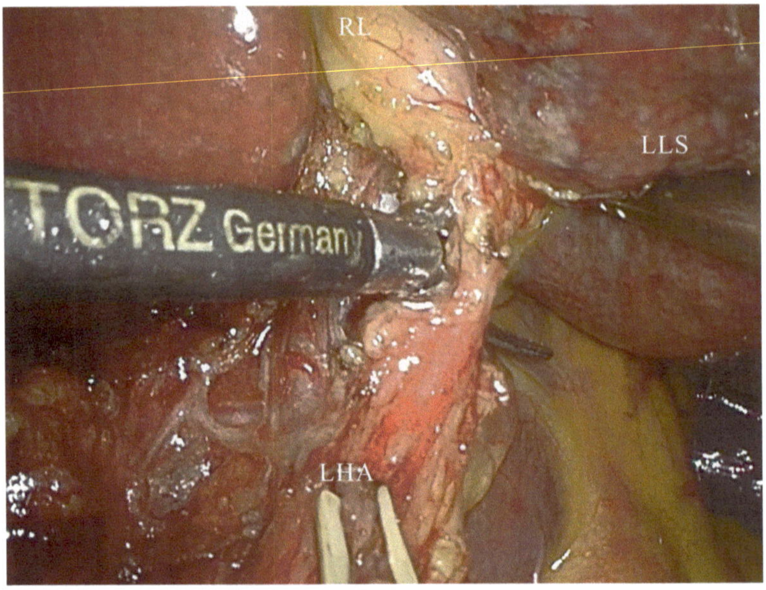

Fig. 3.8 The branch of left hepatic artery (*LHA*) to the left lateral segment (*LLS*) is dissected

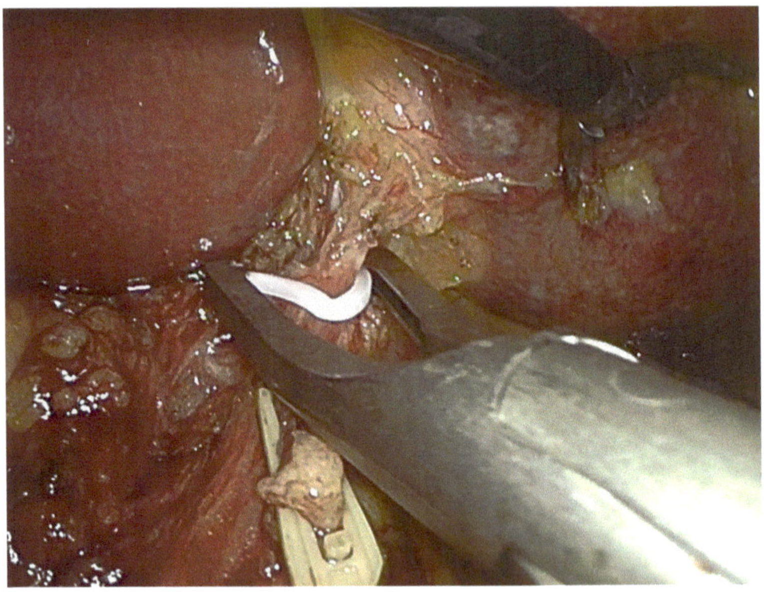

Fig. 3.9 The branch of left hepatic artery is clamped with a nonabsorbable polymer clip

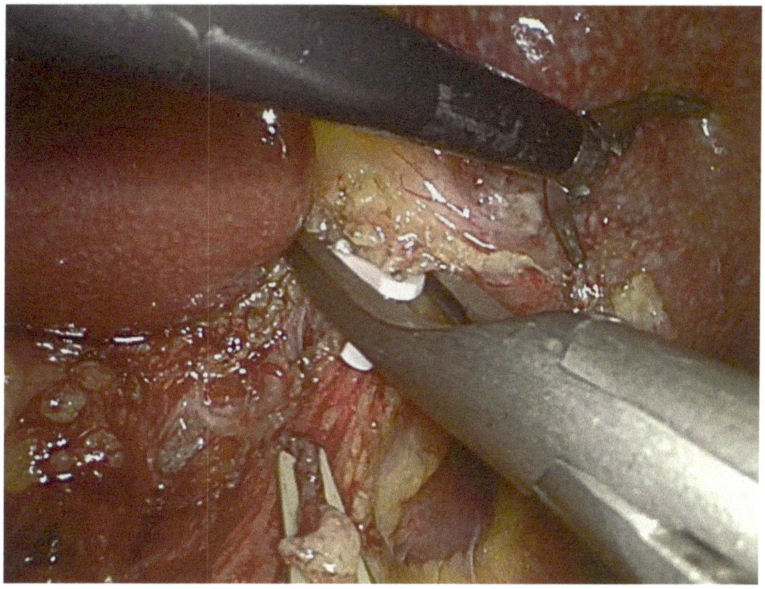

Fig. 3.10 Another nonabsorbable polymer clip is applied on the distal portion of the branch of left hepatic artery

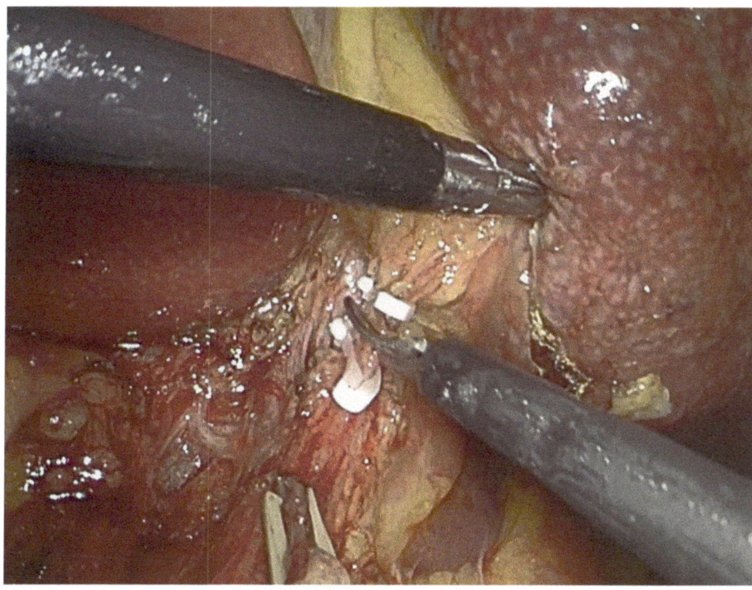

Fig. 3.11 The branch of left hepatic artery is divided

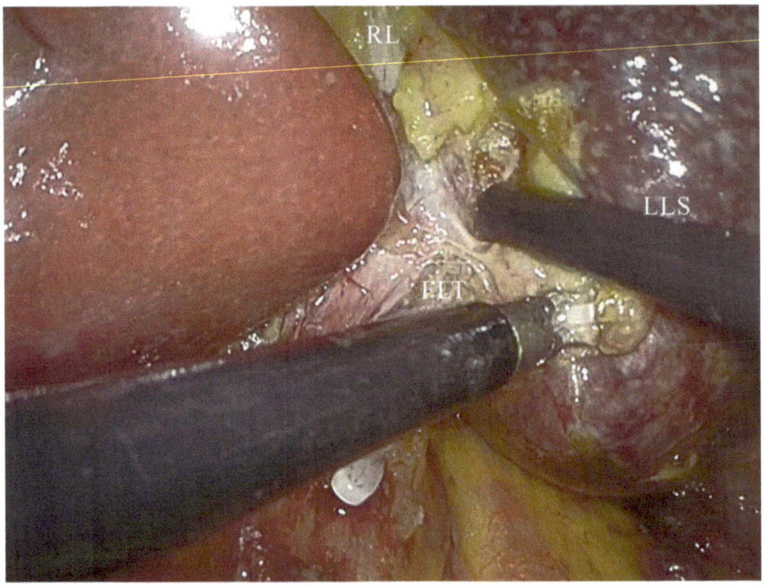

Fig. 3.12 Vessels in the FLT are dissected with LPMOD

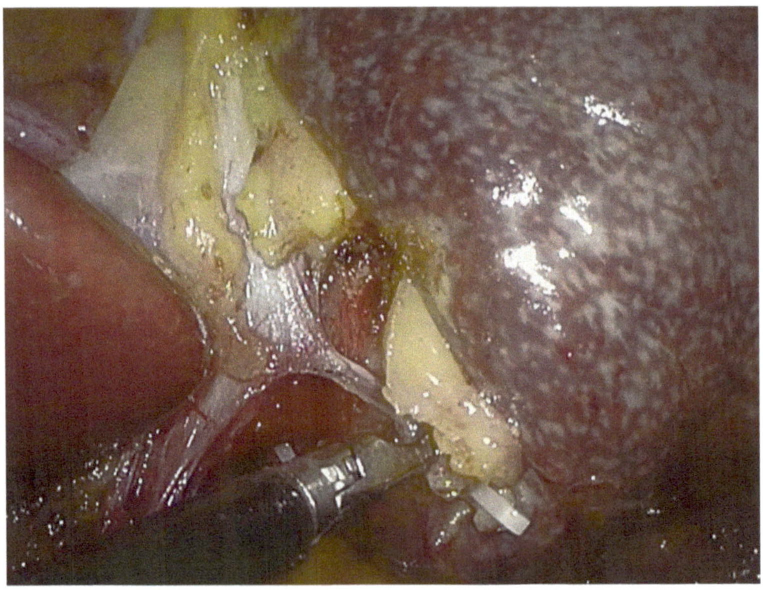

Fig. 3.13 A secondary branch of portal vein (PV) is dissected

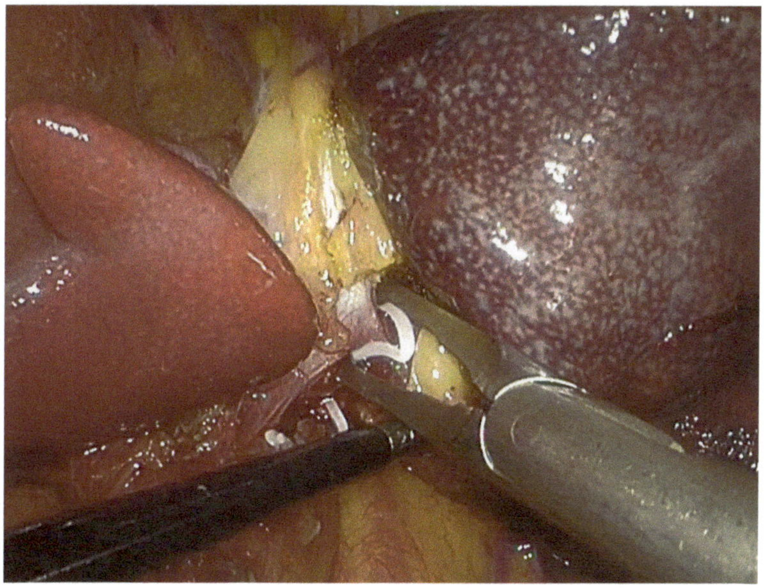

Fig. 3.14 The secondary branch of portal vein is clamped with a nonabsorbable polymer clip

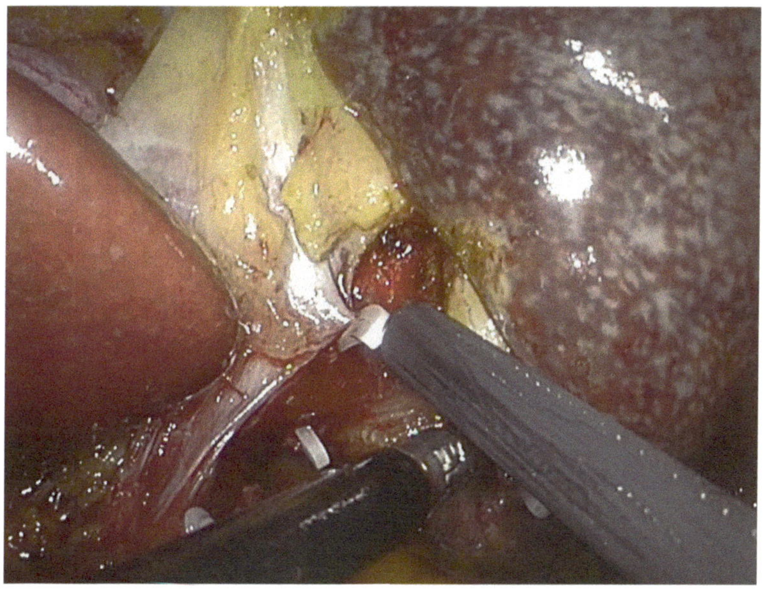

Fig. 3.15 The secondary branch of portal vein is divided

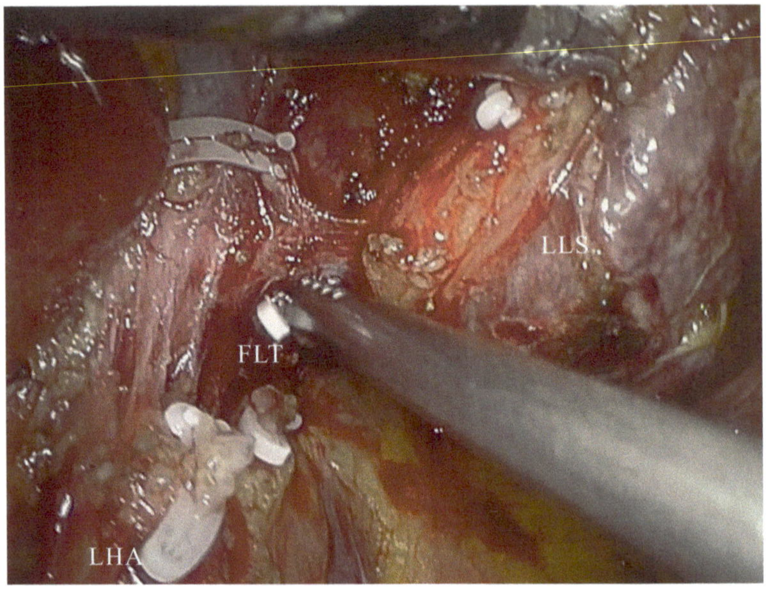

Fig. 3.16 Another secondary branch of portal vein is visualized after the previous one was divided

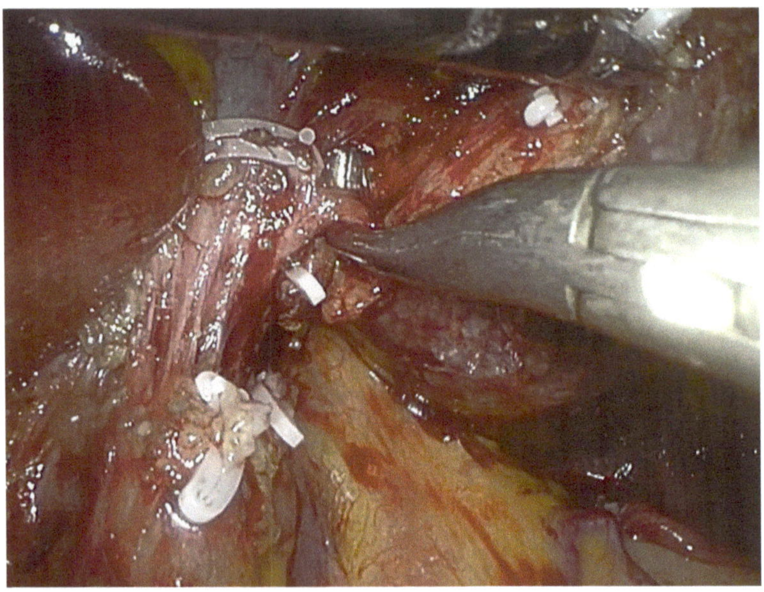

Fig. 3.17 The secondary branch of portal vein is dissected

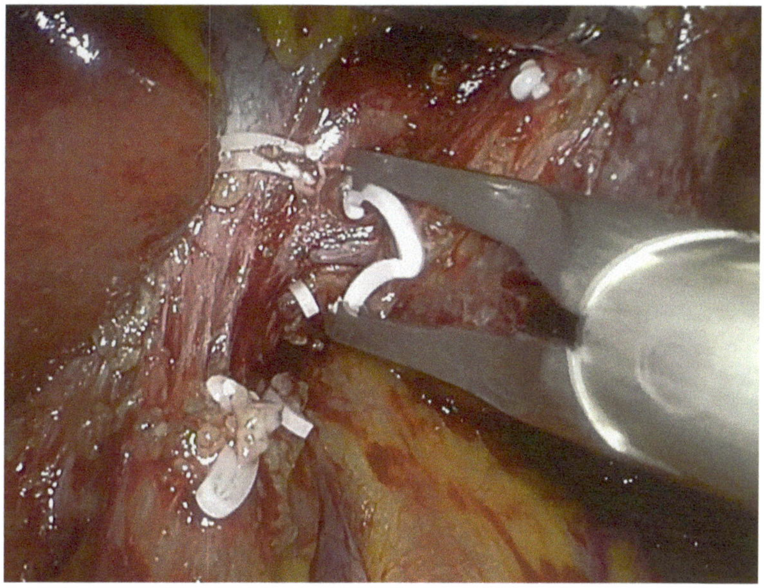

Fig. 3.18 The secondary branch of portal vein is clamped with a nonabsorbable polymer clip

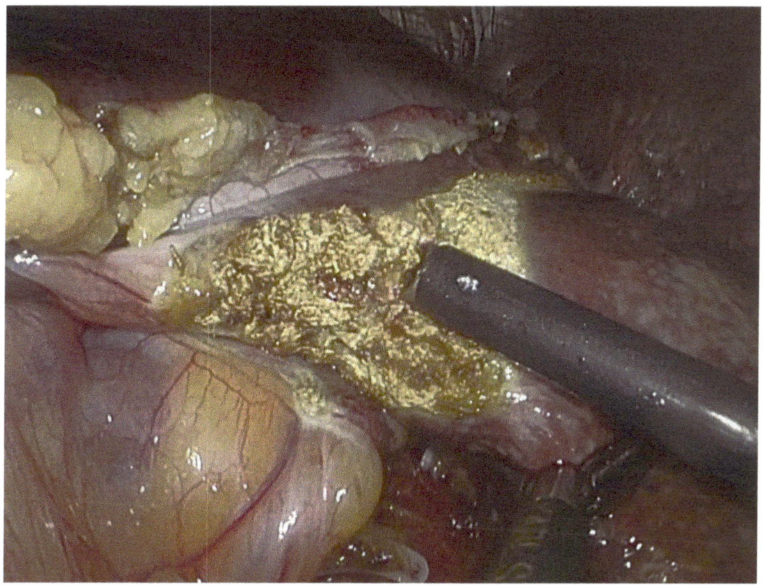

Fig. 3.19 Liver parenchyma is transected with LPMOD along the falciform ligament

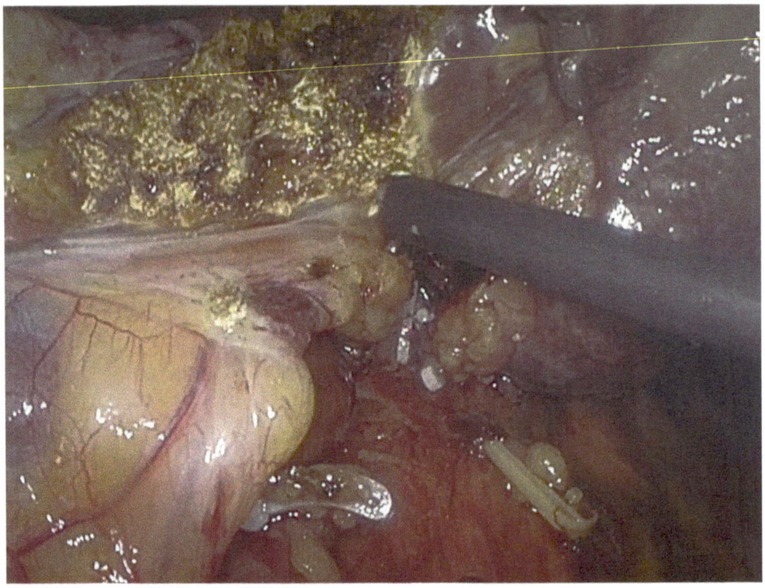

Fig. 3.20 The left lobe of the liver is elevated after the liver parenchyma was transected with LPMOD along the fissure for ligamentum teres

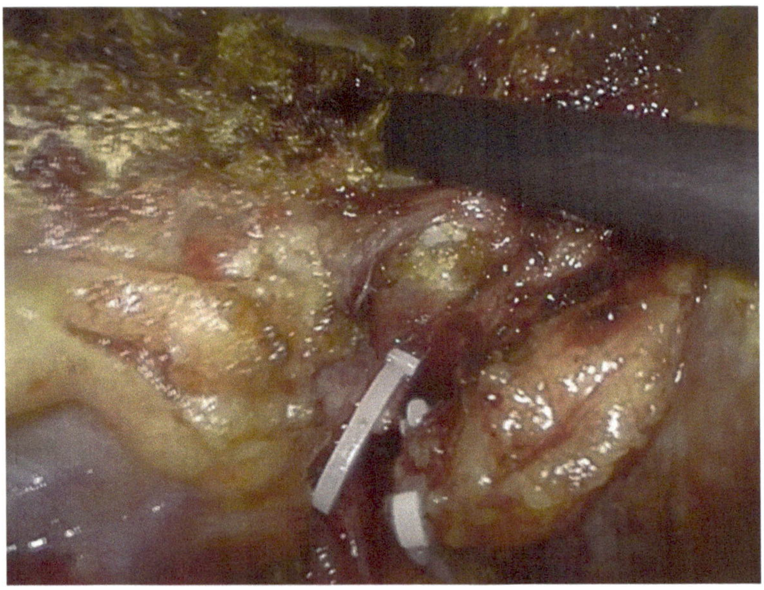

Fig. 3.21 A secondary branch of portal vein is visualized in the transection

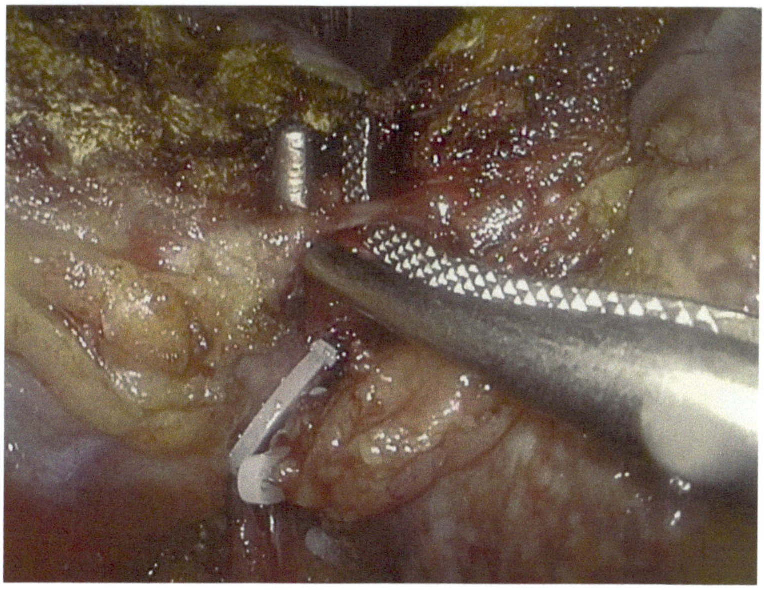

Fig. 3.22 The secondary branch of portal vein is dissected

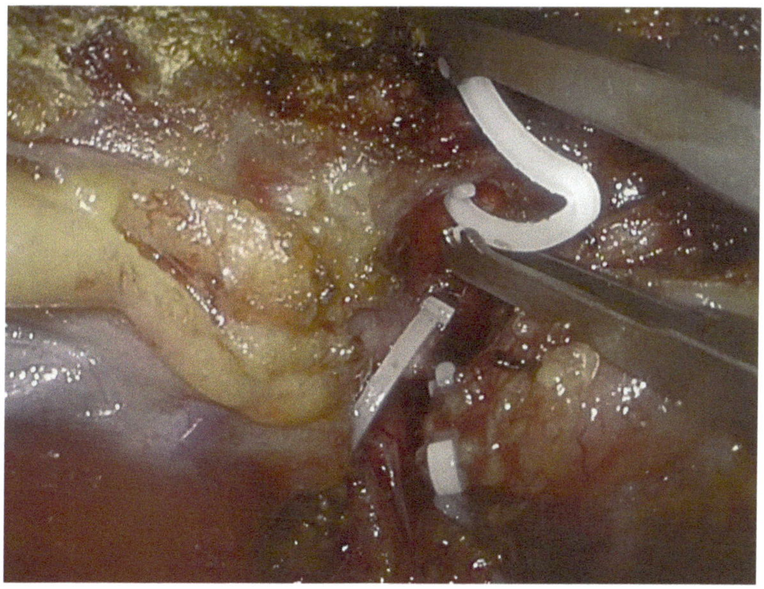

Fig. 3.23 The secondary branch of portal vein is clamped with a nonabsorbable polymer clip

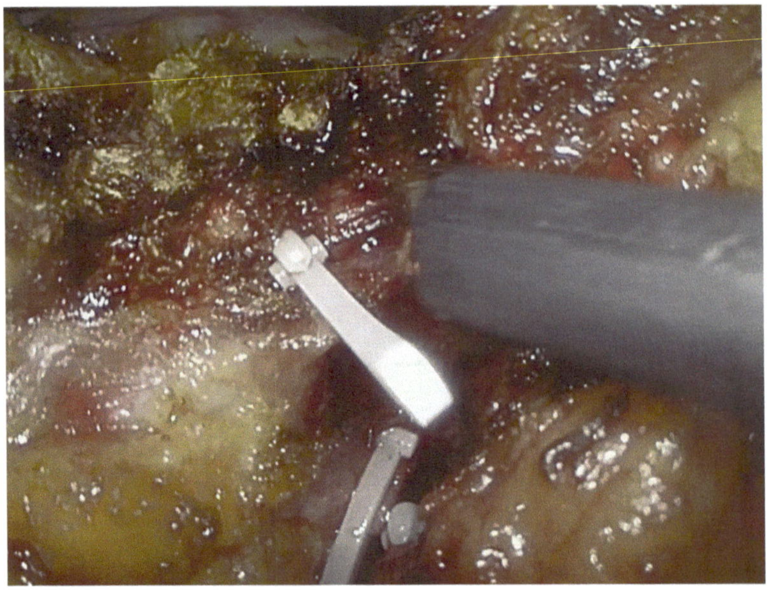

Fig. 3.24 The secondary branch of portal vein is transected

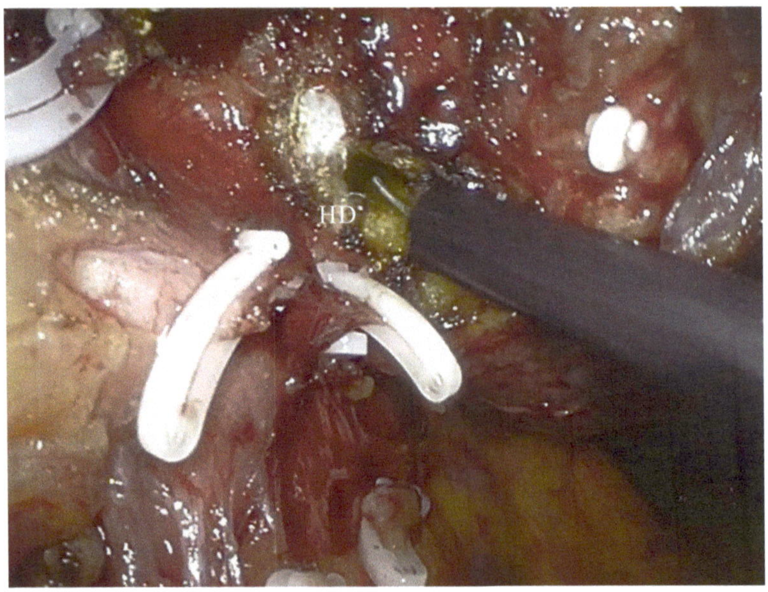

Fig. 3.25 The hepatic duct (*HD*) to the left lateral segment is visualized

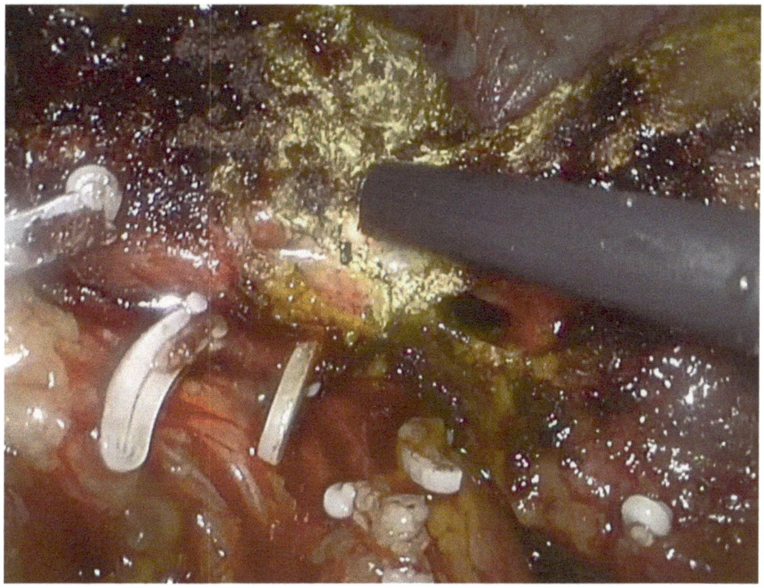

Fig. 3.26 The hepatic duct is transected with LPMOD

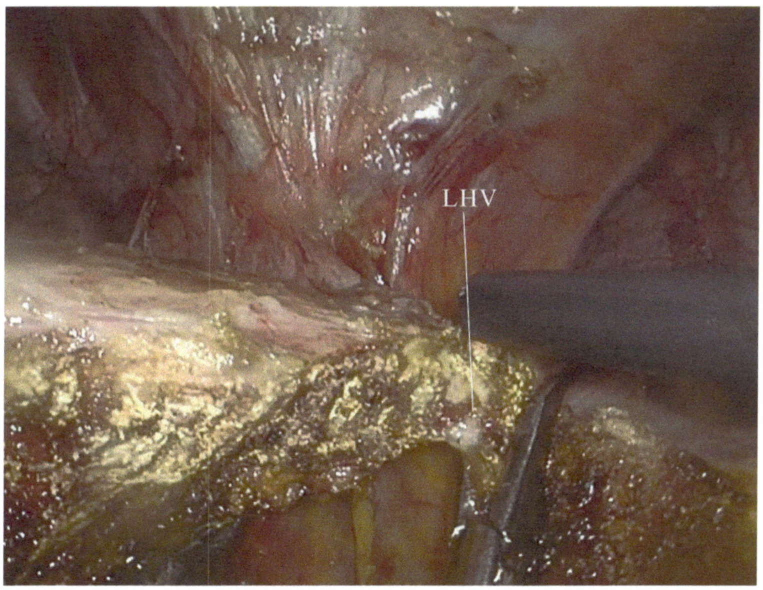

Fig. 3.27 LHV is dissected with LPMOD

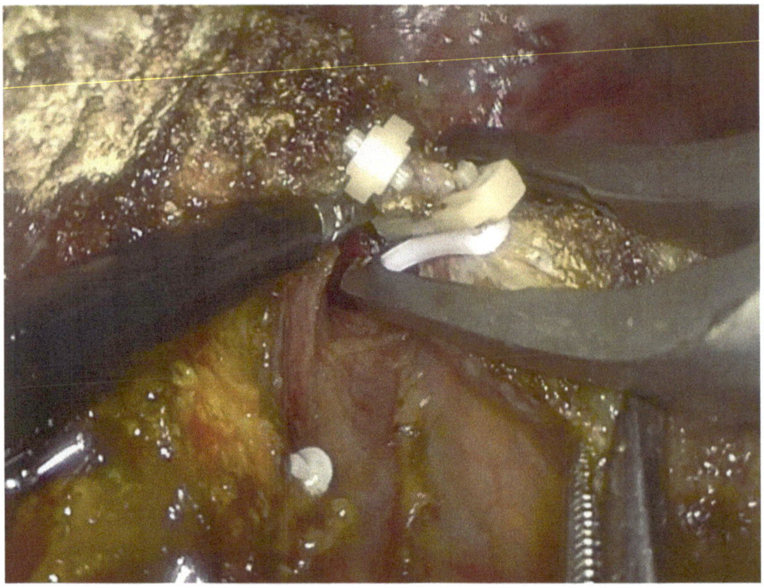

Fig. 3.28 LHV is clamped with clips

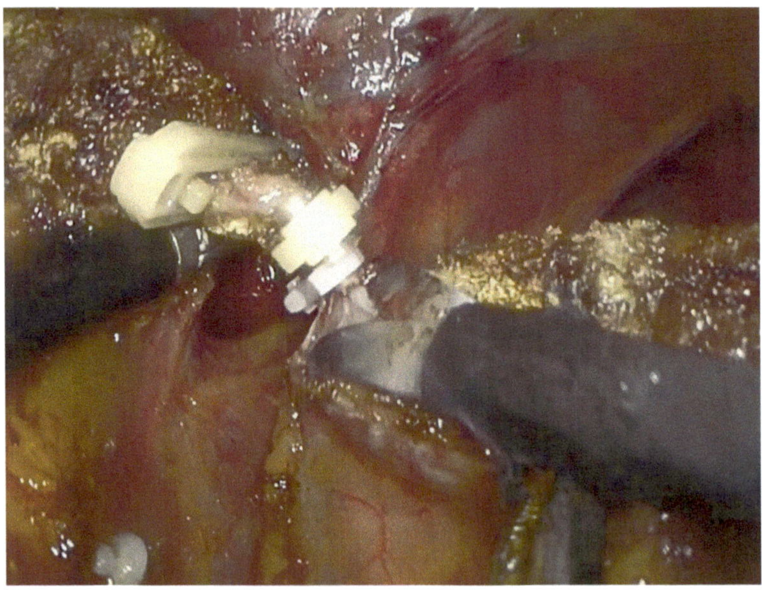

Fig. 3.29 LHV is divided and the left lateral segment is resected

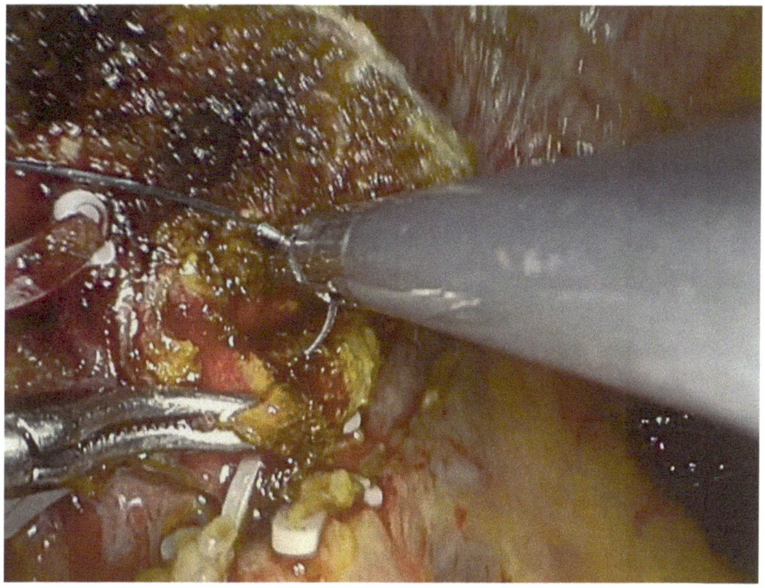

Fig. 3.30 After the left lateral segment was removed, the stump of the left hepatic duct (LHD) is sutured

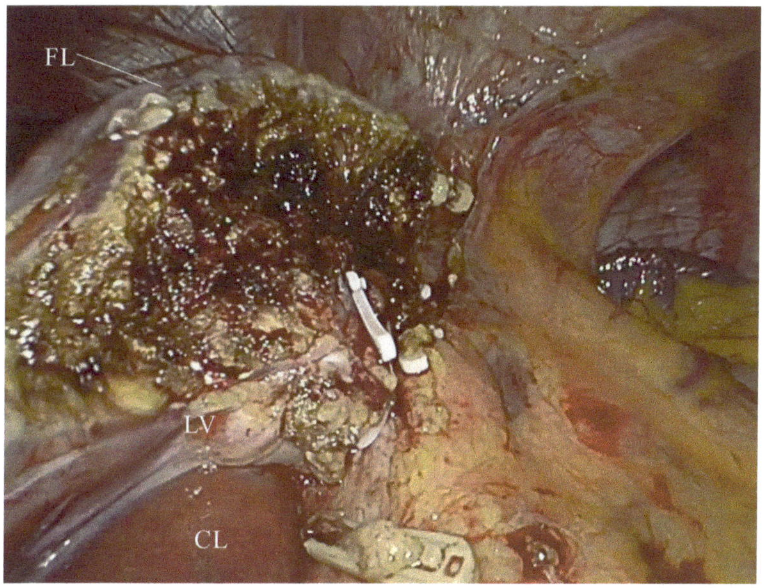

Fig. 3.31 The view of the transection plane

References

Azagra JS, Goergen M, Gilbart E, et al. Laparoscopic anatomical (hepatic) left lateral segmentectomy-technical aspects. Surg Endosc. 1996;10:758–61.

Buell JF, Cherqui D, Geller DA, et al. The international position on laparoscopic liver surgery: the Louisville Statement, 2008. Ann Surg. 2009;250:825–30.

4 Laparoscopic Left Hemihepatectomy

Laparoscopic hemihepatectomy is one of the most difficult laparoscopic surgeries and is rarely performed worldwide. In our institute, laparoscopic left hemihepatectomy has been performed as a routine procedure since 2005. The technique of hepatectomy by curettage and aspiration and the selective left inflow occlusion (Fig. 4.1) are the points of this procedure by which the intraoperative blood loss decreases significantly. Total vascular occlusion is the conventional procedure for controlling intraoperative bleeding in open major liver resection and is used in some laparoscopic liver resections (Dulucq et al. 2005; Descottes et al. 2003; Cherqui et al. 2003, 2006). Laparoscopic selective inflow occlusion is more difficult than the total vascular occlusion, but it can avoid the complications of ischemia-reperfusion injury and gastrointestinal congestion (Sahin et al. 2004; Teoh and Farrell 2003; Malassagne et al. 1998). The selective inflow occlusion does not require fast liver transection to decrease the occlusion time allowing surgeons sufficient time for meticulous dissection.

Gas embolism is a dangerous complication of a laparoscopic surgery. In major hepatectomy, the vena cava could be intermittently partly occluded for the compression or the torsion of inferior vena cava (IVC). The venous pressure of the proximal vena cava decreased significantly, and carbon dioxide could be sucked into the vena cava via tears in hepatic veins, which was described as Venturi effect by Hatano et al. (1990). In such a situation, even a small tear in the hepatic vein may lead to the gas embolism. Before liver transection, occluding the hepatic vein of the lobe to be resected should be a good method to avoid this complication. However, occlusion of the left hepatic vein (LHV) before liver transection is a skill-demanding and riskful procedure, which may lead to unmanageable bleeding and emergency conversion. Therefore, we do not carry it out as a routine procedure. It is only performed on selected patients whose LHV is exposed sufficiently and can be dissected safely.

Electronic supplementary material The online version of this chapter at (doi: 10.1007/978-94-017-9840-2_4) contains supplementary material, which is available to authorized users.

X. Cai, *Laparoscopic Hepatectomy: Atlas and Techniques*,
DOI 10.1007/978-94-017-9840-2_4,

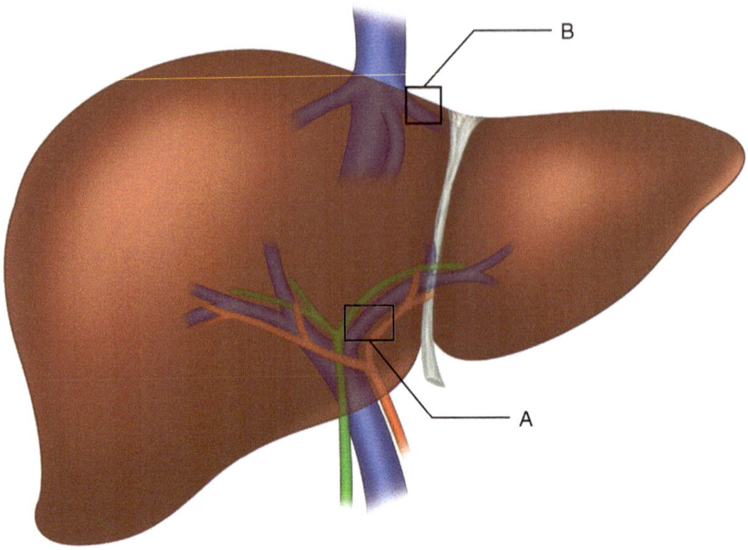

Fig. 4.1 Vascular control in laparoscopic left hemihepatectomy. (*A*) Selective left inflow occlusion; (*B*) Occlusion of left hepatic vein

4.1 Indications and Contraindications

The indications include liver tumors in the left lobe or left intrahepatic bile duct stones with irreversible diseases (biliary stricture, severe parenchymal fibrosis or atrophy) requiring left hemihepatectomy and liver function of Child A to B classification. The contraindications include malignant tumor involving porta hepatis, history of biliary surgeries such as exploration of common bile duct or cholangiojejunostomy (cholecystectomy is not regarded as a contraindication), extrahepatic bile duct stricture, or acute suppurative cholangitis.

4.2 Patient Position and Trocars' Position

Patients are placed in the supine position under general anesthesia. Three surgeons are needed in the operation. As shown in Fig. 4.2, the senior surgeon stands on the left side of the patient, one assistant surgeon stands on the right side of the senior surgeon controlling the aspiration device, and the other assistant surgeon stands on right side of the patient. Four entries are made. A supraumbilical 10-mm trocar is inserted as the observation port. A 12-mm trocar below the left costal margin is inserted as the main manipulation port. And two 5-mm trocars are inserted at the right flank area as assistant manipulation ports.

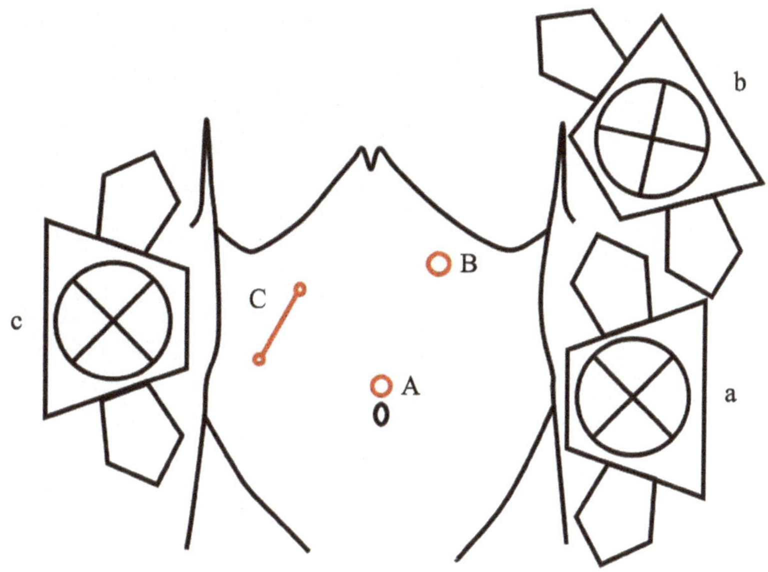

Fig. 4.2 The trocars' position and surgeons' position. (*A*) Observation port; (*B*) Main manipulation port; (*C*) Two assistant ports and the incision for removing specimen; (**a**) The senior surgeon stands on the left side of the patient; (**b**) One assistant surgeon stands on the right side of the senior surgeon controlling the aspiration device; (**c**) The other assistant surgeon stands on the right side of the patient

4.3 Laparoscopic Left Hemihepatectomy with Selective Left Inflow Occlusion and Occlusion of Left Hepatic Vein

See Figs. 4.3, 4.4, 4.5, 4.6, 4.7, 4.8, 4.9, 4.10, 4.11, 4.12, 4.13, 4.14, 4.15, 4.16, 4.17, 4.18, 4.19, 4.20, 4.21, 4.22, 4.23, 4.24, 4.25, 4.26, 4.27, 4.28, 4.29, 4.30, 4.31, 4.32, 4.33, 4.34, 4.35, 4.36, 4.37, 4.38, 4.39, 4.40, 4.41, 4.42, 4.43, 4.44, 4.45, 4.46, 4.47, and Video 4.1.

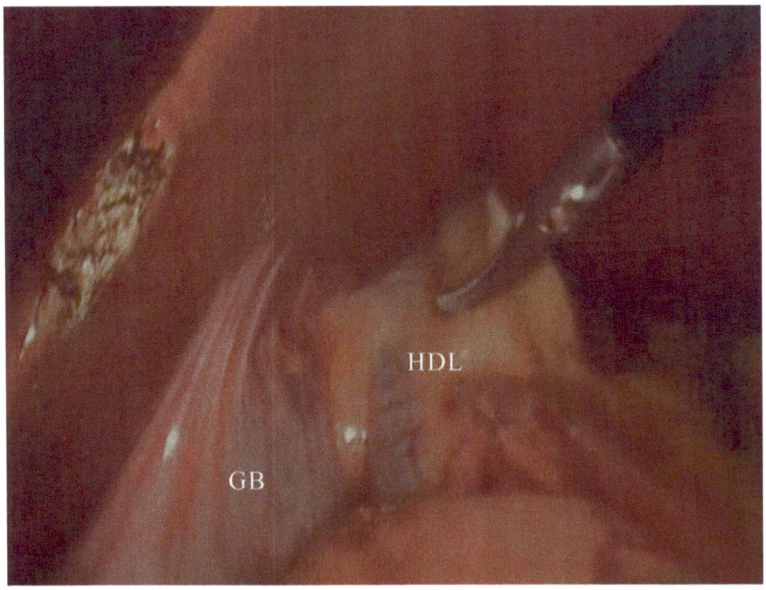

Fig. 4.3 The liver is mobilized upward by the traction of the round ligament (RL), and the hepatoduodenal ligament (*HDL*) is visualized

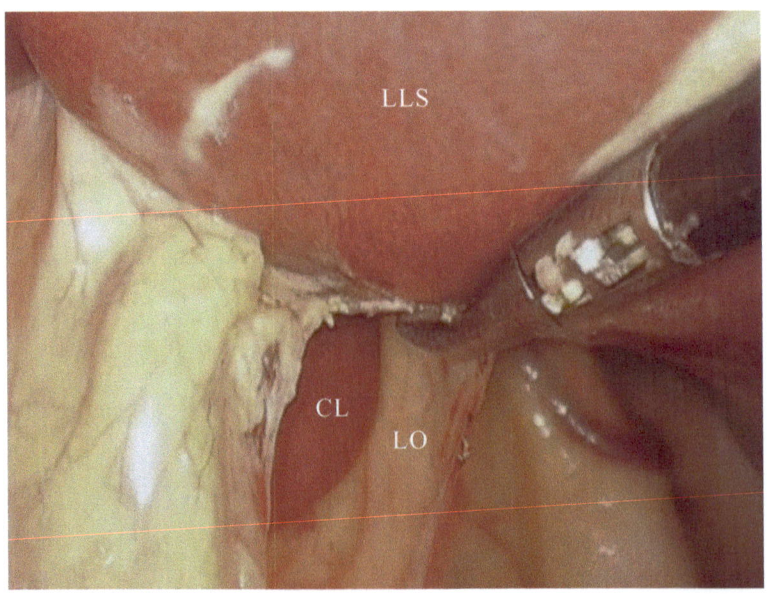

Fig. 4.4 The lesser omentum (*LO*) is divided and the caudate lobe (*CL*) of the liver is visualized

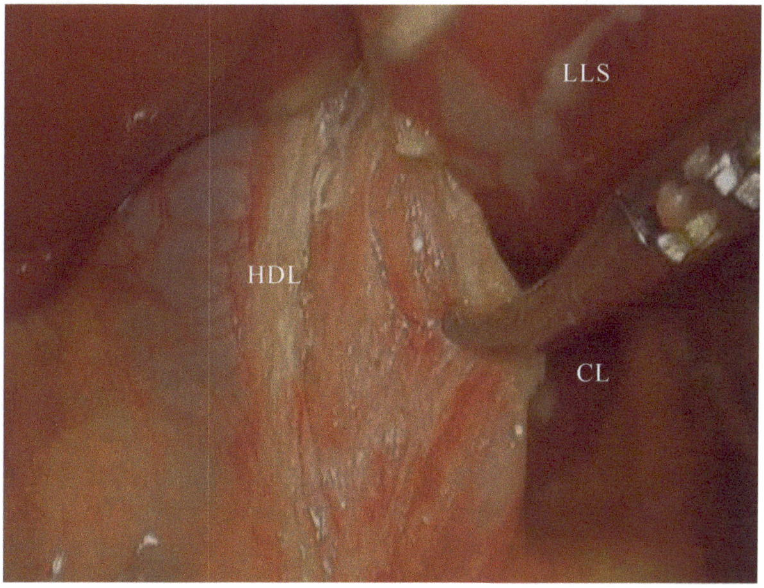

Fig. 4.5 HDL is dissected with a forceps, LPMOD, or the tip of aspiration tube

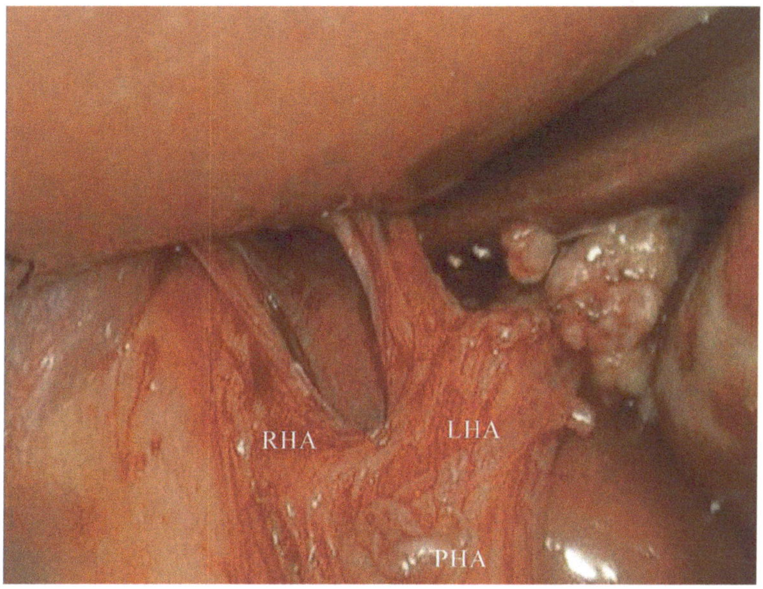

Fig. 4.6 The left hepatic artery (*LHA*) is dissected

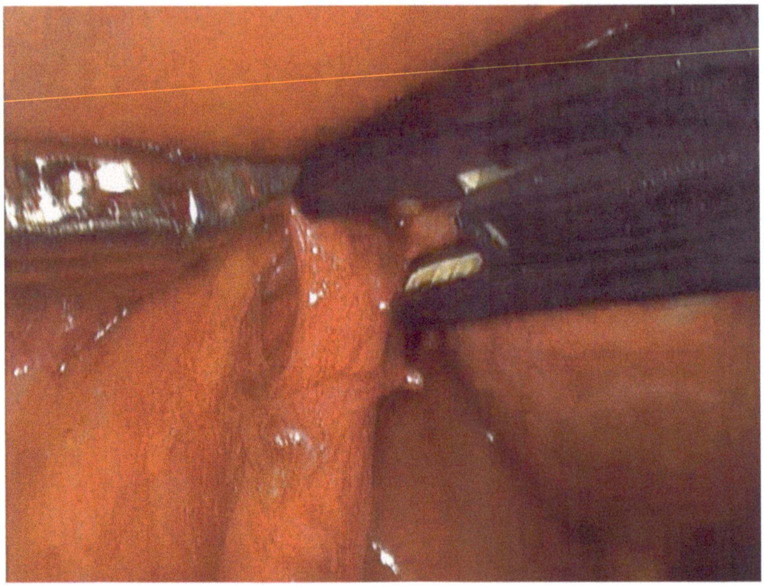

Fig. 4.7 The LHA is clamped with an absorbable clip

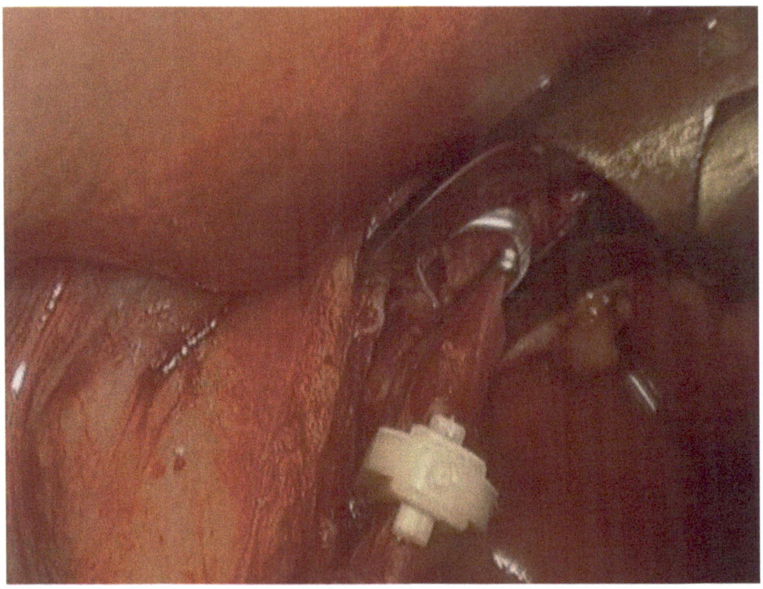

Fig. 4.8 Titanic clips are applied on the distal portion of the LHA

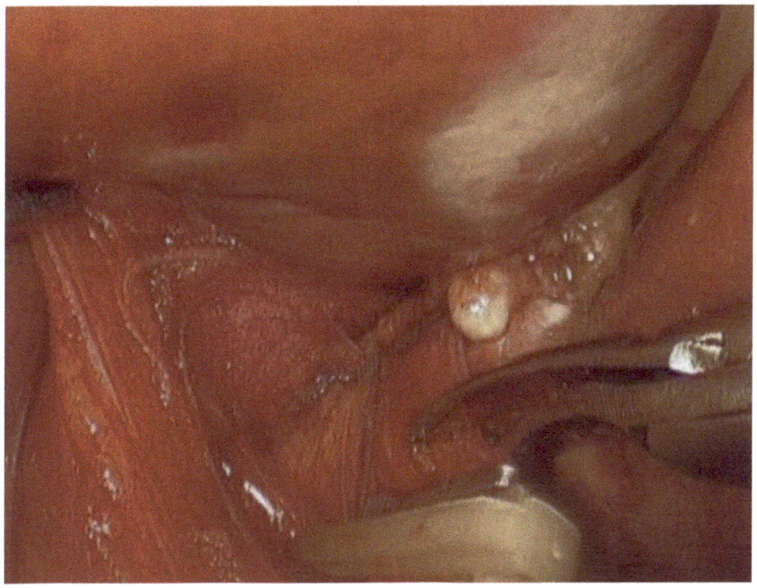

Fig. 4.9 The LHA is divided

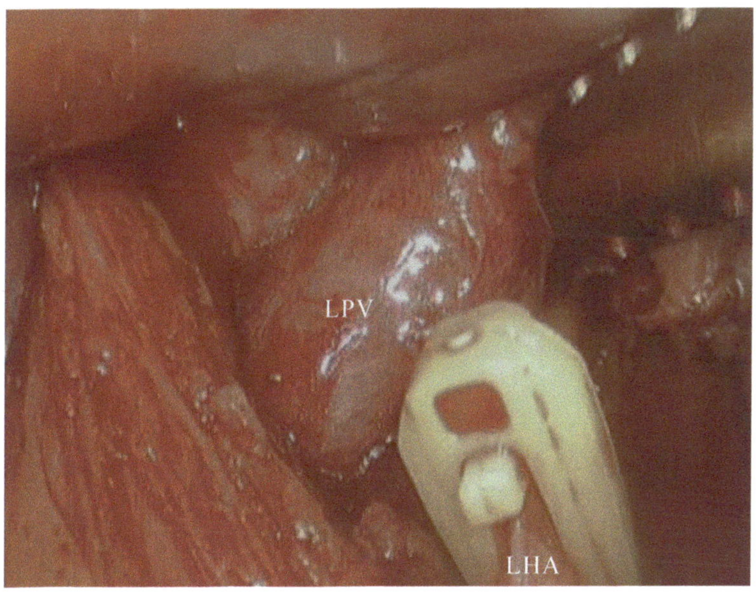

Fig. 4.10 After the LHA was divided, the left branch of portal vein (*LPV*) is visualized

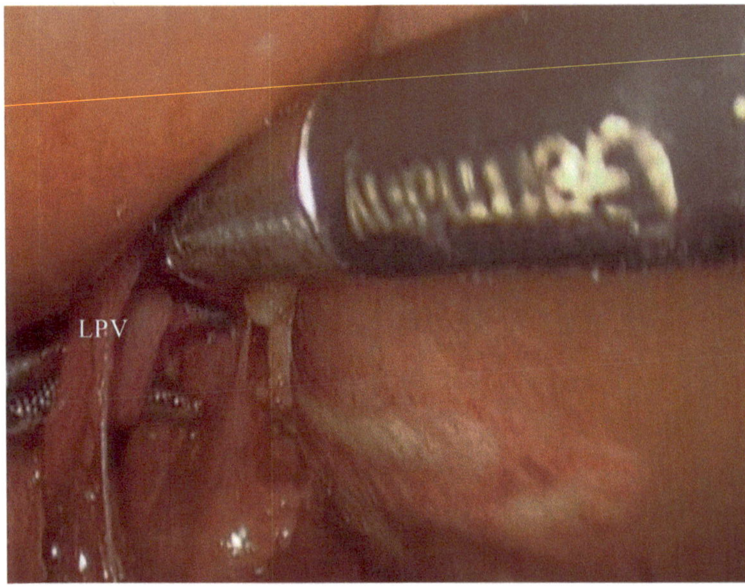

Fig. 4.11 The LPV is freed

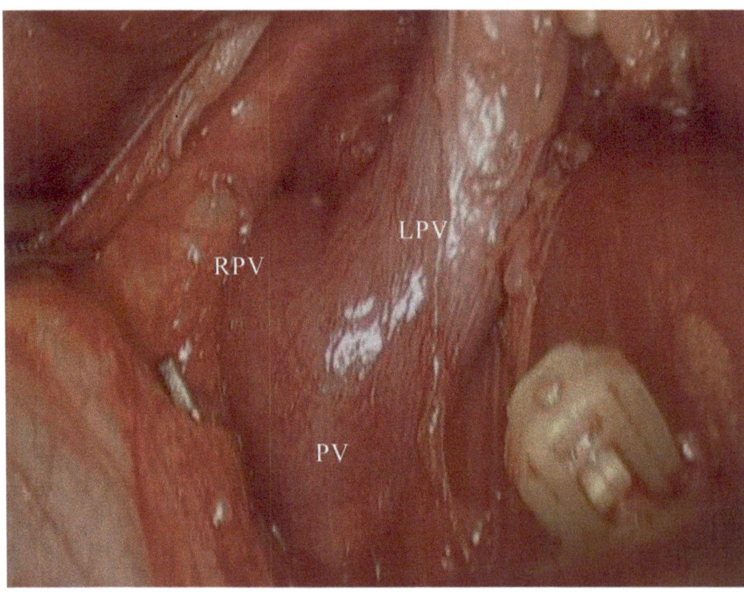

Fig. 4.12 The right branch of portal vein (*RPV*), as well as the portal vein (*PV*), is visualized, and the bifurcation is identified before the execution of the selective inflow occlusion

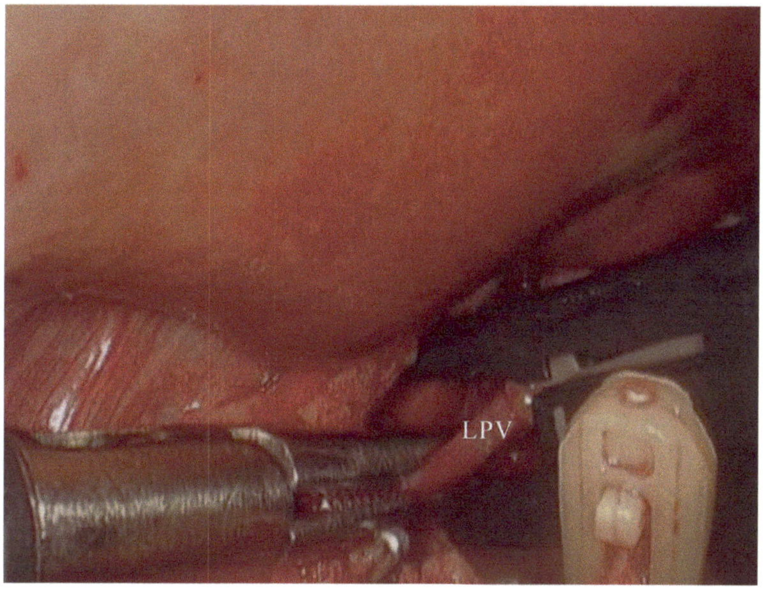

Fig. 4.13 The selective inflow occlusion is executed by applying an absorbable clip on the LPV

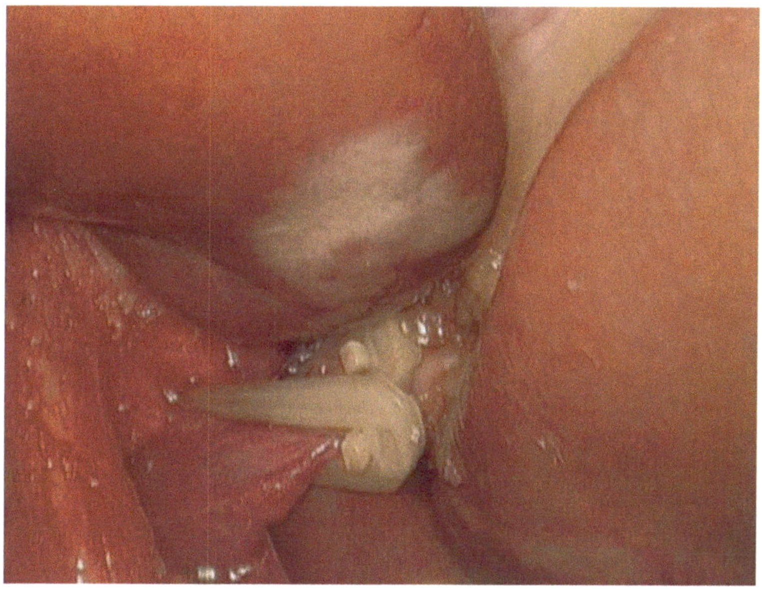

Fig. 4.14 The LPV is clamped with absorbable clips, and the selective left inflow occlusion is completed

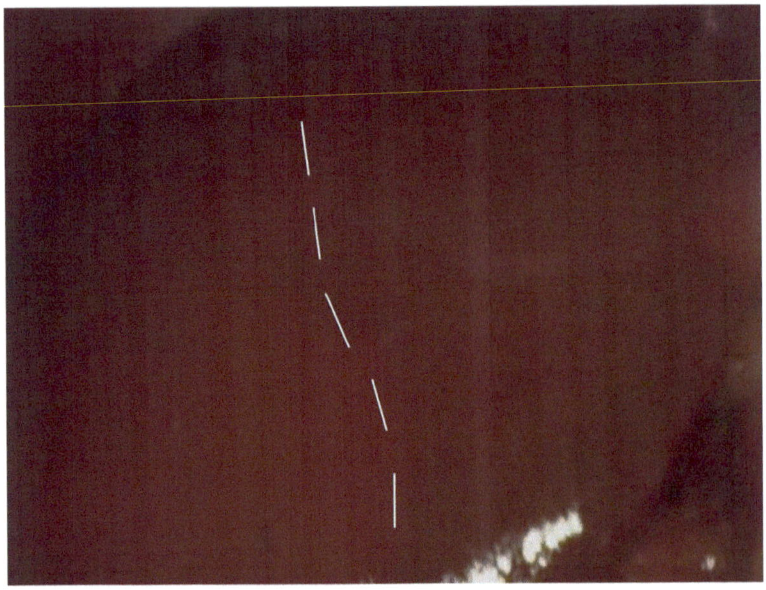

Fig. 4.15 A ischemic *line* can be visualized on the liver's surface

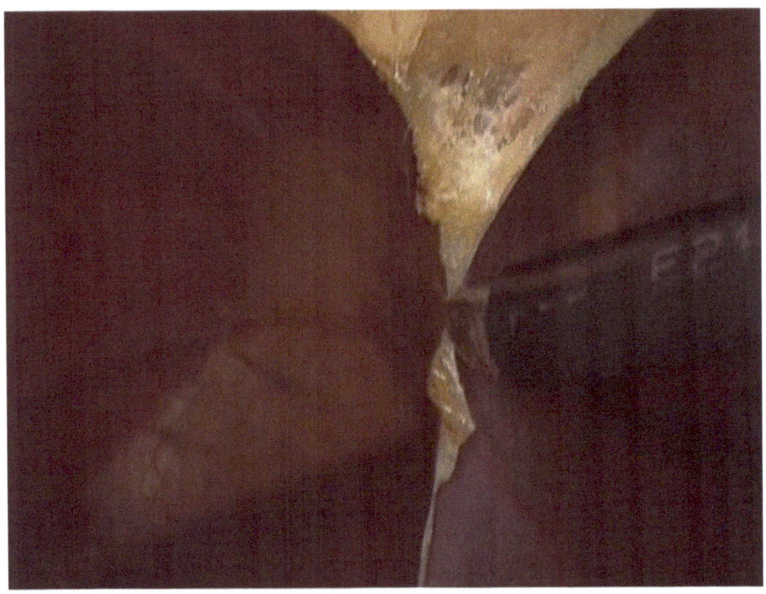

Fig. 4.16 The round ligament and the falciform ligament (FL) are divided with LPMOD

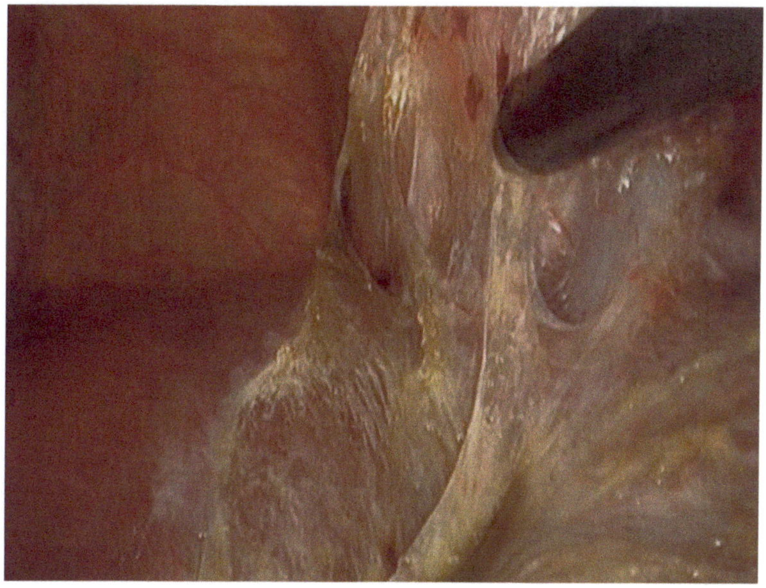

Fig. 4.17 The inferior vena cava is dissected with LPMOD

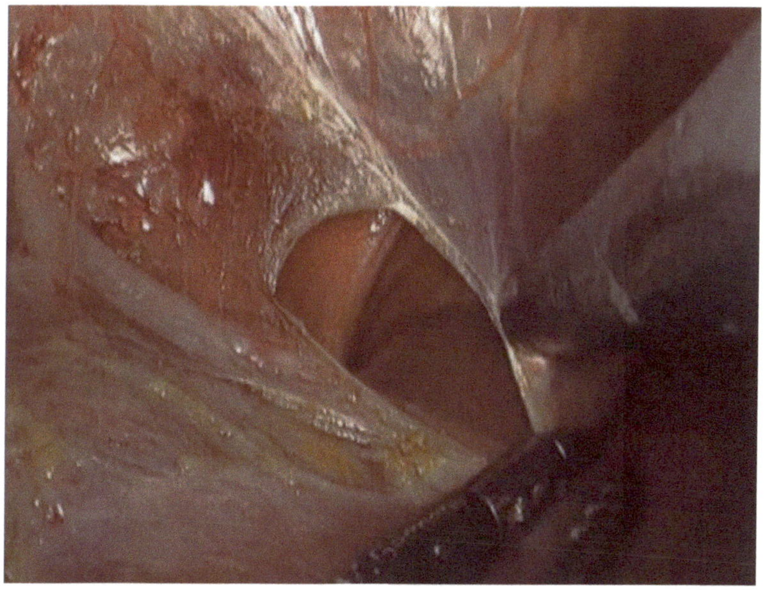

Fig. 4.18 The left lobe (LL) of the liver is pressed downward with a laparoscopic grasping forceps, and the left coronary ligament (LCL) is divided with LPMOD

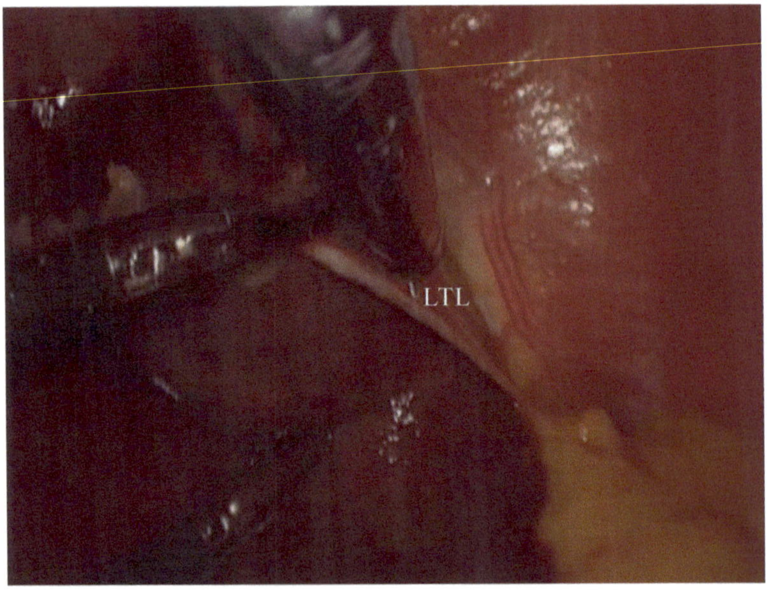

Fig. 4.19 The left lobe is mobilized to the right, and the left triangle ligament (*LTL*) is divided with LPMOD

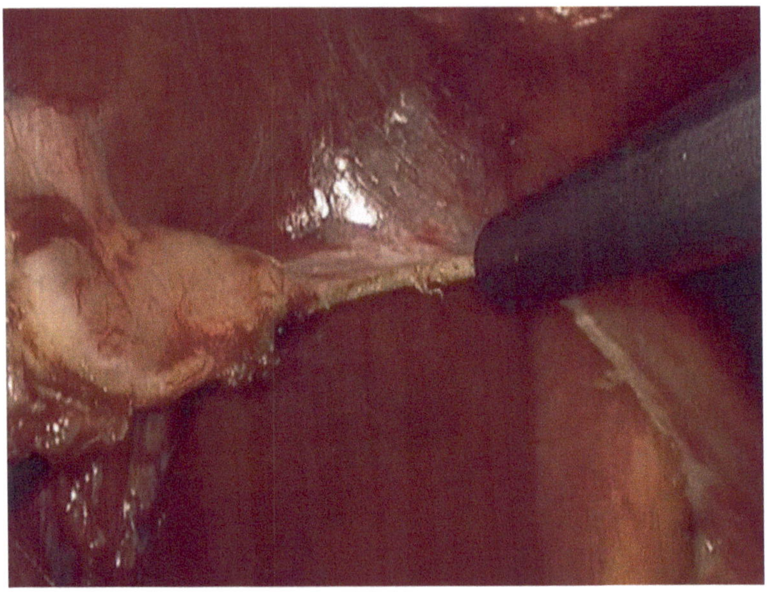

Fig. 4.20 The left lobe of the liver is mobilized to the right and LO is divided

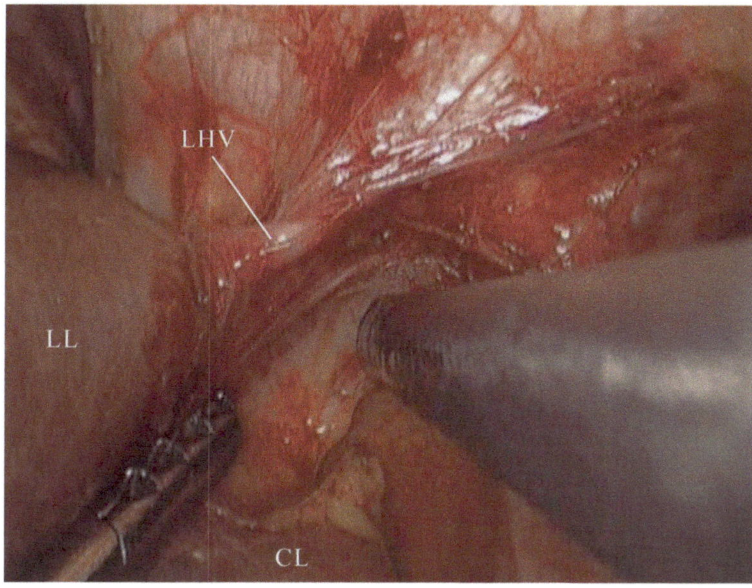

Fig. 4.21 The LL of the liver is mobilized downward and the LHV is dissected with the LPMOD

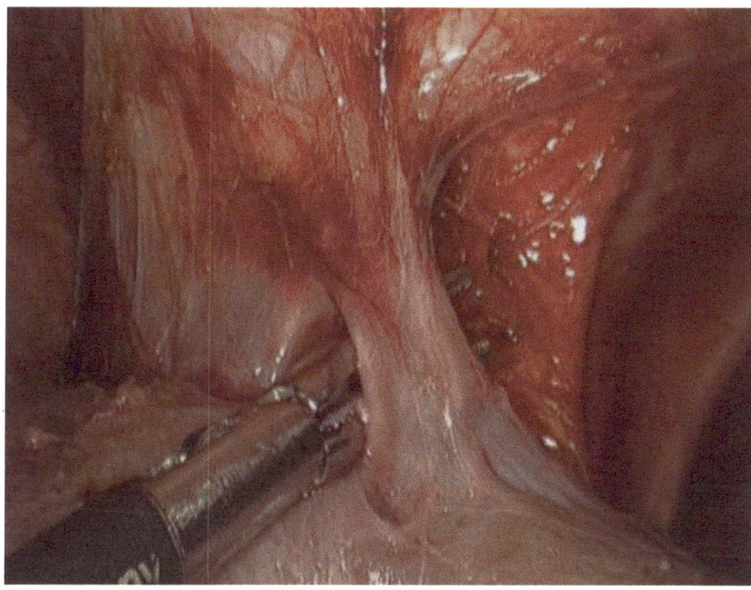

Fig. 4.22 The LHV is freed

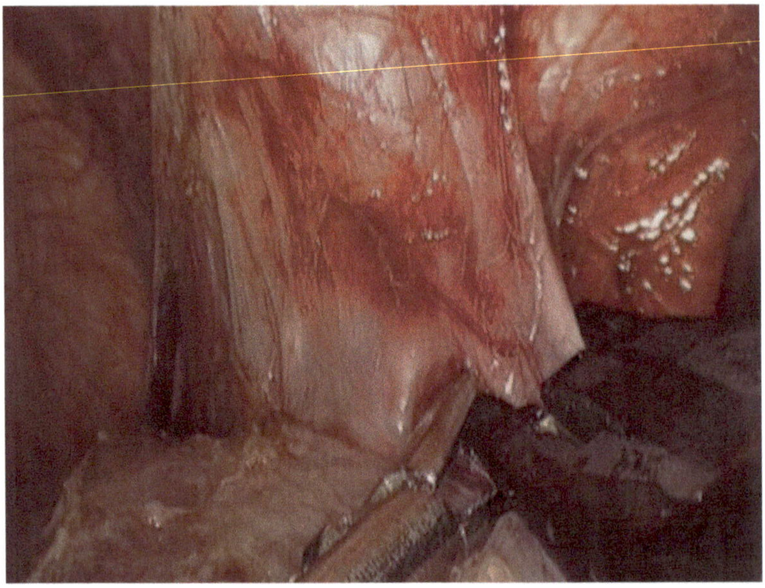

Fig. 4.23 The LHV is clamped with an absorbable clip

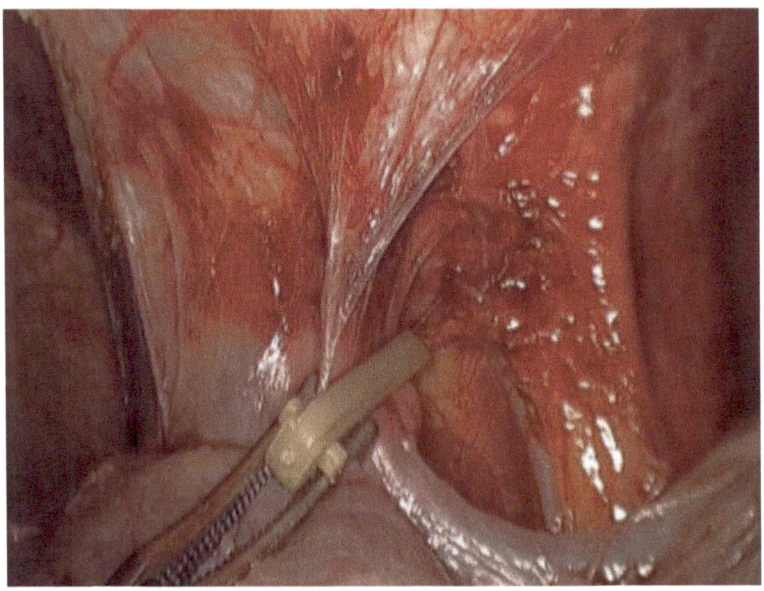

Fig. 4.24 The view of the LHV after being occluded

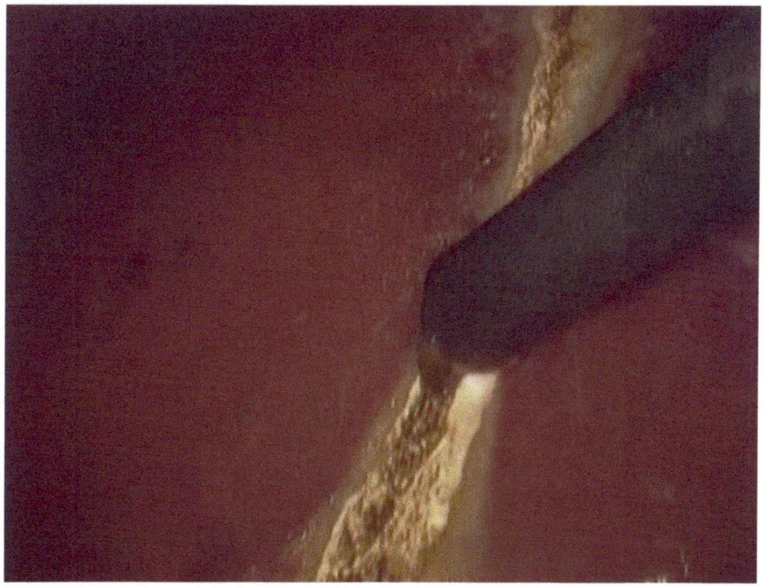

Fig. 4.25 A transection line is marked on the liver surface along the ischemic line

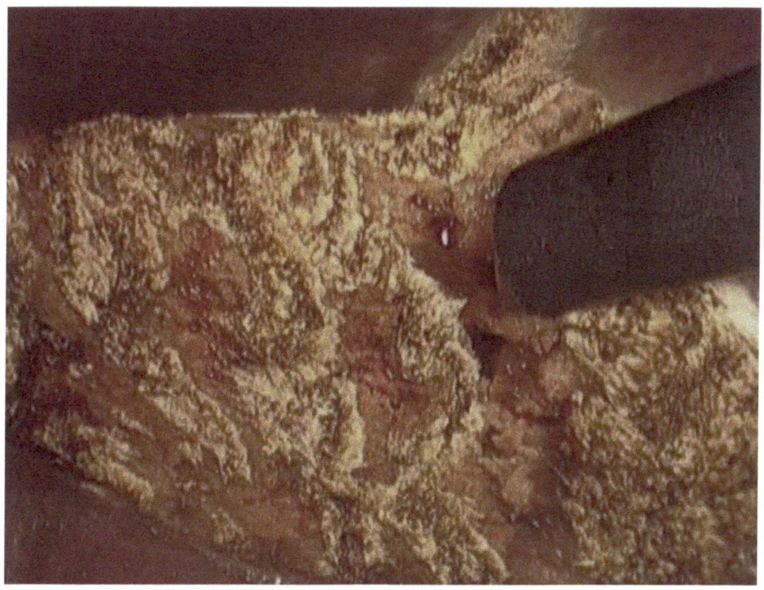

Fig. 4.26 Liver parenchyma is transected with LPMOD

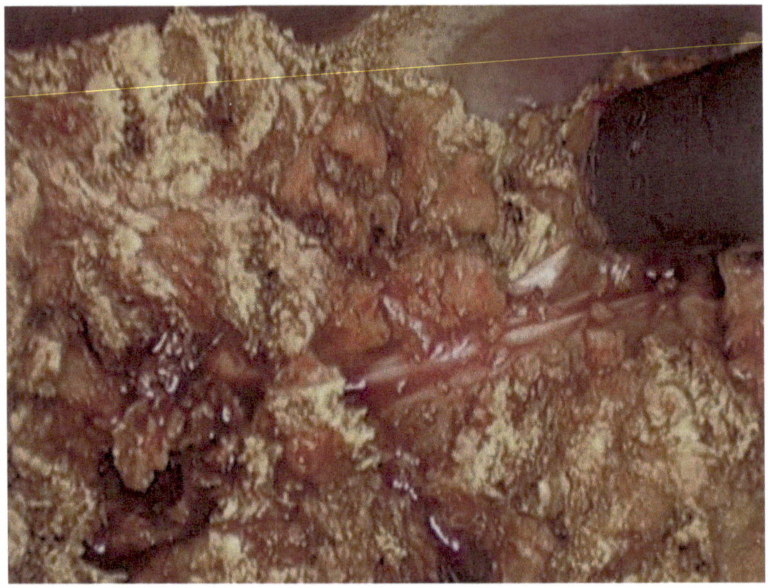

Fig. 4.27 Small vessels are visualized in the transection of the liver parenchyma

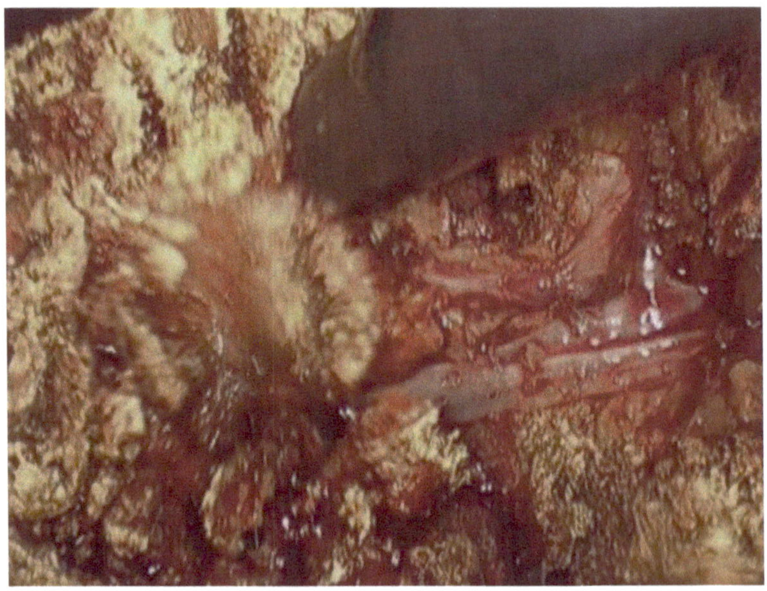

Fig. 4.28 The vessels are dissected with LPMOD

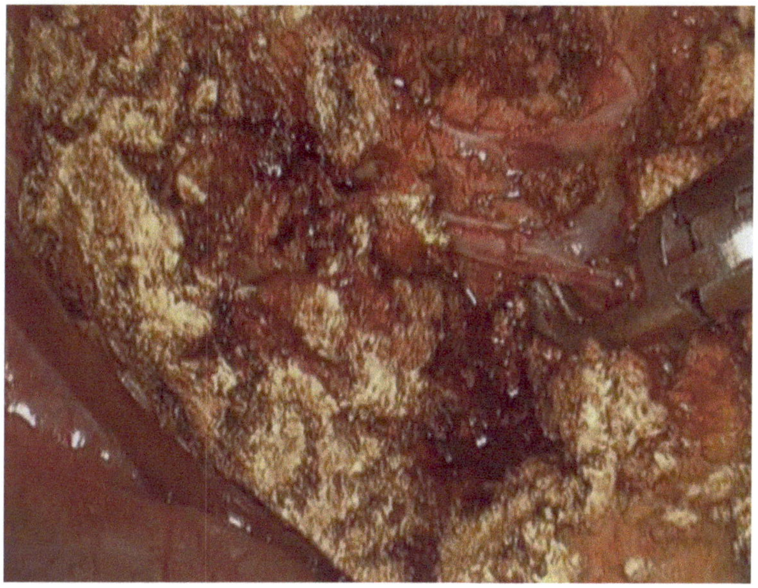

Fig. 4.29 The vessels are freed with a curved dissecting forceps

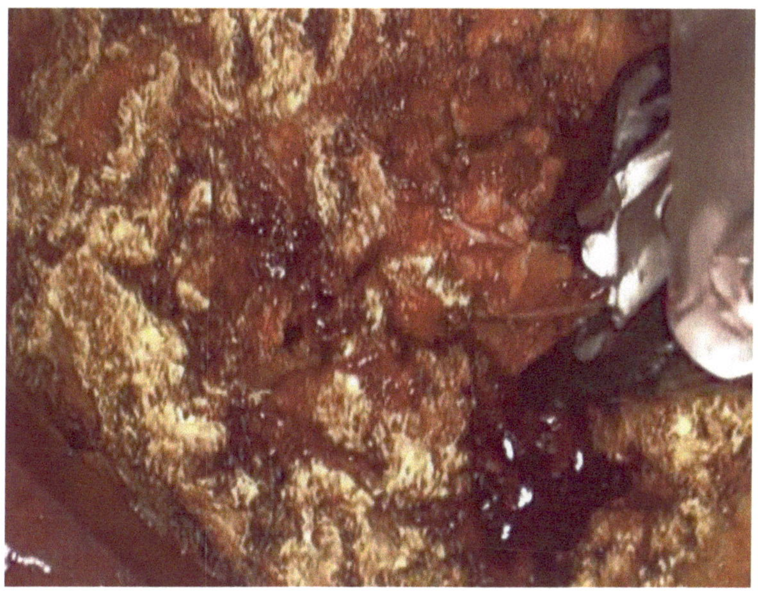

Fig. 4.30 The vessels are clamped with titanic clips

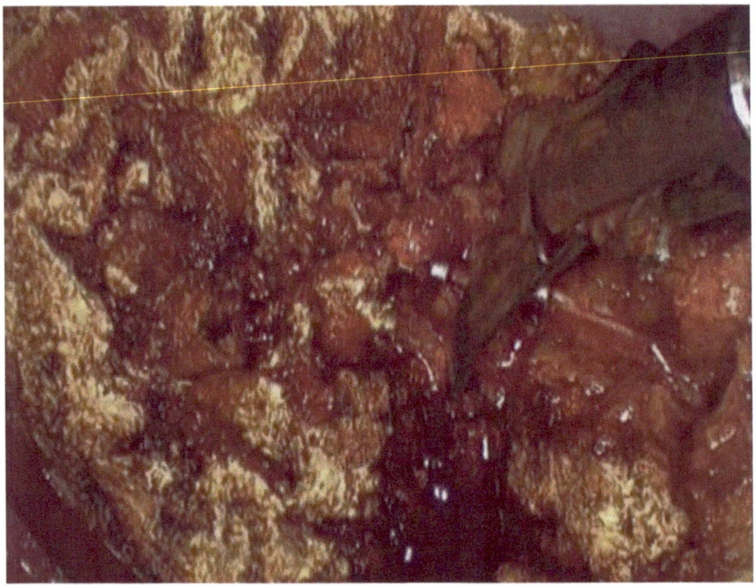

Fig. 4.31 The vessels are divided

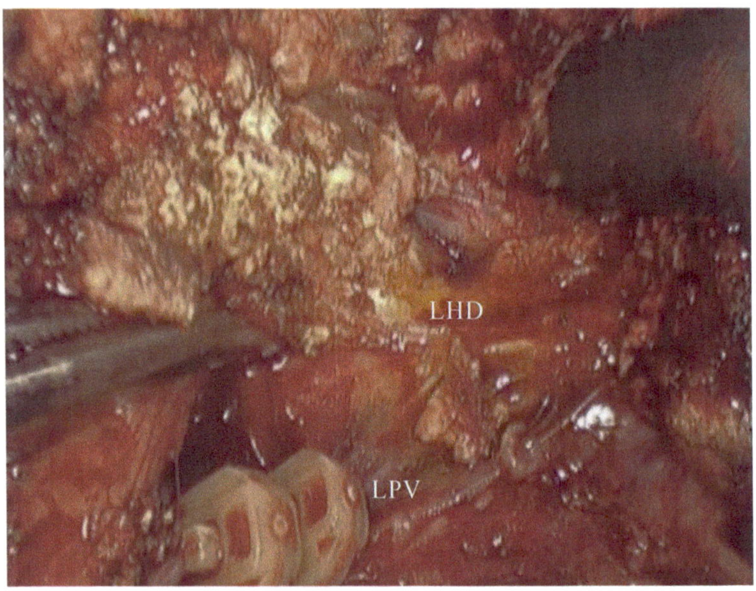

Fig. 4.32 The left hepatic duct (*LHD*) is visualized in the transection of the liver parenchyma and is dissected with LPMOD

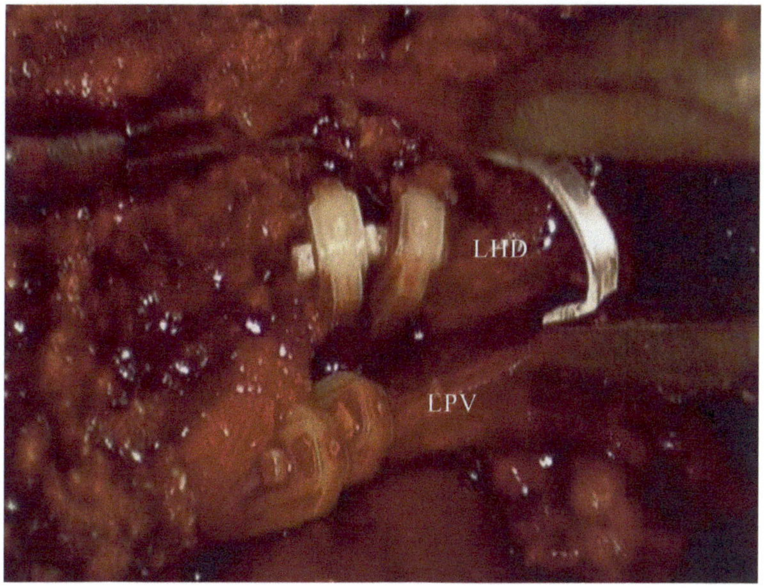

Fig. 4.33 The LHD is clamped with absorbable clips

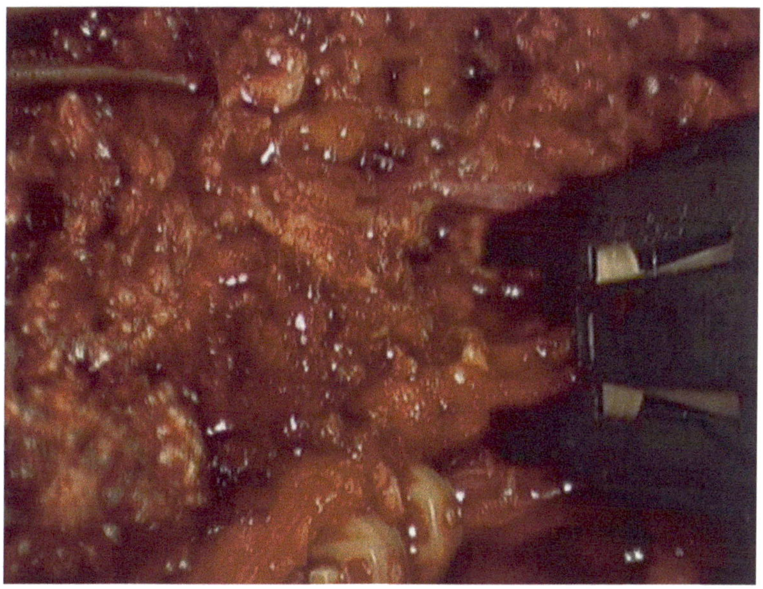

Fig. 4.34 A titanic clip is applied on the distal portion of the LHD

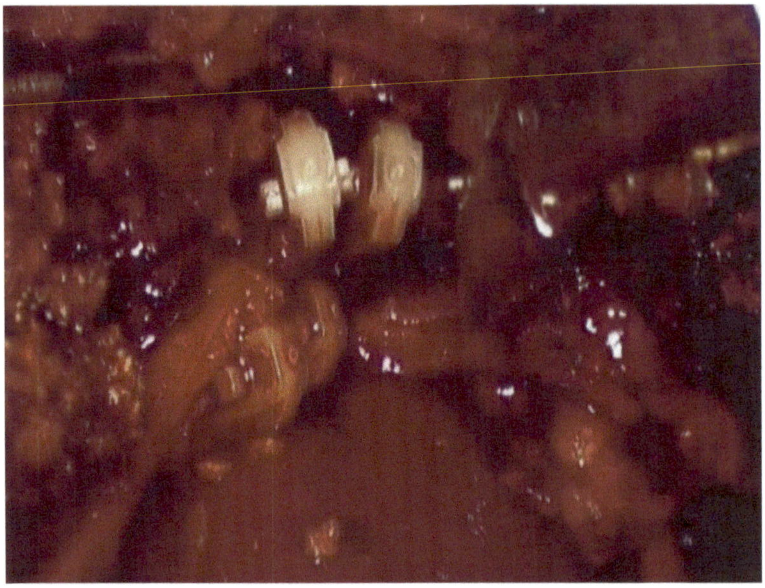

Fig. 4.35 The LHD is divided

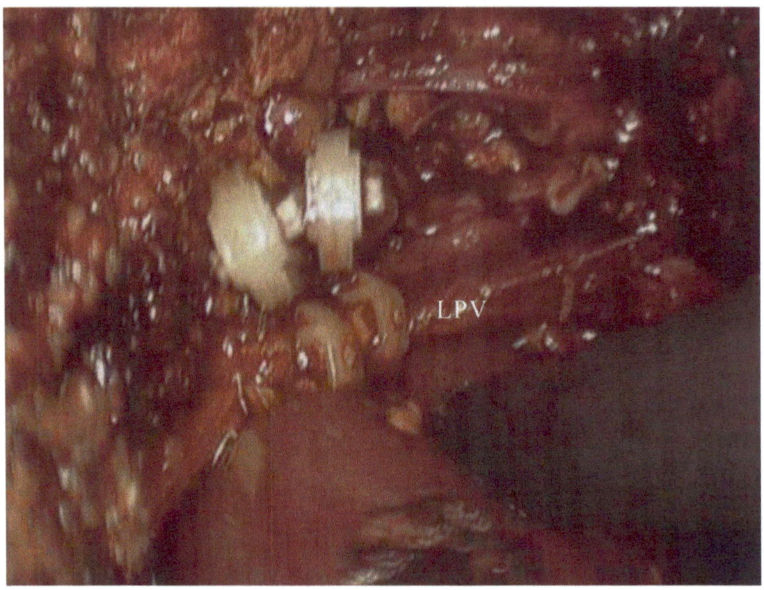

Fig. 4.36 The LPV which was occluded before liver transection is clearly exposed after the division of the LHD

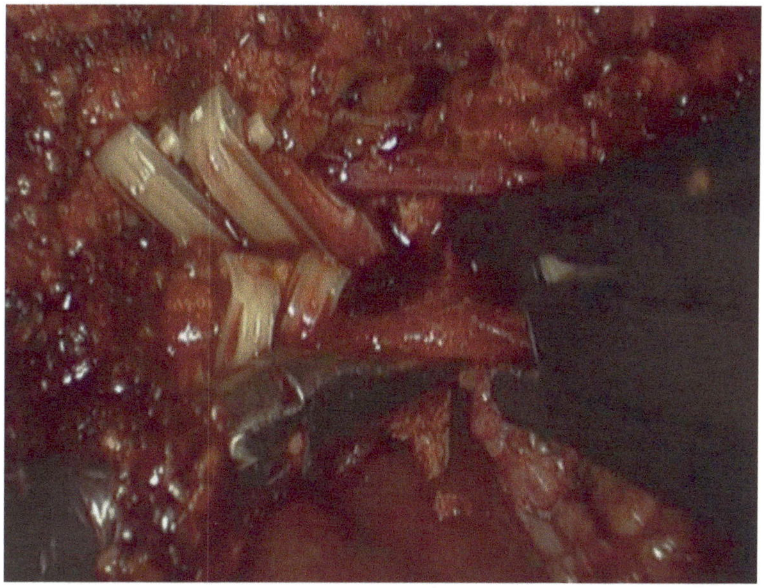

Fig. 4.37 An absorbable clip is applied on the distal portion of the LPV

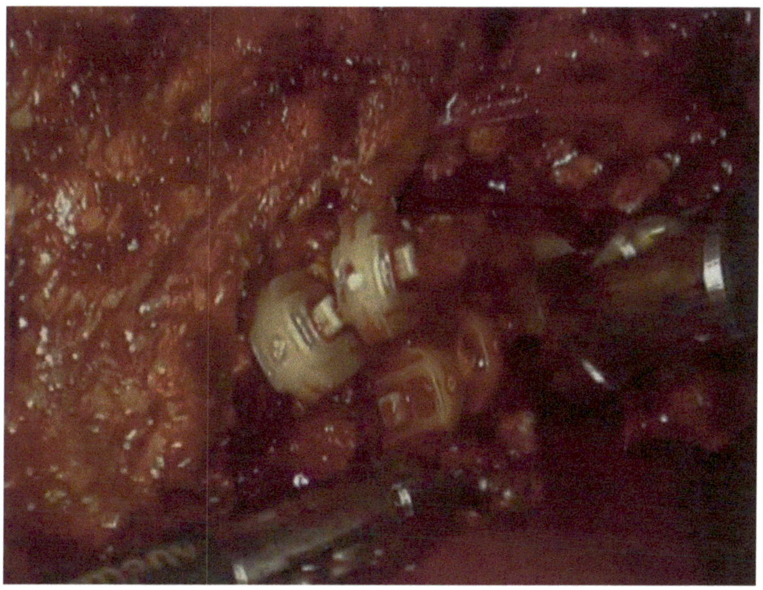

Fig. 4.38 The LPV is divided

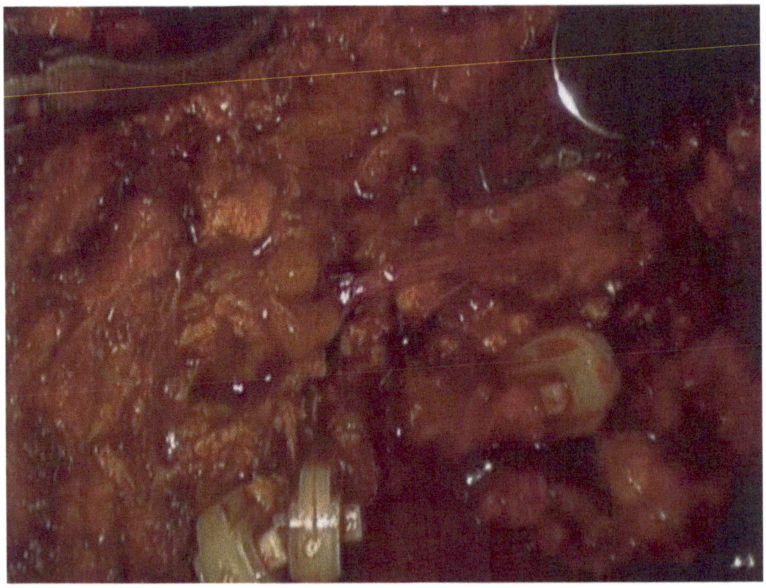

Fig. 4.39 A branch of middle hepatic vein (MHV) is dissected

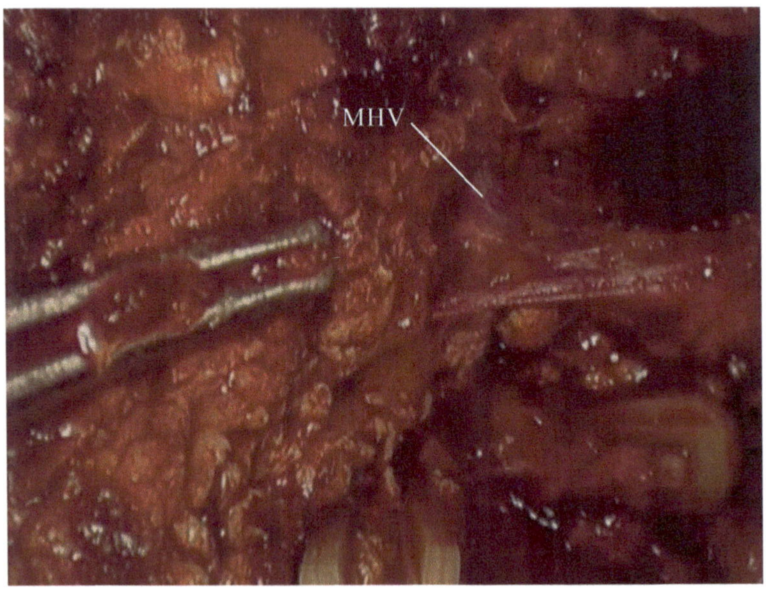

Fig. 4.40 The MHV is visualized after further dissection

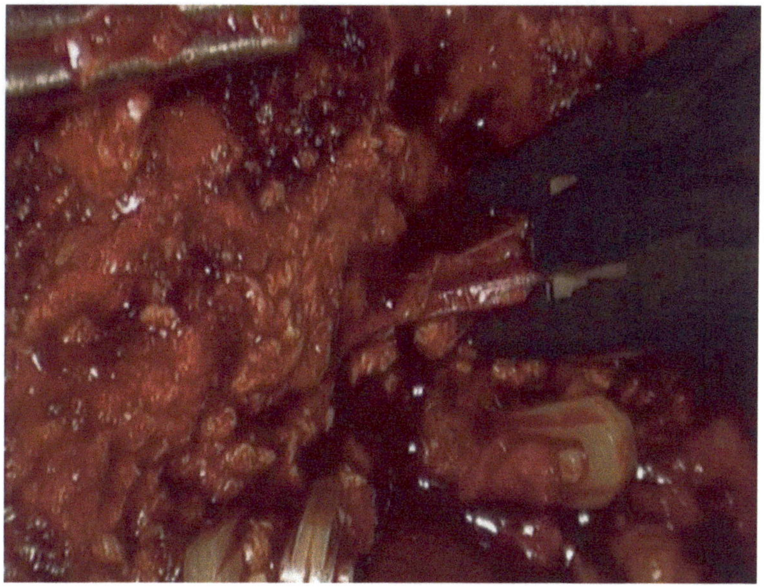

Fig. 4.41 The branch of MHV is clamped with an absorbable clip

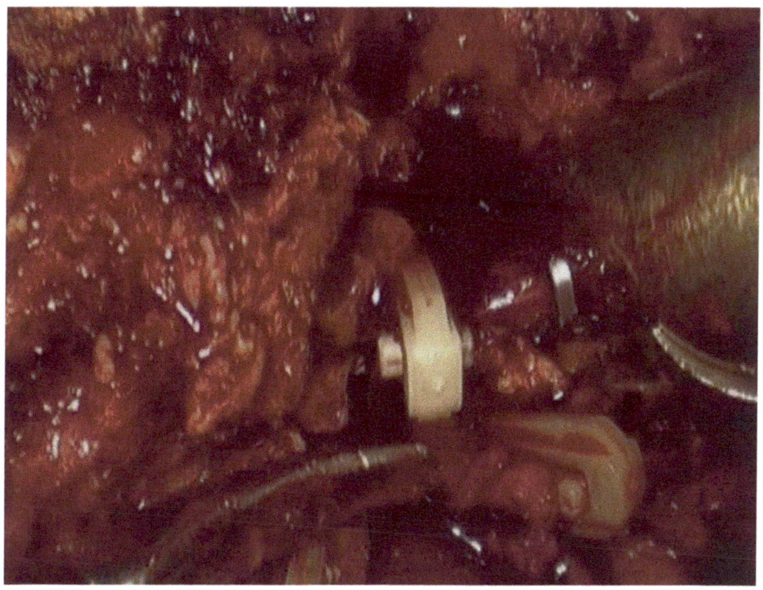

Fig. 4.42 A titanic clip is applied on the distal portion of the branch of MHV

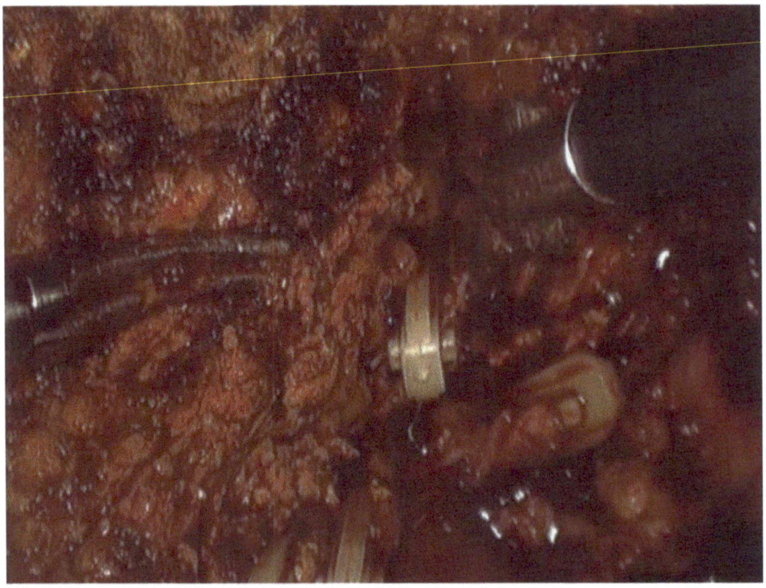

Fig. 4.43 The branch of MHV is divided

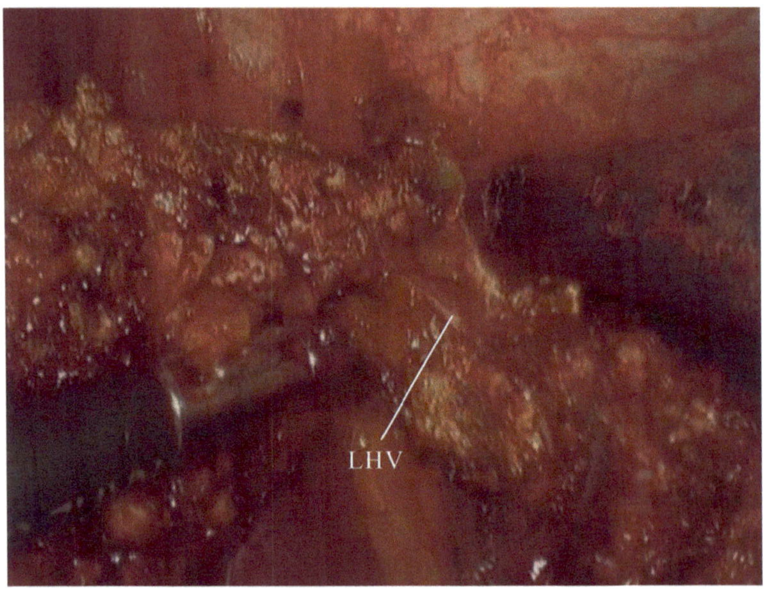

Fig. 4.44 The LHV which was occluded before liver transection is visualized in the transection of the liver parenchyma

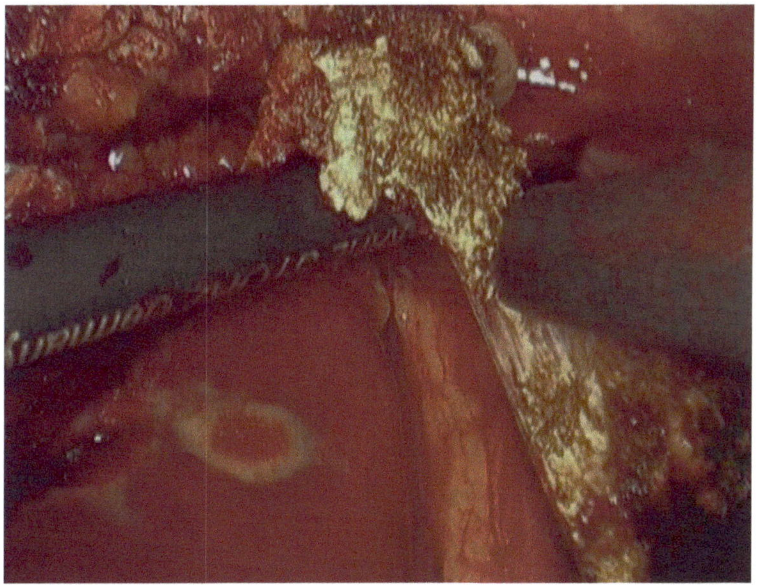

Fig. 4.45 The LHV is transected with LPMOD without applying clips

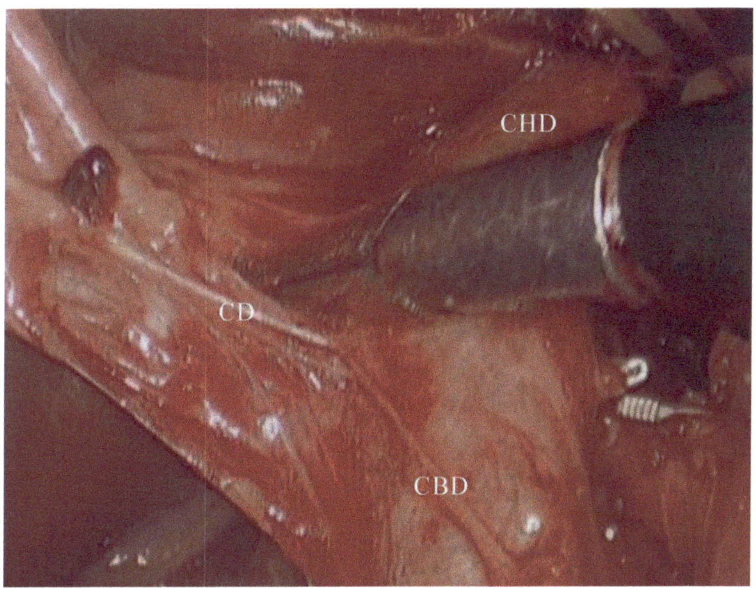

Fig. 4.46 The cystic duct (*CD*), common hepatic duct (*CHD*), and common bile duct (*CBD*) are dissected, and the gallbladder (GB) which was used for traction is to be resected

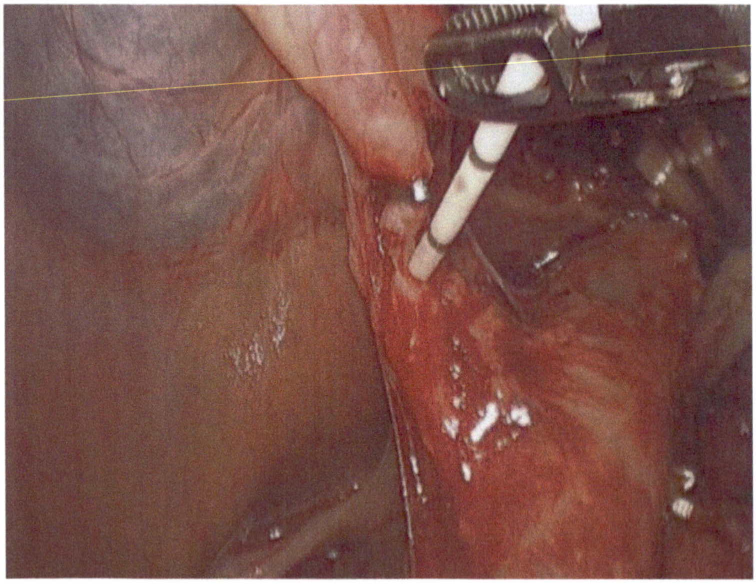

Fig. 4.47 Before the gallbladder is resected, cholangiography is performed to rule out potential biliary leakage on the transection plane

4.4 Laparoscopic Left Hemihepatectomy with Selective Left Inflow Occlusion

See Figs. 4.48, 4.49, 4.50, 4.51, 4.52, 4.53, 4.54, 4.55, 4.56, 4.57, 4.58, 4.59, 4.60, 4.61, 4.62, 4.63, 4.64, 4.65, 4.66, 4.67, 4.68, 4.69, 4.70, 4.71, 4.72, 4.73, 4.74, 4.75, 4.76, 4.77, 4.78, 4.79, 4.80, 4.81, 4.82, 4.83, 4.84, 4.85, 4.86, 4.87, 4.88, 4.89, 4.90, 4.91, 4.92, and Video 4.2.

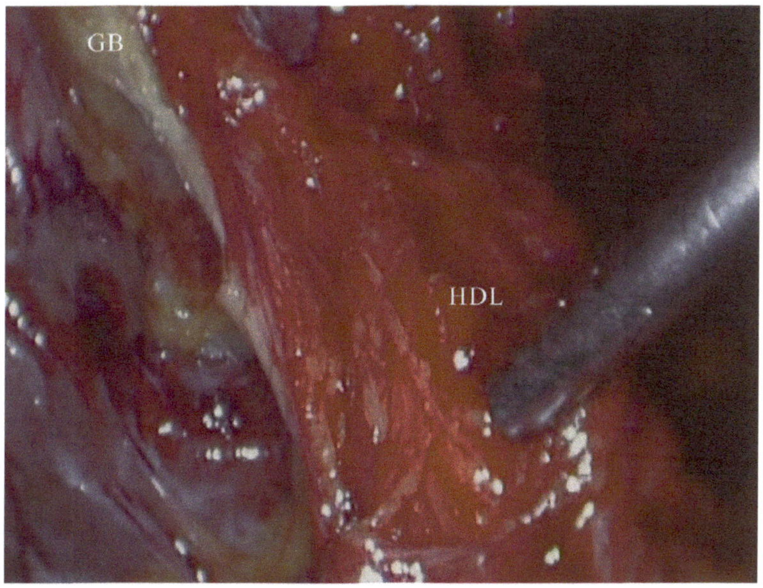

Fig. 4.48 The liver is mobilized upward by the traction of the round ligament (RL) and the gallbladder, and the hepatoduodenal ligament (*HDL*) is dissected

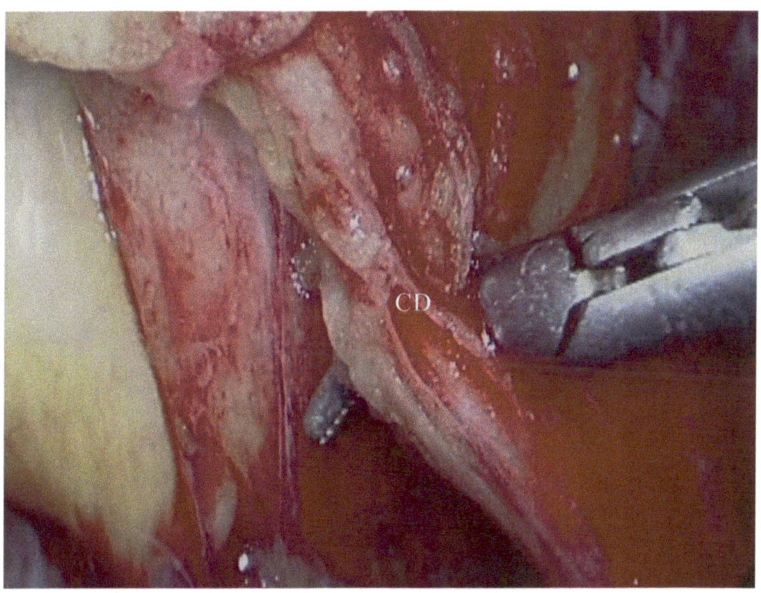

Fig. 4.49 The CD is dissected

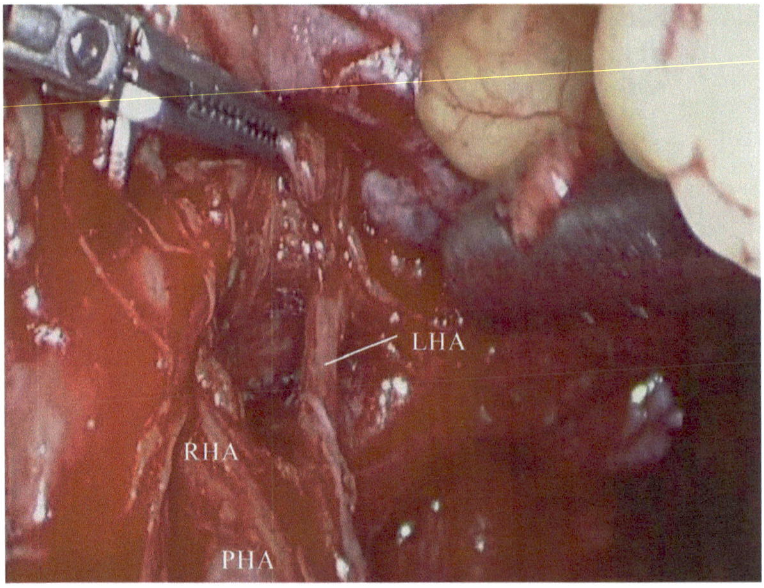

Fig. 4.50 The LHA is dissected

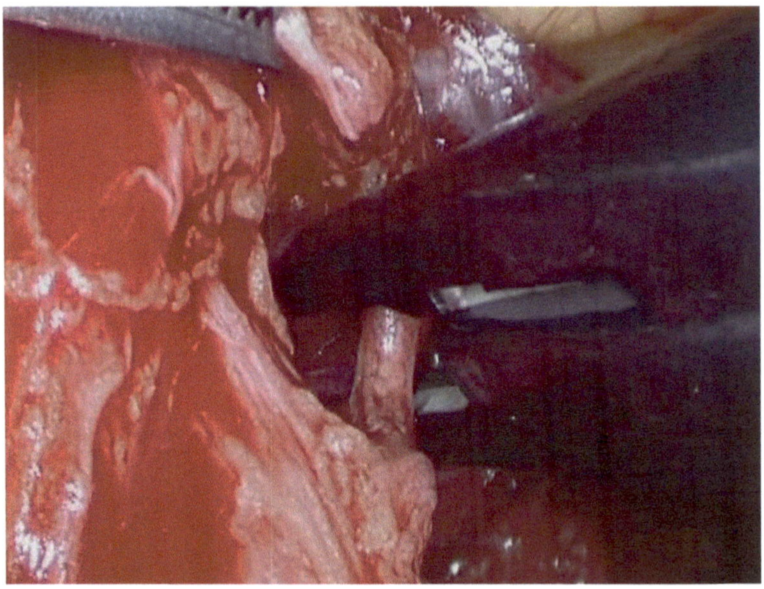

Fig. 4.51 The LHA is clamped with an absorbable clip

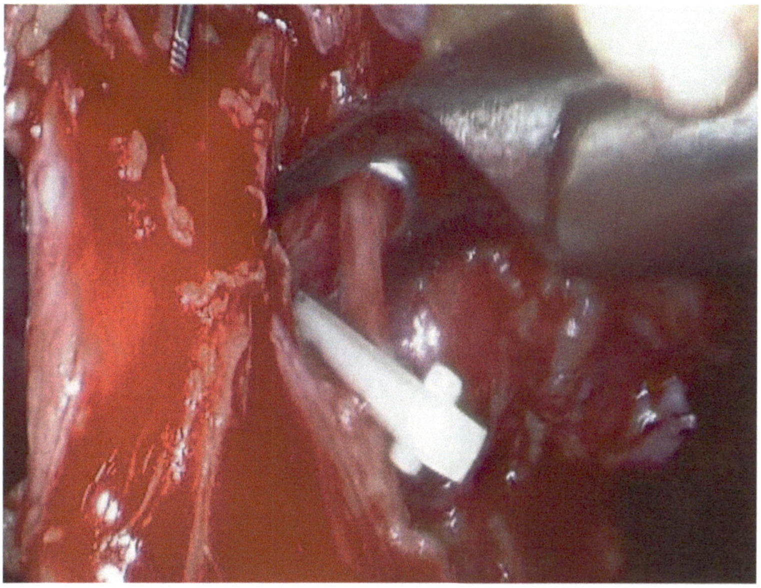

Fig. 4.52 A titanic clip is applied on the distal portion of the LHA

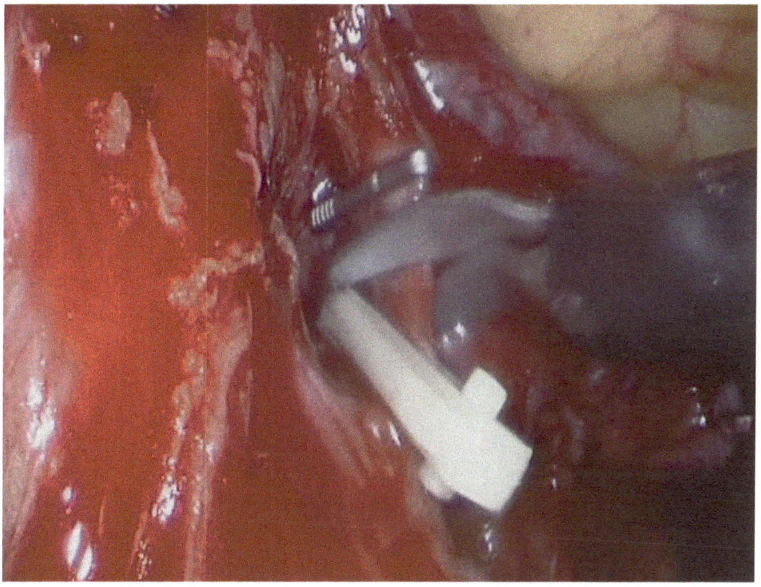

Fig. 4.53 The LHA is divided

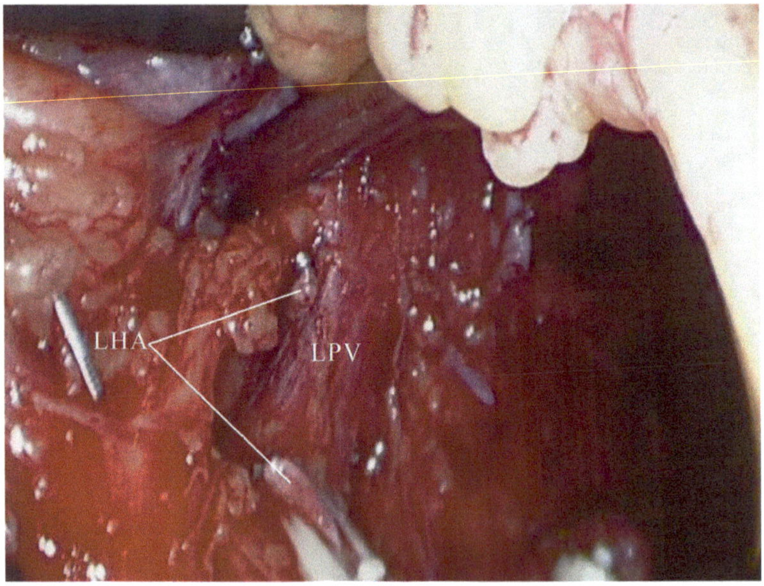

Fig. 4.54 The LPV is visualized after the LHA was divided

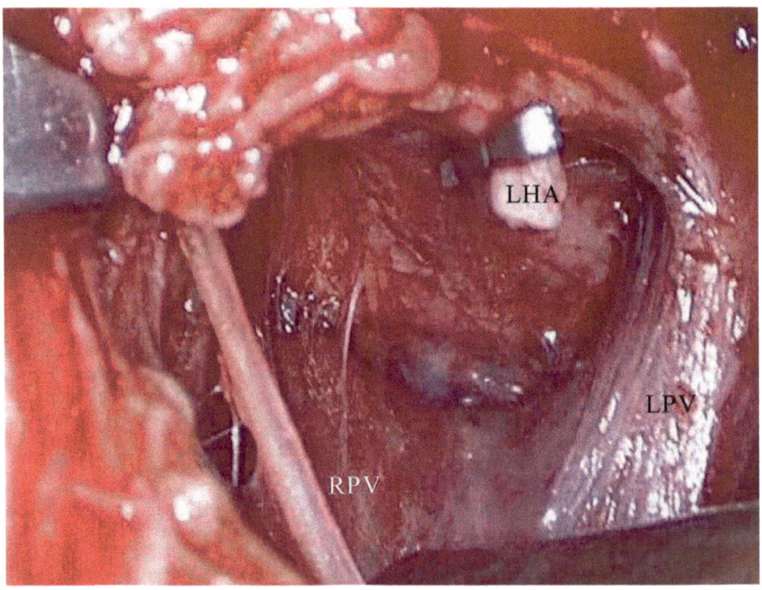

Fig. 4.55 The bifurcation of portal vein (*BPV*) is visualized after the meticulous dissection

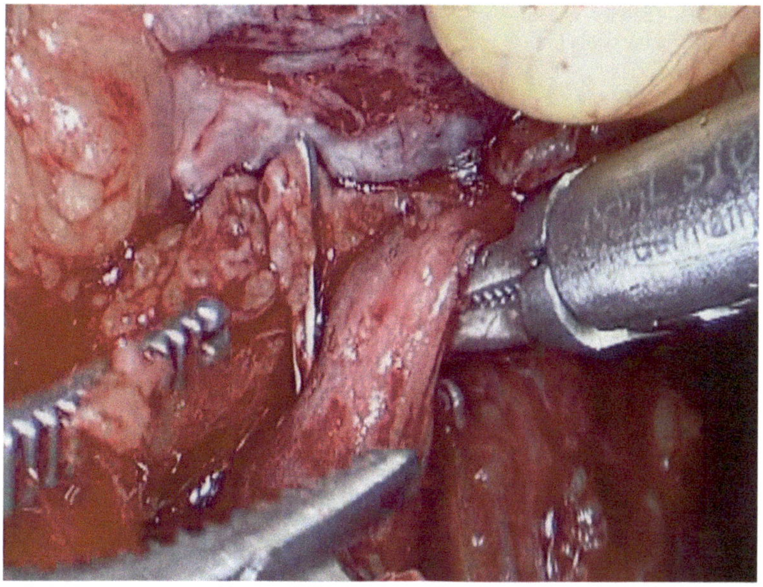

Fig. 4.56 The LPV is freed

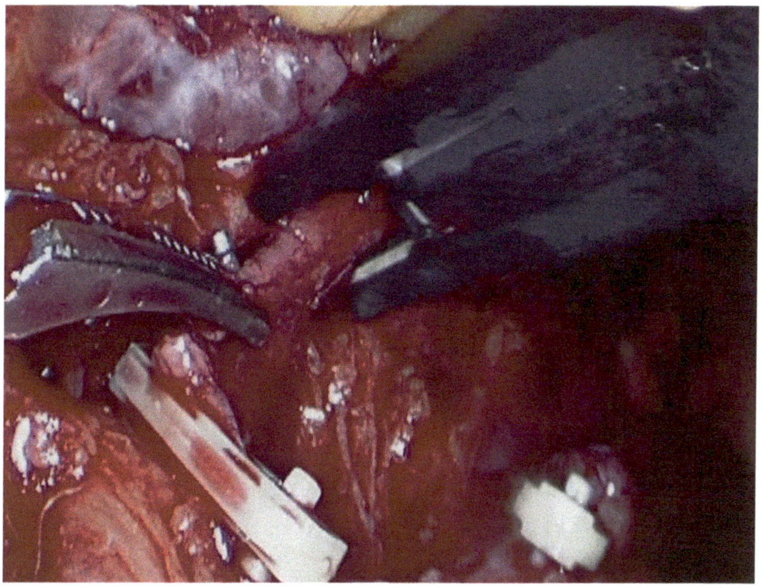

Fig. 4.57 The LPV is clamped with an absorbable clip

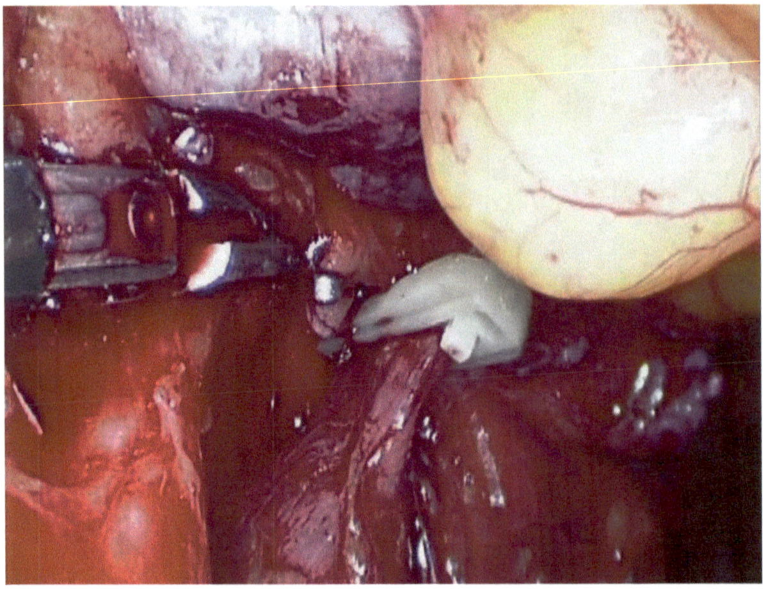

Fig. 4.58 The view of the LPV after being occluded

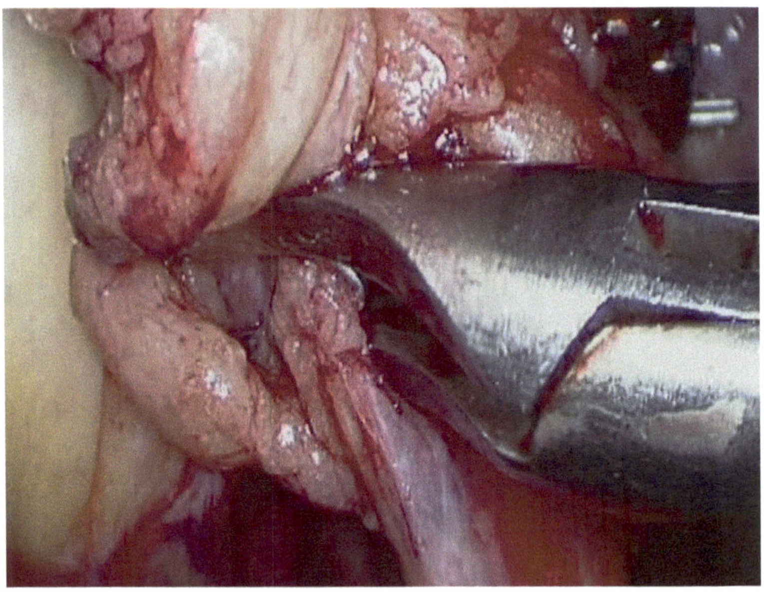

Fig. 4.59 The cystic duct is dissected and is clamped with a titanic clip

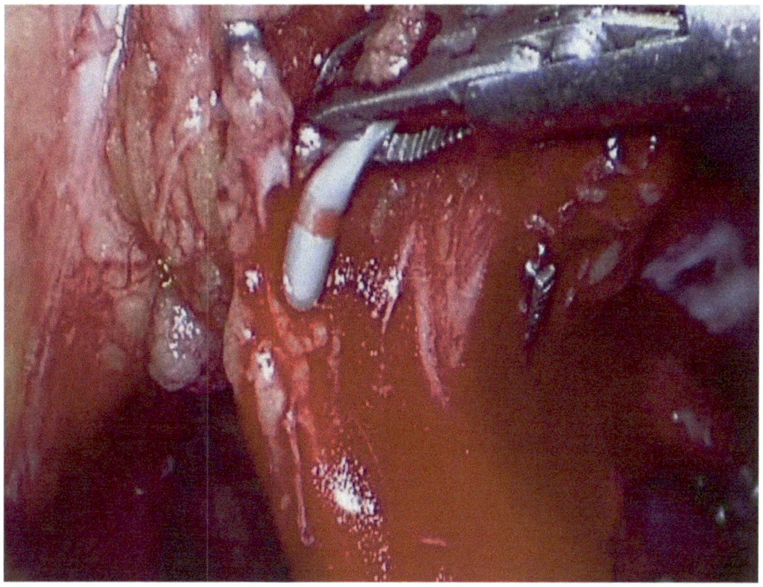

Fig. 4.60 Cholangiography is performed by injecting contrast through the cystic duct

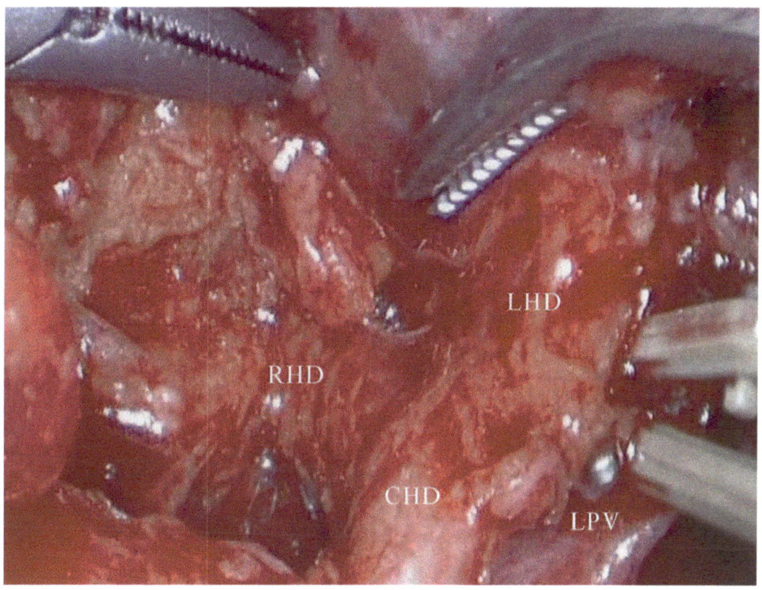

Fig. 4.61 The LHD, the right hepatic duct (*RHD*), and the CHD are identified according to the image of cholangiography

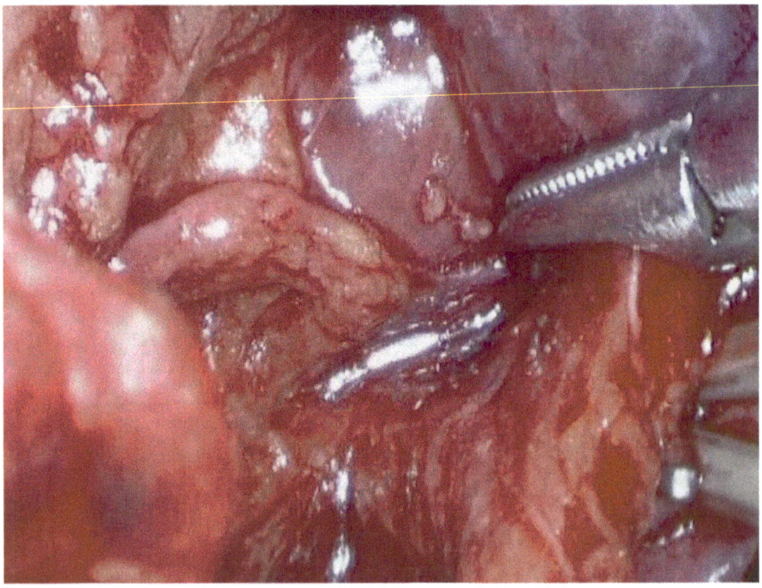

Fig. 4.62 The LHD is dissected

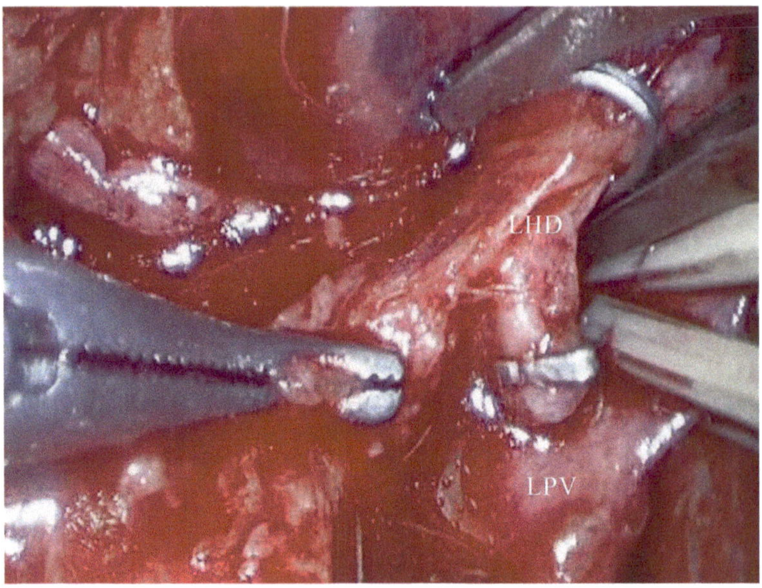

Fig. 4.63 The LHD is clamped with a titanic clip

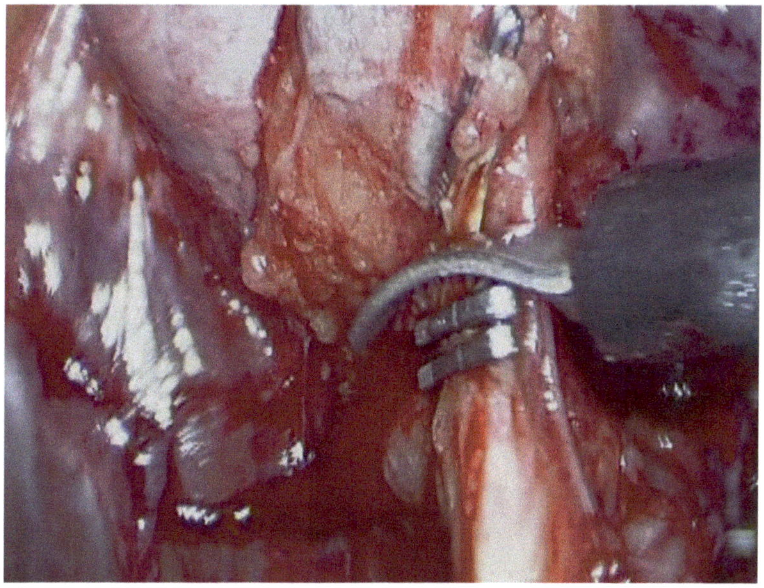

Fig. 4.64 The cystic duct is divided, after being clamped with titanic clips

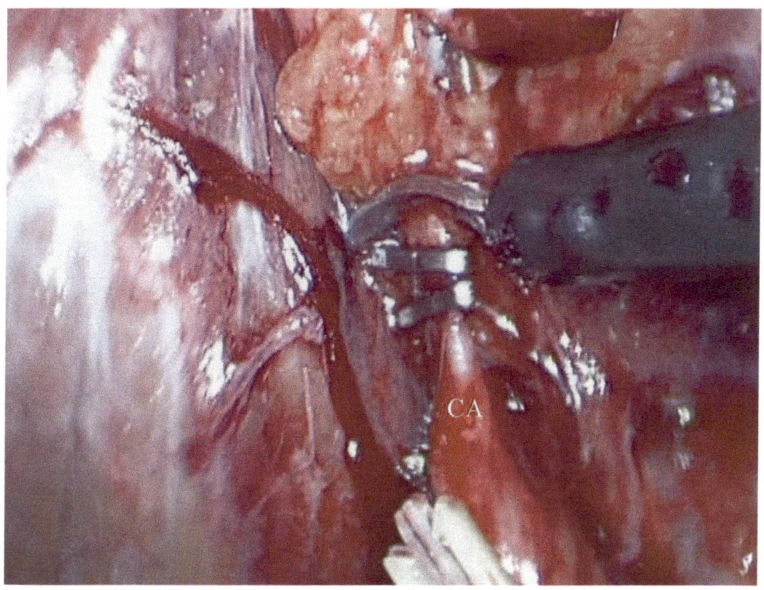

Fig. 4.65 After being clamped with titanic clips, the cystic artery (*CA*) is divided

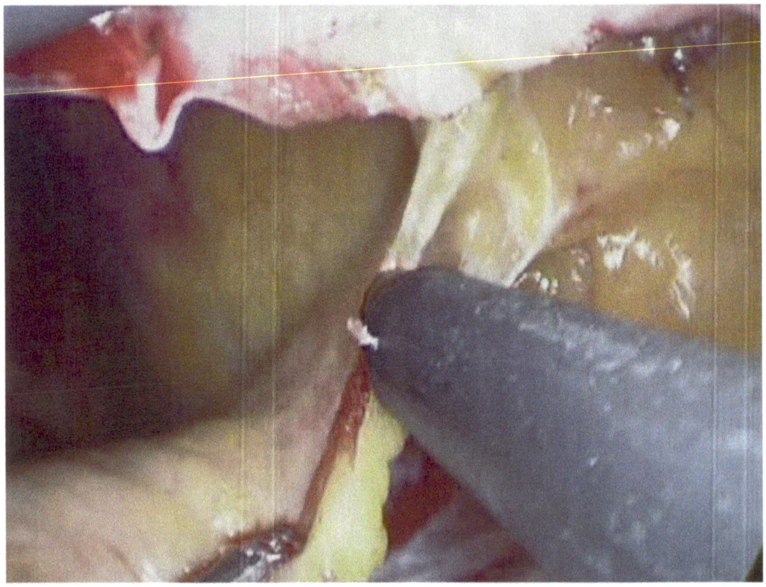

Fig. 4.66 The round ligament and the falciform ligament are divided with LPMOD

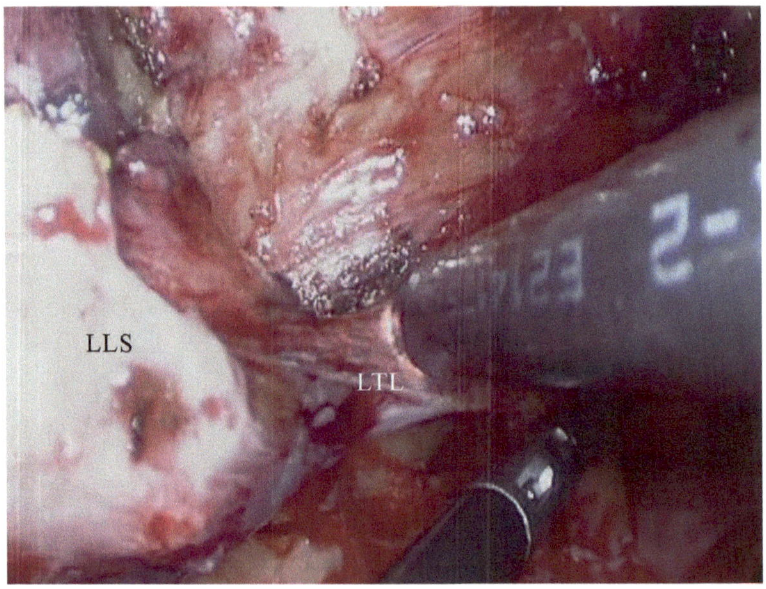

Fig. 4.67 The left lobe of the liver is mobilized to the right, and the LTL is divided with LPMOD

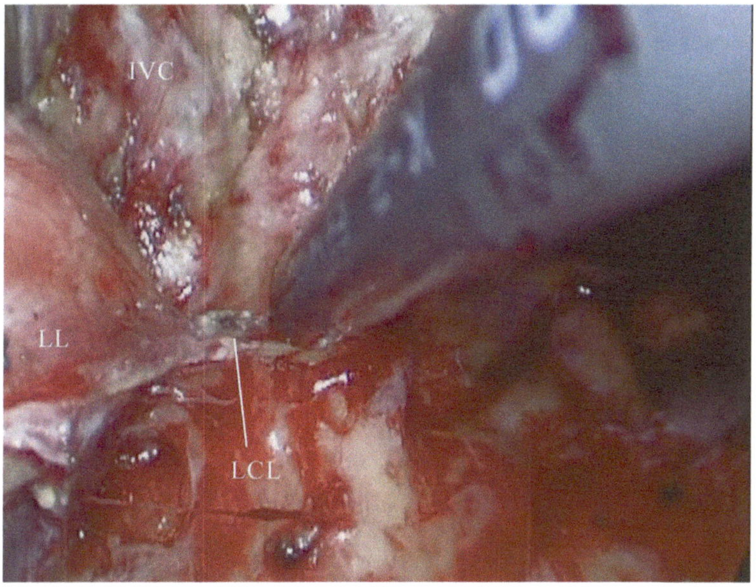

Fig. 4.68 The LCL is divided with LPMOD

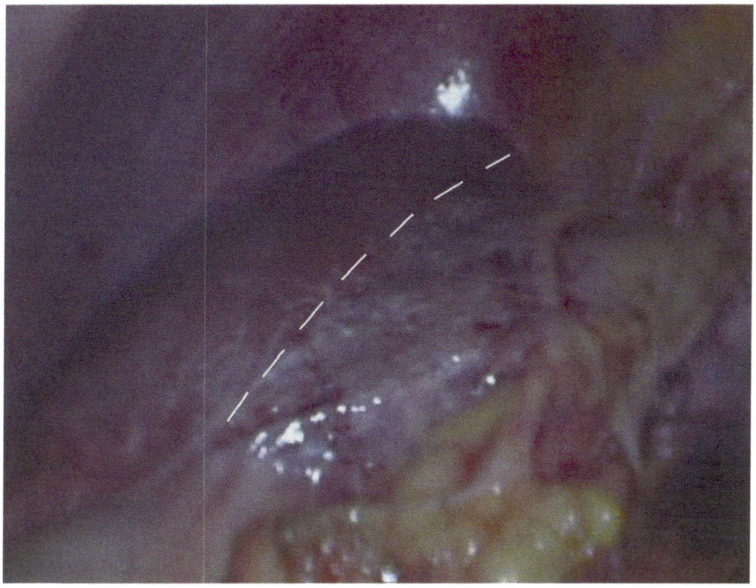

Fig. 4.69 An ischemic *line* is visualized on the liver surface

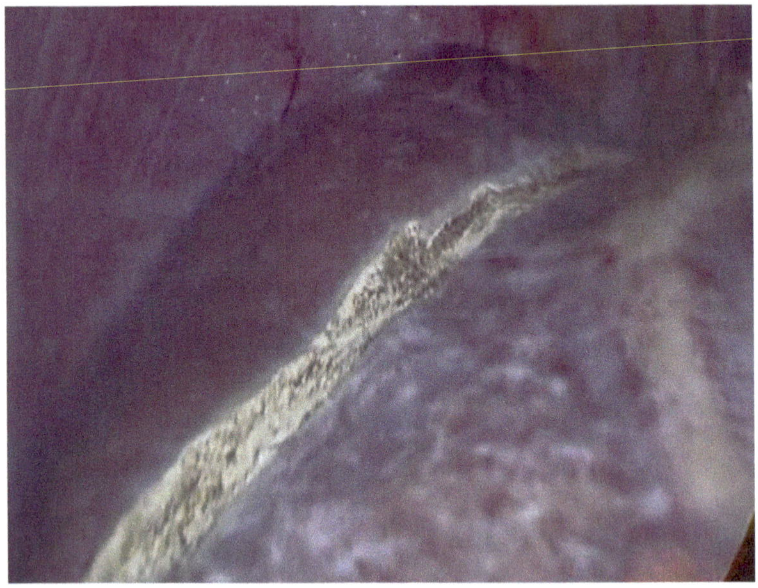

Fig. 4.70 The transection line was marked on the liver surface along the ischemic line

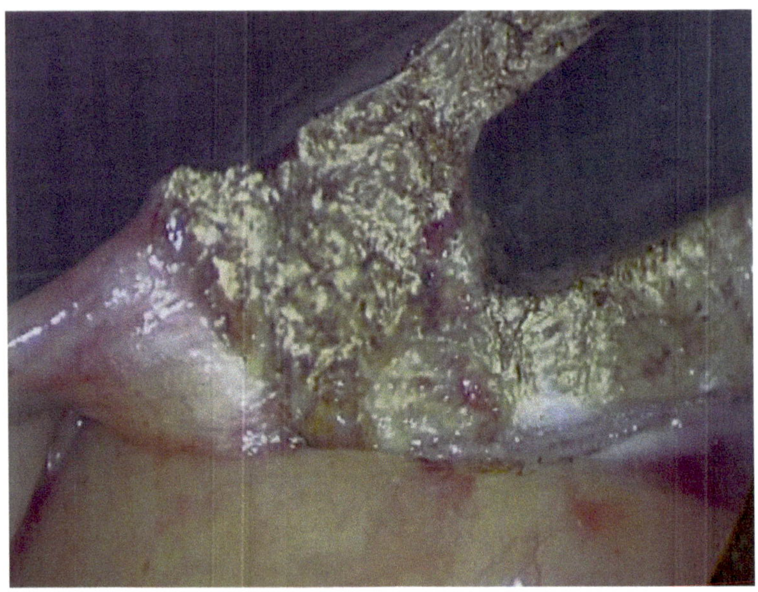

Fig. 4.71 Liver parenchyma is transected with LPMOD

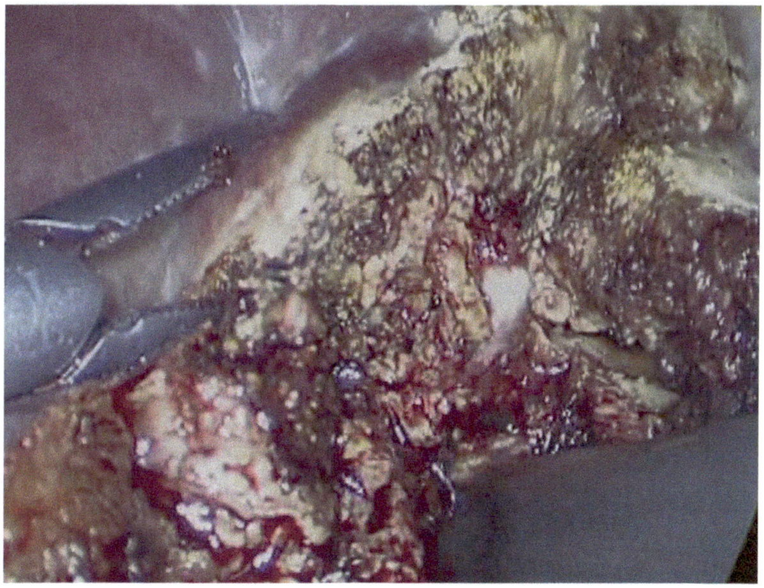

Fig. 4.72 A small vessel is visualized in the transection of the liver parenchyma

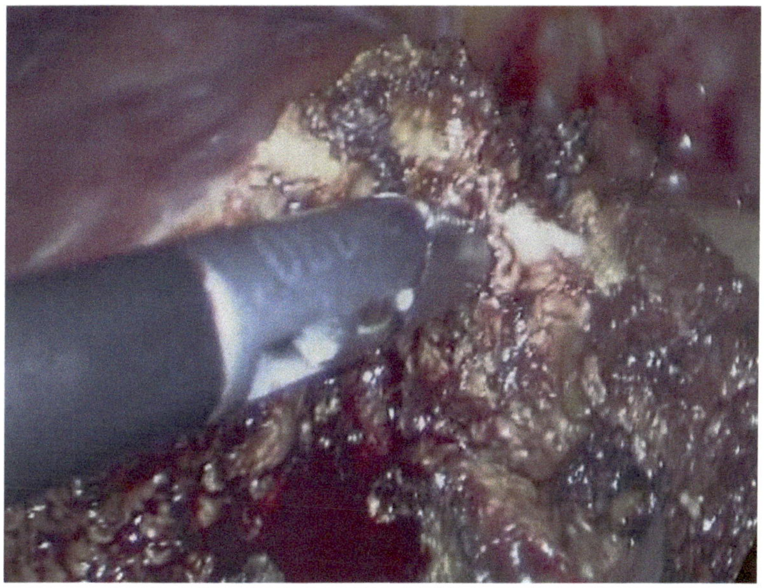

Fig. 4.73 The small vessel is freed

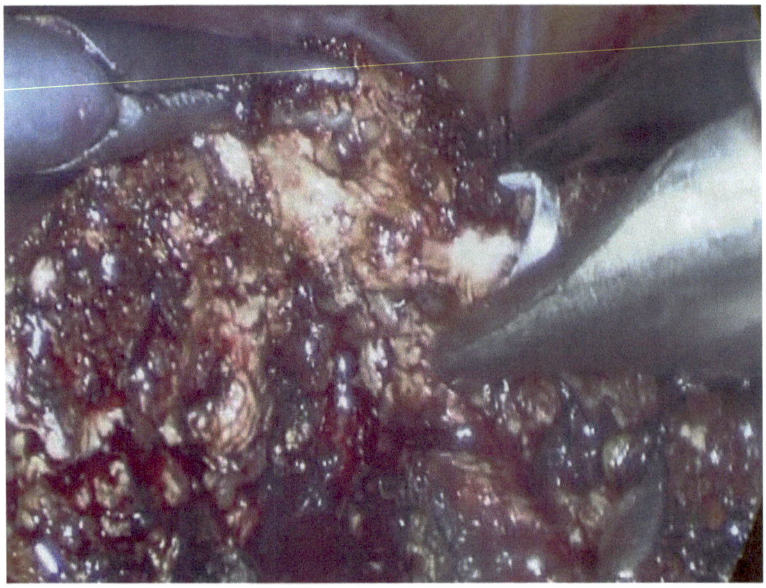

Fig. 4.74 The small vessel is clamped with titanic clips

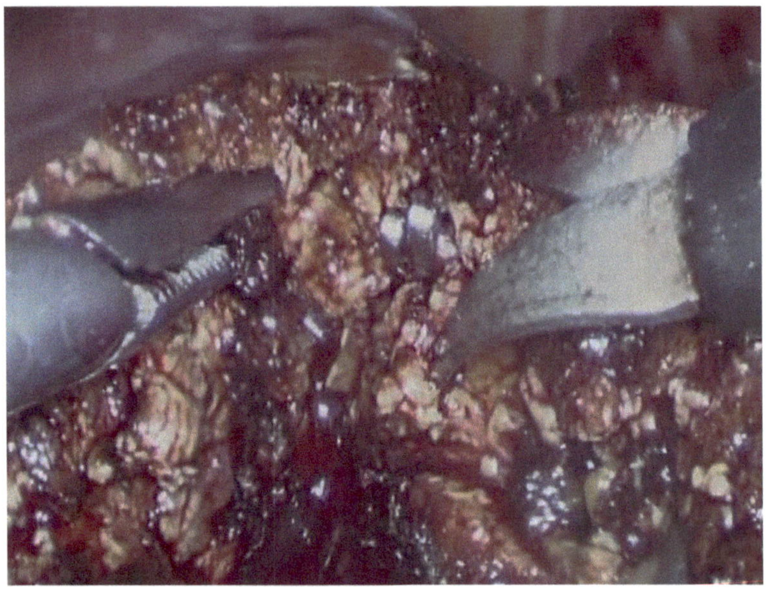

Fig. 4.75 The small vessels are transected

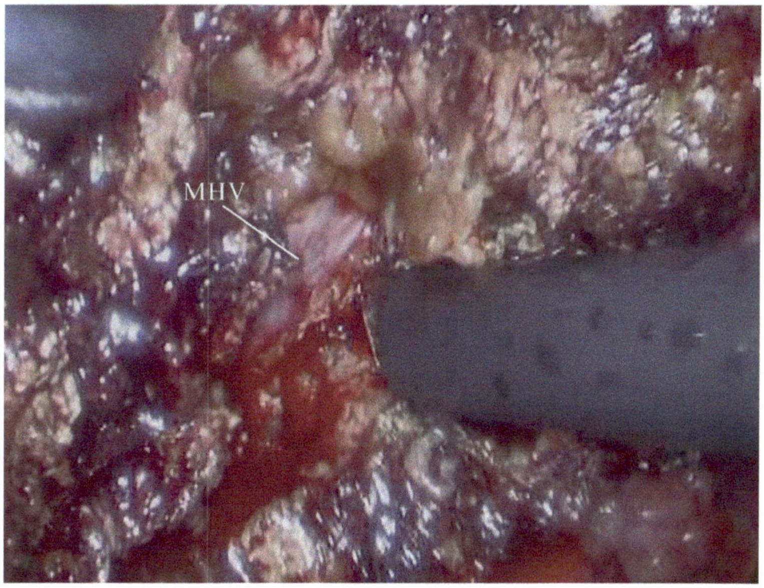

Fig. 4.76 The MHV is visualized in the transection of the liver parenchyma

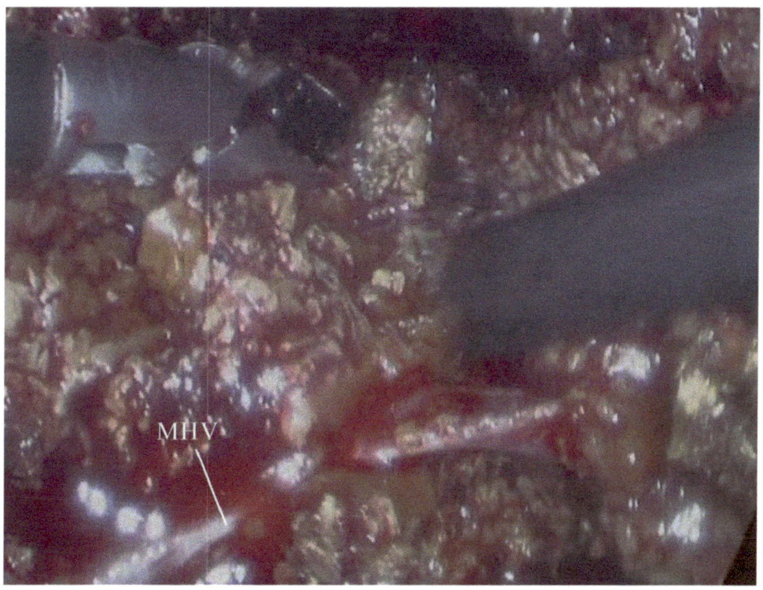

Fig. 4.77 Liver parenchyma is transected along the MHV, and a branch of MHV is dissected with LPMOD

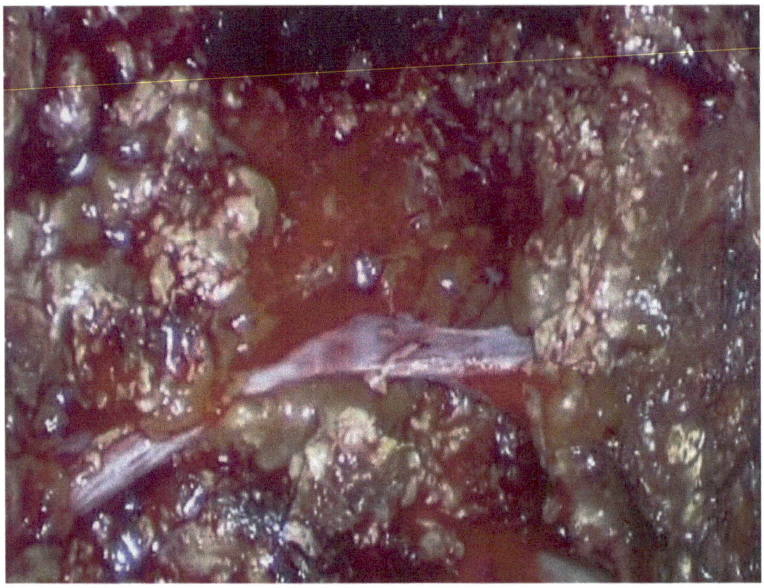

Fig. 4.78 The view of the MHV and a branch of the MHV

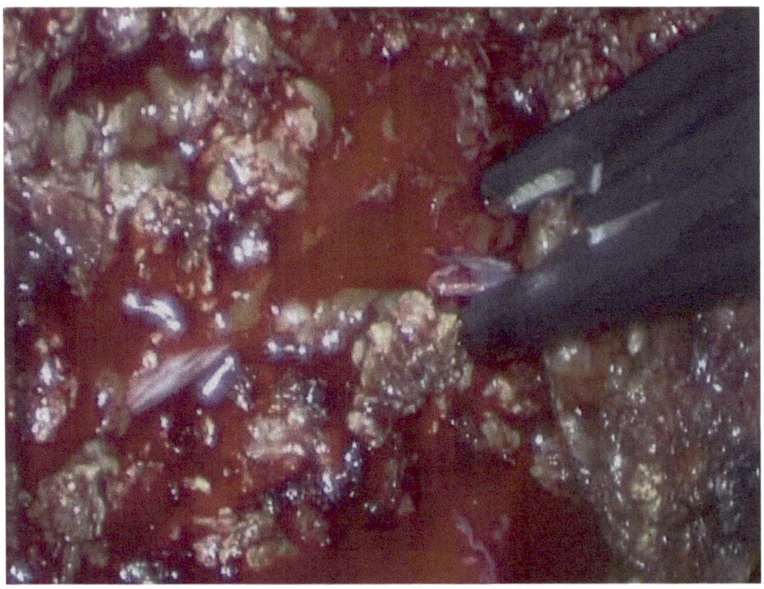

Fig. 4.79 The branch of MHV is clamped with a titanic clip

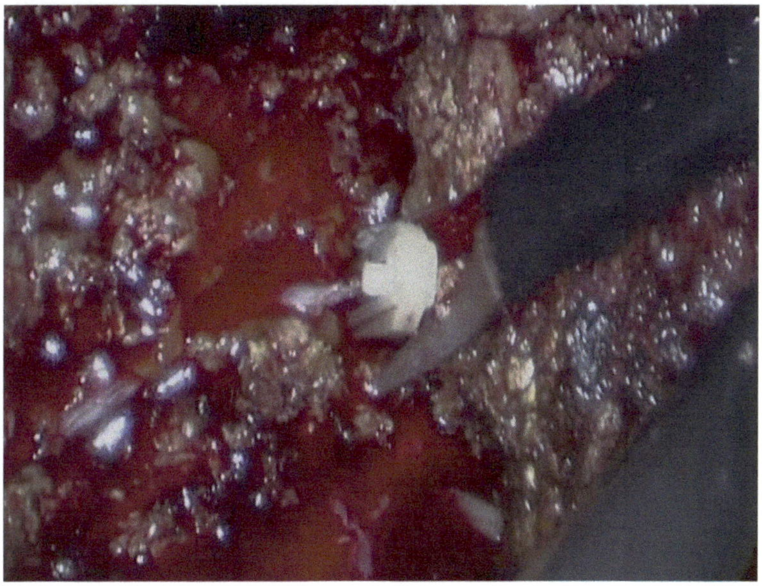

Fig. 4.80 The branch of MHV is divided

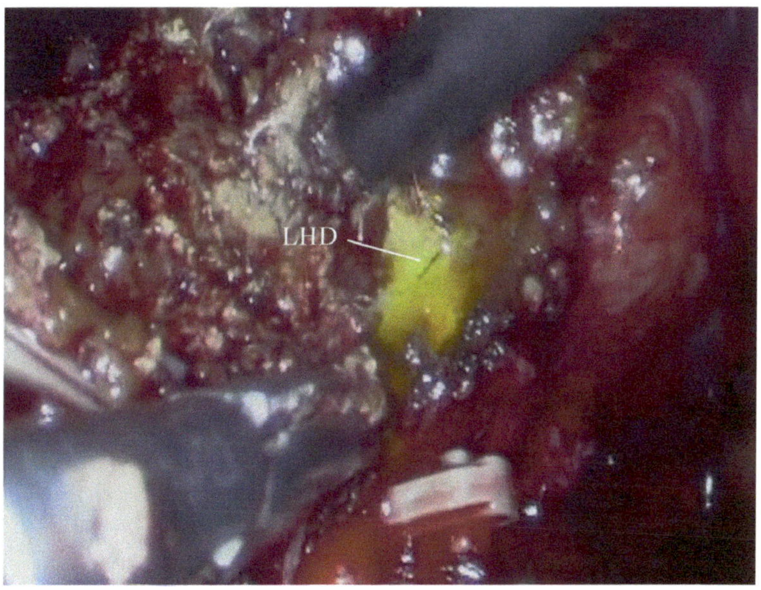

Fig. 4.81 The LHD which was already clamped outside the liver parenchyma is visualized and is transected with LPMOD

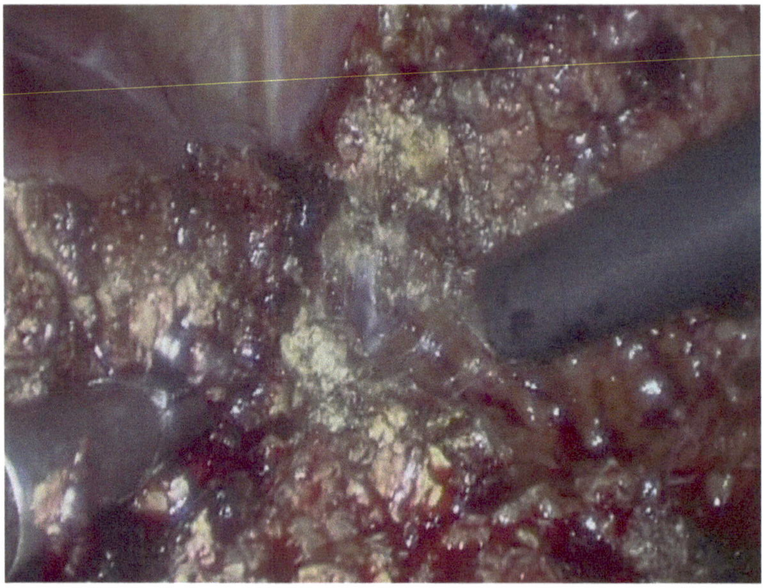

Fig. 4.82 Another branch of MHV is visualized in the transection of the liver parenchyma

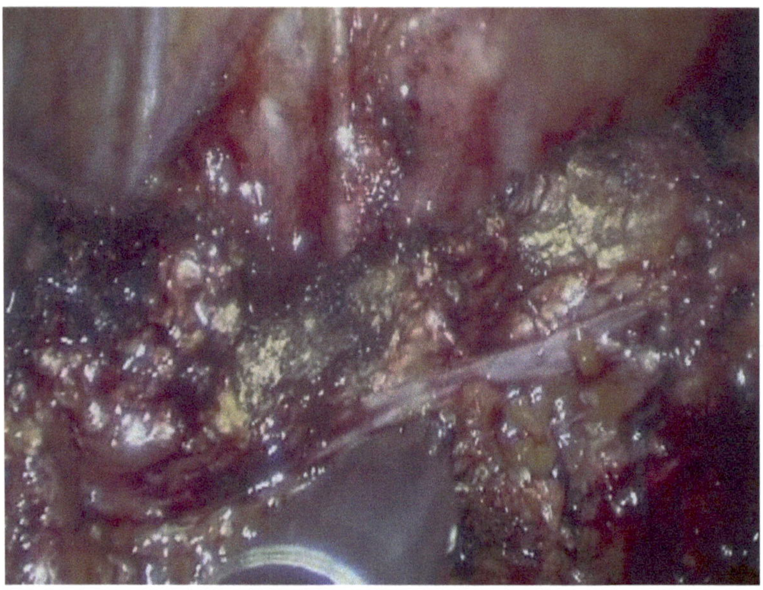

Fig. 4.83 The branch of MHV is dissected

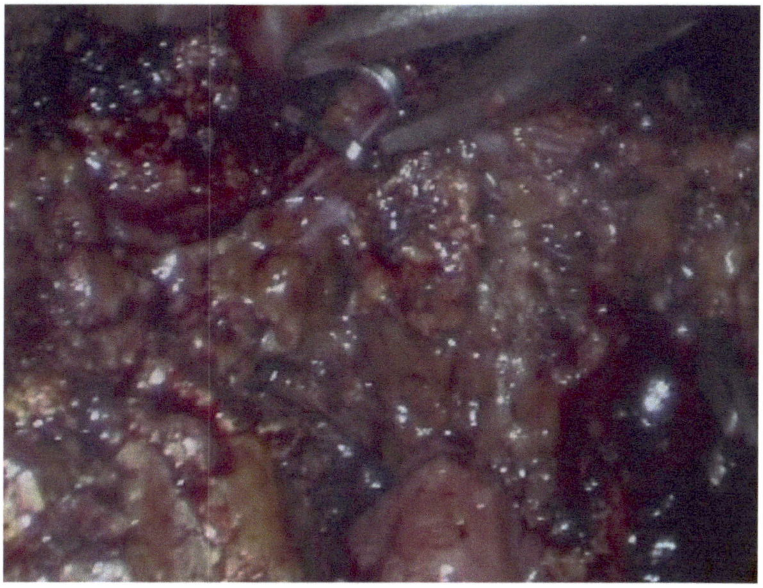

Fig. 4.84 The branch of MHV is clamped with titanic clips

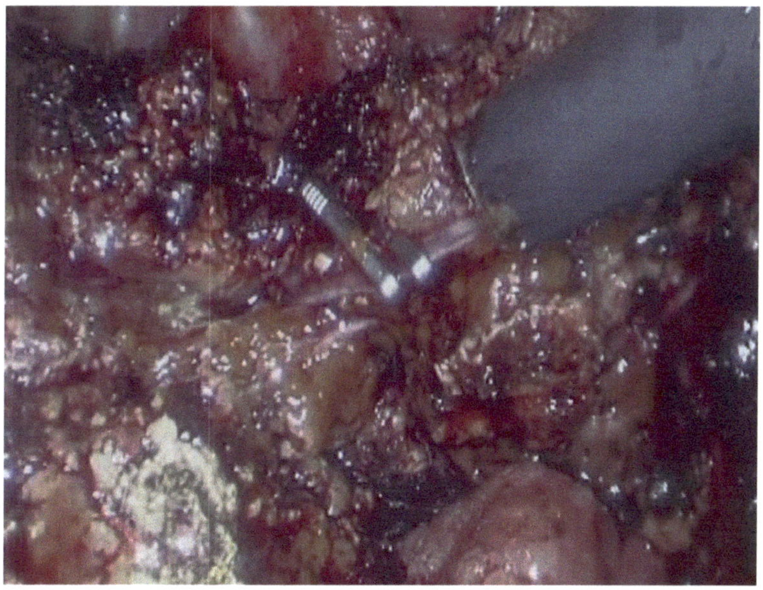

Fig. 4.85 The branch of MHV is divided with LPMOD

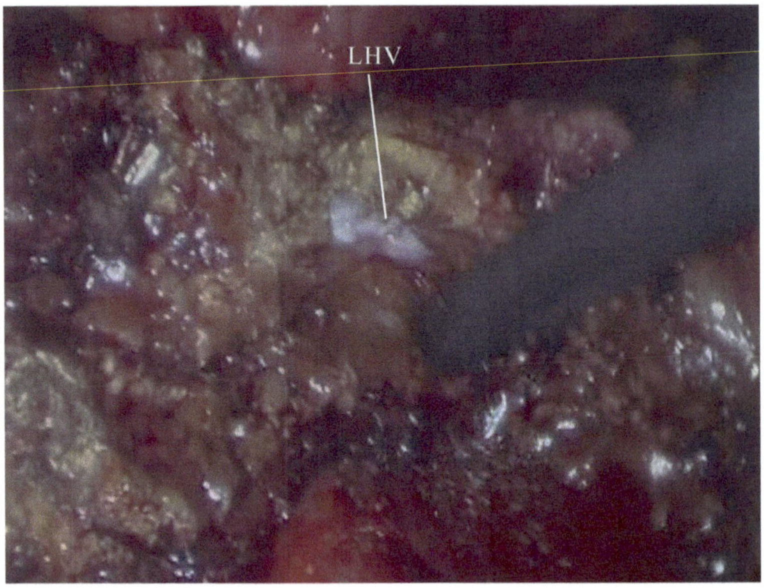

Fig. 4.86 The LHV is visualized in the transection of the liver parenchyma

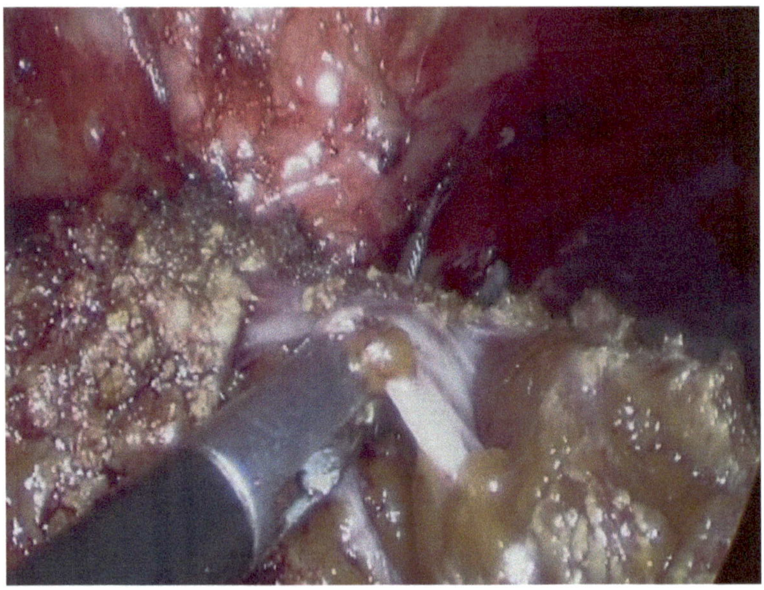

Fig. 4.87 The LHV is dissected

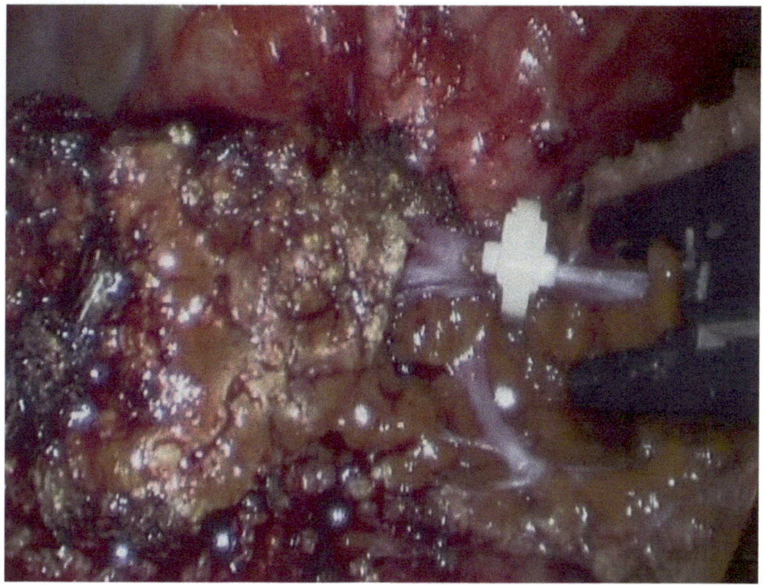

Fig. 4.88 The LHV is clamped with absorbable clips

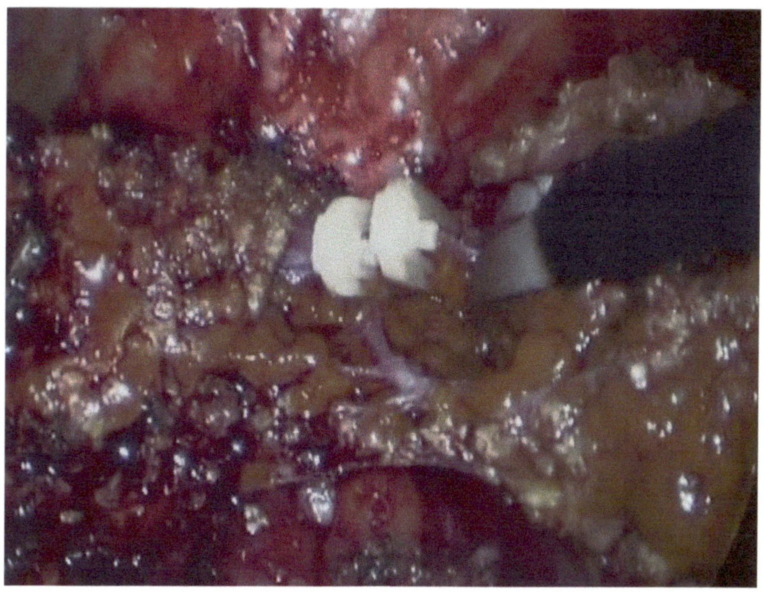

Fig. 4.89 The LHV is divided

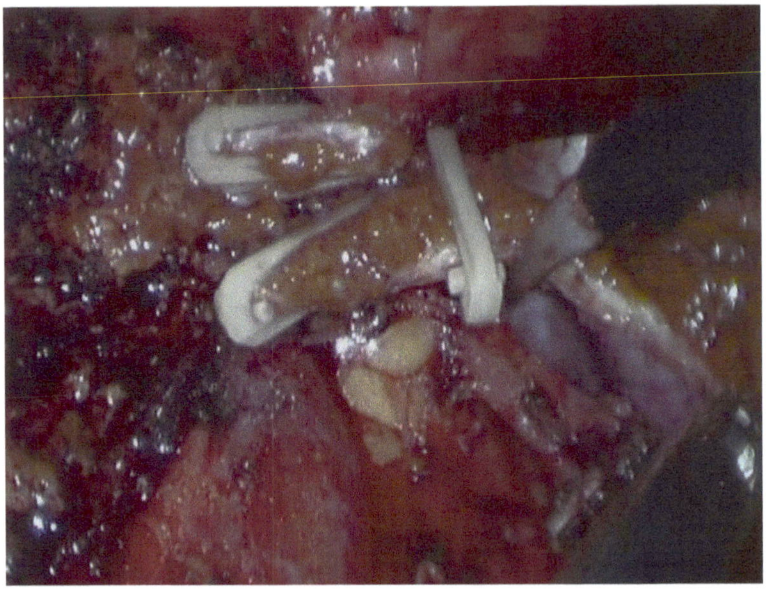

Fig. 4.90 The remaining liver parenchyma and the liver capsule are clamped and are divided

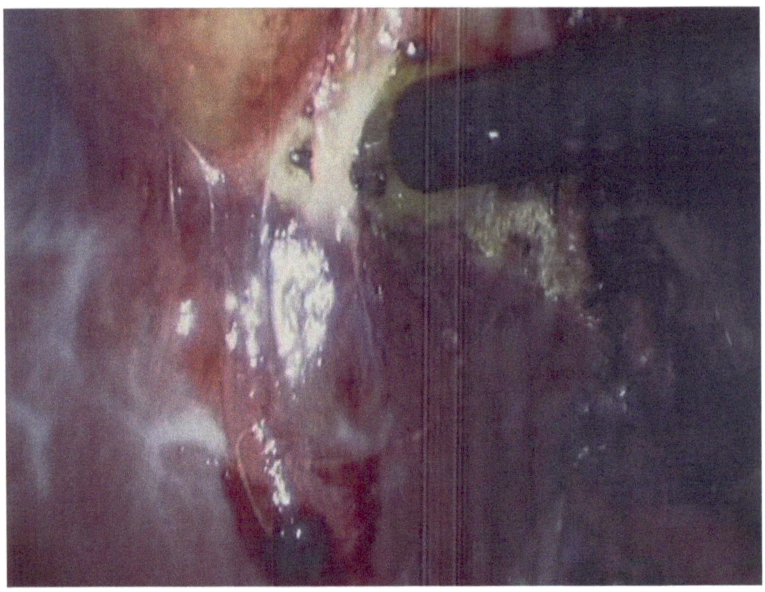

Fig. 4.91 The gallbladder which was used for liver traction is resected

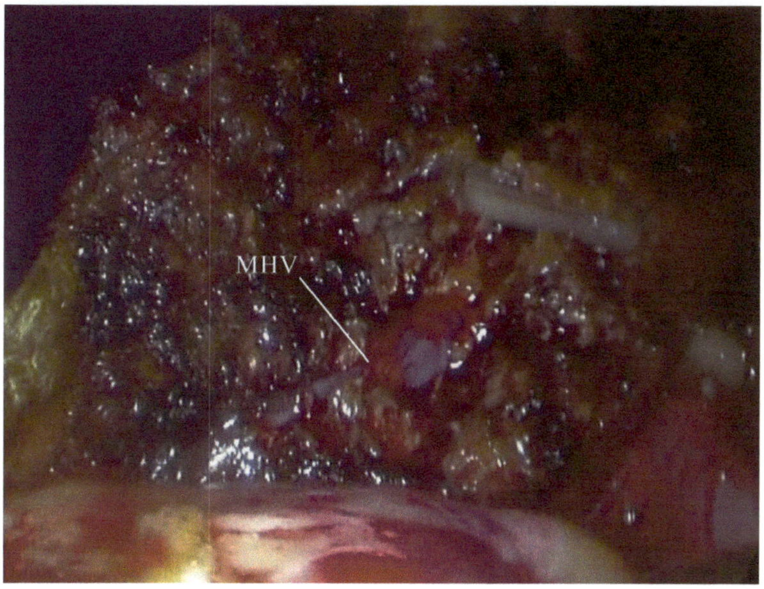

Fig. 4.92 The MHV can be visualized on the transection plane after the left lobe was removed

References

Cherqui D, Laurent A, Tayar C, et al. Laparoscopic versus open left lateral hepatic lobectomy: a case-control study. J Am Coll Surg. 2003;196:236–42.

Cherqui D, Laurent A, Tayar C, et al. Laparoscopic liver resection for peripheral hepatocellular carcinoma in patients with chronic liver disease: midterm results and perspectives. Ann Surg. 2006;243:499–506.

Descottes B, Glineur D, Lachachi F, et al. Laparoscopic liver resection of benign liver tumors. Surg Endosc. 2003;17:23–30.

Dulucq JL, Wintringer P, Stabilini C, et al. Laparoscopic liver resections: a single center experience. Surg Endosc. 2005;19:886–91.

Hatano Y, Murakawa M, Segawa H, et al. Venous air embolism during hepatic resection. Anesthesiology. 1990;73:1282–5.

Malassagne B, Cherqui D, Alon R, et al. Safety of selective vascular clamping for major hepatectomies. J Am Coll Surg. 1998;187:482–6.

Sahin M, Avsar FM, Ozel H, et al. The effects of dimethyl sulfoxide on liver damage caused by ischemia-reperfusion. Transplant Proc. 2004;36:2590–2.

Teoh NC, Farrell GC. Hepatic ischemia reperfusion injury: pathogenic mechanisms and basis for hepatoprotection. J Gastroenterol Hepatol. 2003;18:891–902.

5 Laparoscopic Right Hemihepatectomy

Laparoscopic right hemihepatectomy is one of the most difficult laparoscopic surgeries. The first series of laparoscopic right hemihepatectomy was reported by O'Rourke N in 2004 (O'Rourke and Fielding 2004). To this day, it is still not considered as a conventional surgery by the majority of institutes of hepato-biliary-pancreatic surgery worldwide. The major reasons hindering the development of this procedure could include the limited space for mobilizing the right lobe, difficulties in managing short hepatic veins and right hepatic pedicle, and the possibility of massive bleeding in liver transection.

In our institute, the technique of hepatectomy by curettage and aspiration and the selective inflow occlusion were routinely carried out in major liver resections that facilitate this procedure much more. Laparoscopic selective inflow occlusion could nearly have the same effect as total vascular occlusion but avoid the complications of ischemia-reperfusion injury and gastrointestinal congestion (Sahin et al. 2004; Malassagne et al. 1998; Teoh and Farrell 2003) and the requirement for fast liver transection. It is supposed to be an ideal technique for bleeding control in laparoscopic major liver resection including the right hemihepatectomy. The supine position is adopted in this procedure, and patients are usually tilted 30–45° left side down that can partly solve the problem of limited space for mobilizing the right lobe.

Electronic supplementary material The online version of this chapter at (doi: 10.1007/978-94-017-9840-2_5) contains supplementary material, which is available to authorized users.

X. Cai, *Laparoscopic Hepatectomy: Atlas and Techniques*,
DOI 10.1007/978-94-017-9840-2_5,

5.1 Indications and Contraindications

The indications include liver tumors in the right lobe or right intrahepatic bile duct stones with irreversible diseases (biliary stricture or severe parenchymal fibrosis or atrophy) requiring right hemihepatectomy and liver function of Child A to B classification. The contraindications include malignant tumors involving porta hepatis, history of biliary surgeries such as exploration of common bile duct (CBD) or cholangiojejunostomy (cholecystectomy is not regarded as a contraindication), extrahepatic bile duct stricture, or acute suppurative cholangitis.

5.2 Patient Position and Trocars' Position

Patients are placed in the supine position under general anesthesia. Three surgeons are needed in the operation. The senior surgeon stands on the left side of the patient, one assistant surgeon stands on the right side of the senior surgeon controlling the aspiration device, and the other assistant surgeon stands on the right side of the patient. Four entries are made. A supraumbilical 10-mm trocar is inserted as the observation port. A subxiphoid 12-mm trocar is inserted as the main manipulation port. And two 5-mm trocars are inserted at the right flank area as assistant manipulation ports (Fig. 5.1).

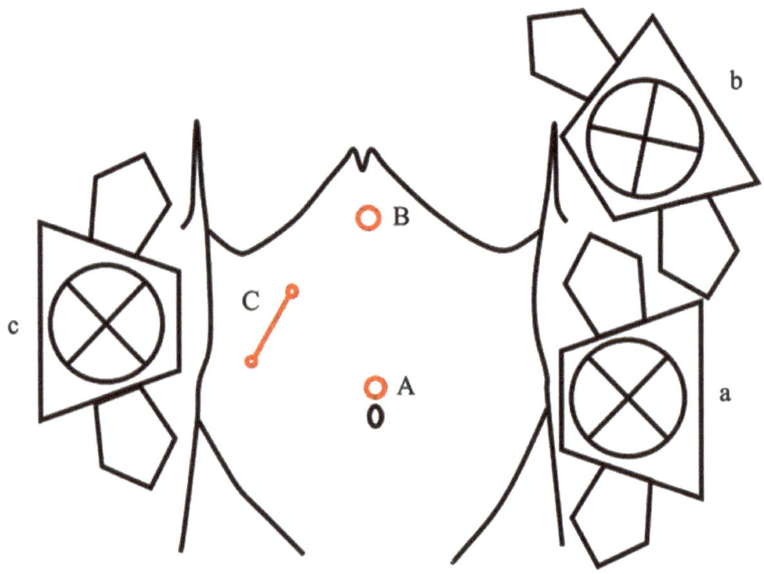

Fig. 5.1 The trocars' position and surgeons' position. (*A*) Observation port; (*B*) Main manipulation port; (*C*) Two assistant ports and the incision for removing specimen; (**a**) The senior surgeon stands on the left side of the patient; (**b**) One assistant surgeon stands on the right side of the senior surgeon controlling the aspiration device; (**c**) The other assistant surgeon stands on the right side of the patient

5.3 Laparoscopic Right Hemihepatectomy with Selective Right Inflow Occlusion

See Figs. 5.2, 5.3, 5.4, 5.5, 5.6, 5.7, 5.8, 5.9, 5.10, 5.11, 5.12, 5.13, 5.14, 5.15, 5.16, 5.17, 5.18, 5.19, 5.20, 5.21, 5.22, 5.23, 5.24, 5.25, 5.26, 5.27, 5.28, 5.29, 5.30, 5.31, 5.32, 5.33, 5.34, 5.35, 5.36, 5.37, 5.38, 5.39, 5.40, 5.41, 5.42, 5.43, 5.44, 5.45, 5.46, 5.47, 5.48, 5.49, 5.50, 5.51, 5.52, 5.53, 5.54, 5.55, 5.56, 5.57, 5.58, 5.59, and Video 5.1.

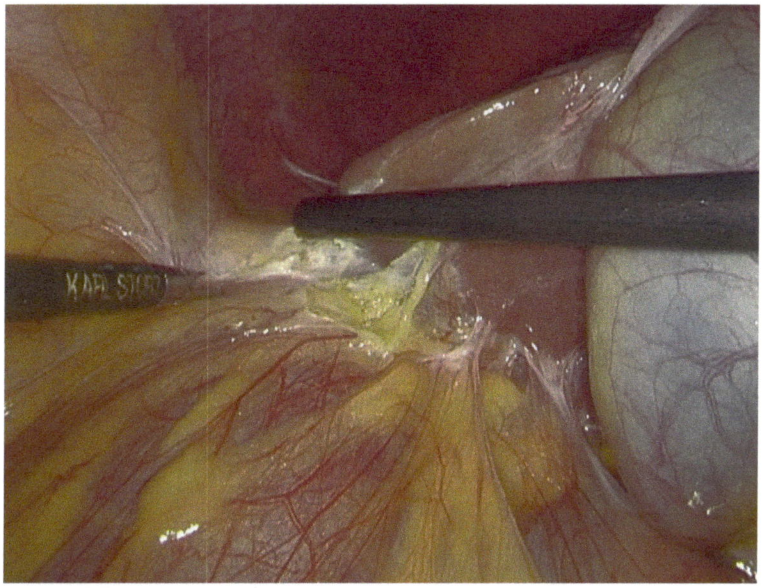

Fig. 5.2 The liver is mobilized upward, and the hepatocolic ligament (HCL) is divided with LPMOD

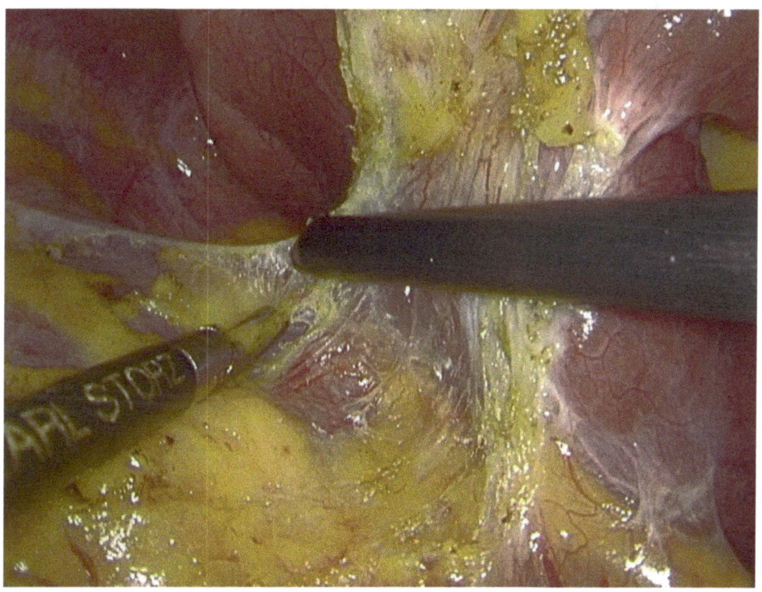

Fig. 5.3 The right lobe of the liver (RLL) is mobilized upward, and the hepatorenal ligament (HRL) is divided with LPMOD

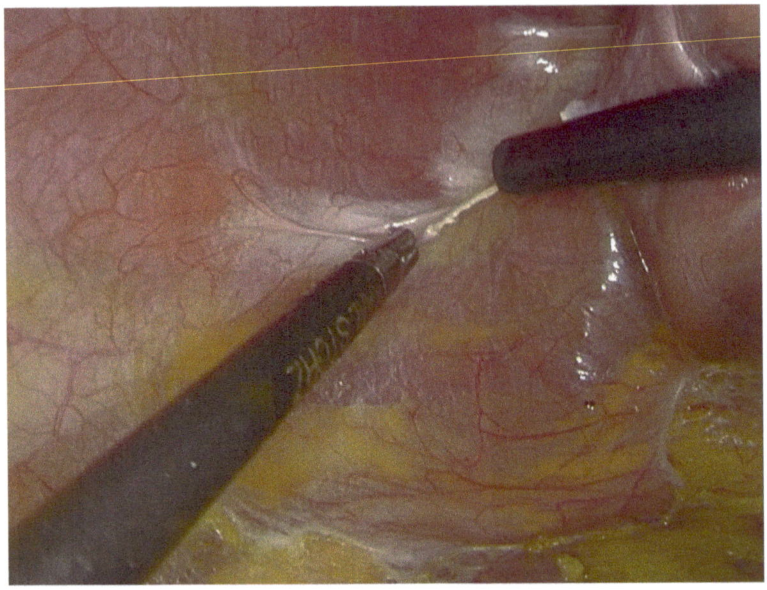

Fig. 5.4 The right lobe is mobilized to the left and the right triangle ligament (RTL) is divided with LPMOD

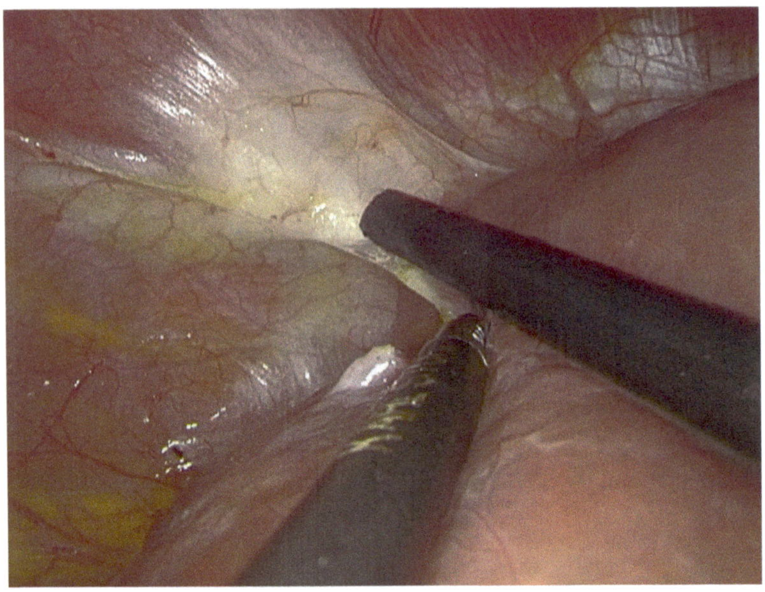

Fig. 5.5 The right lobe is mobilized downward and the right coronary ligament (RCL) is divided with LPMOD

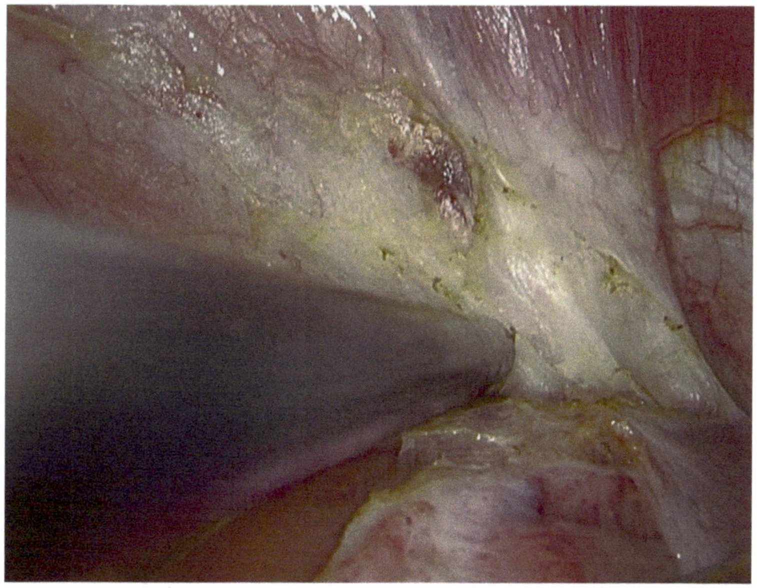

Fig. 5.6 The bare area of the liver is dissected with LPMOD

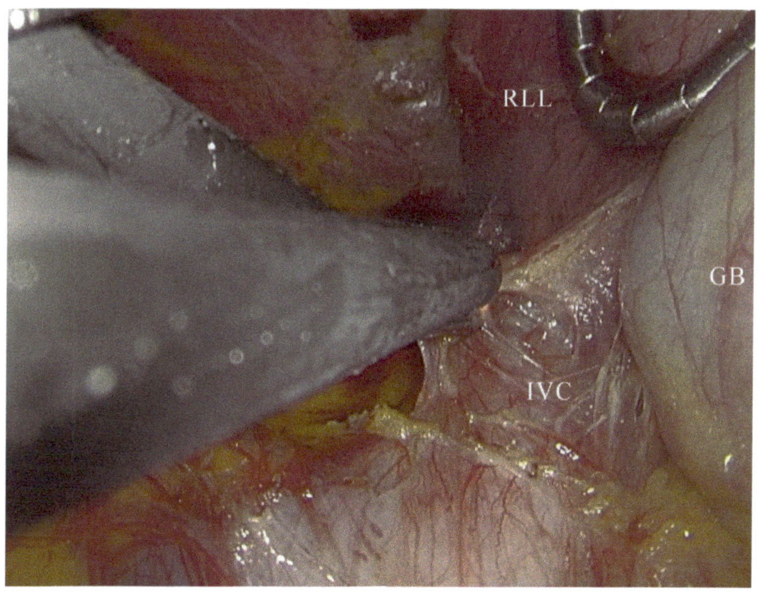

Fig. 5.7 RLL is mobilized to the left. The fossa for the inferior vena cava (*IVC*) is dissected

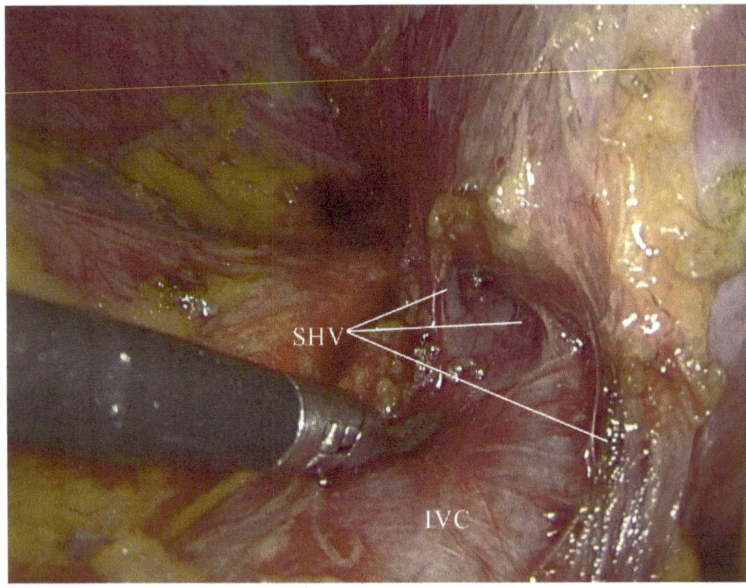

Fig. 5.8 Short hepatic veins (*SHVs*) are visualized

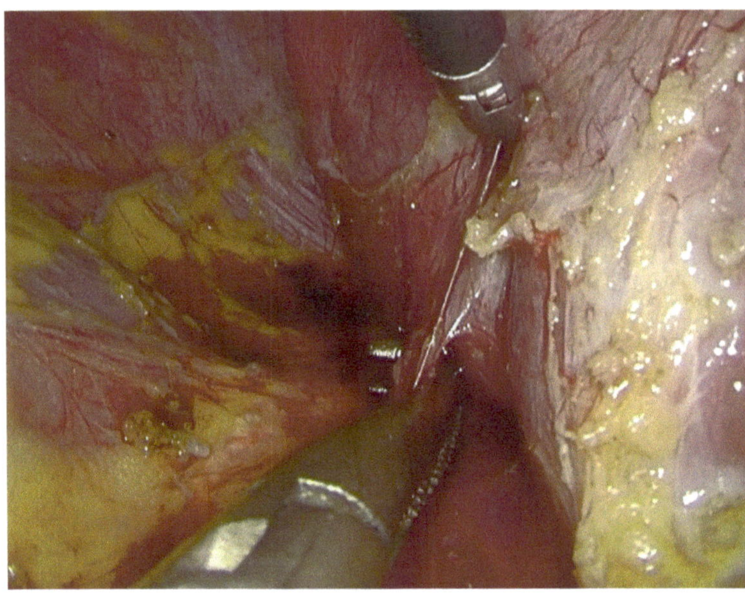

Fig. 5.9 One short hepatic vein (SHV) is dissected

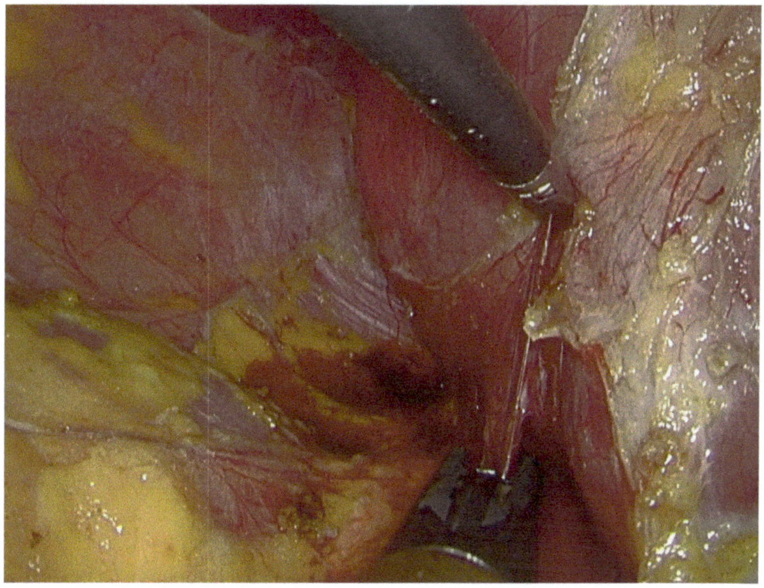

Fig. 5.10 The short hepatic vein is clamped with an absorbable clip

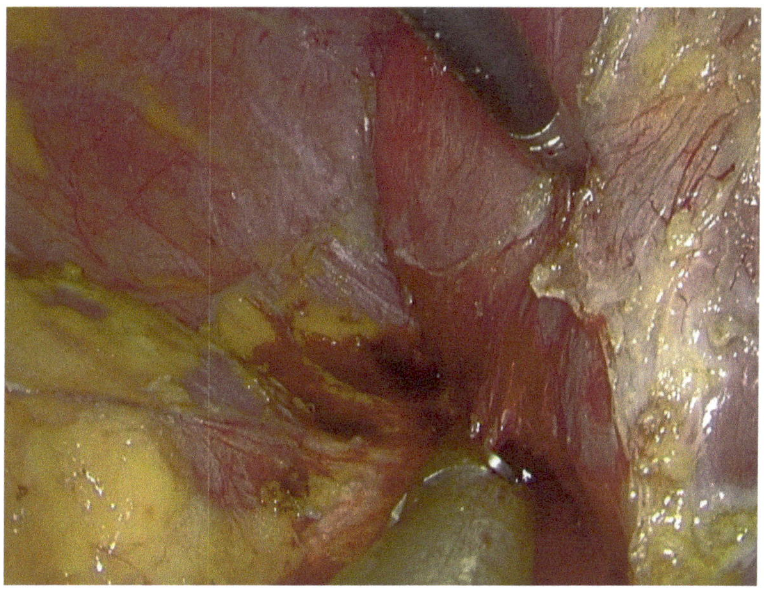

Fig. 5.11 A titanic clip is applied on the distal portion of the short hepatic vein

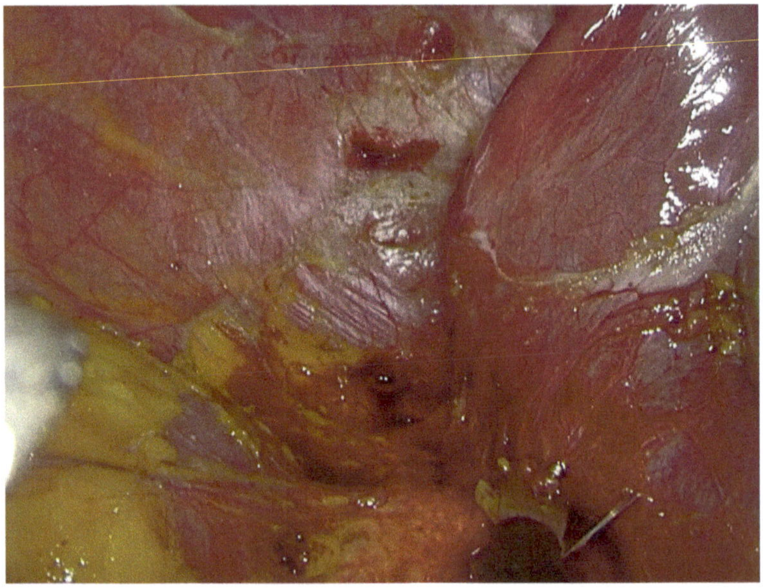

Fig. 5.12 The short hepatic vein is divided

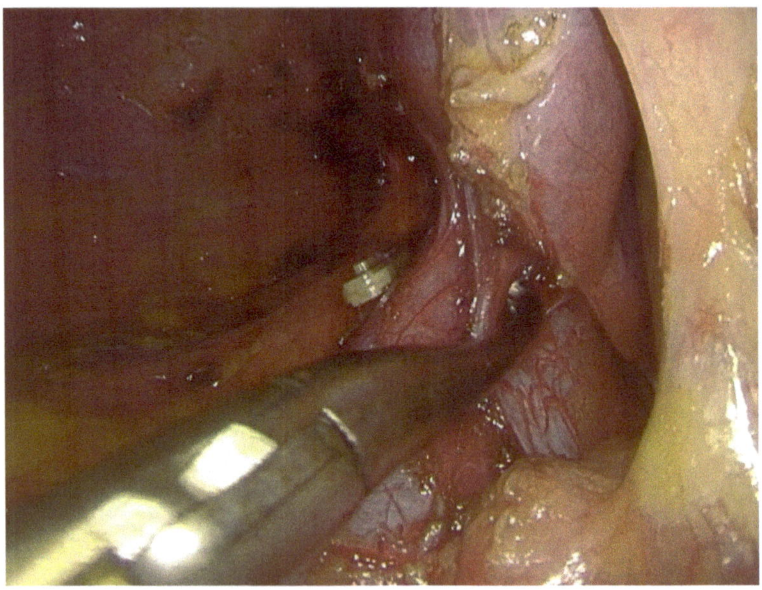

Fig. 5.13 Another short hepatic vein is dissected

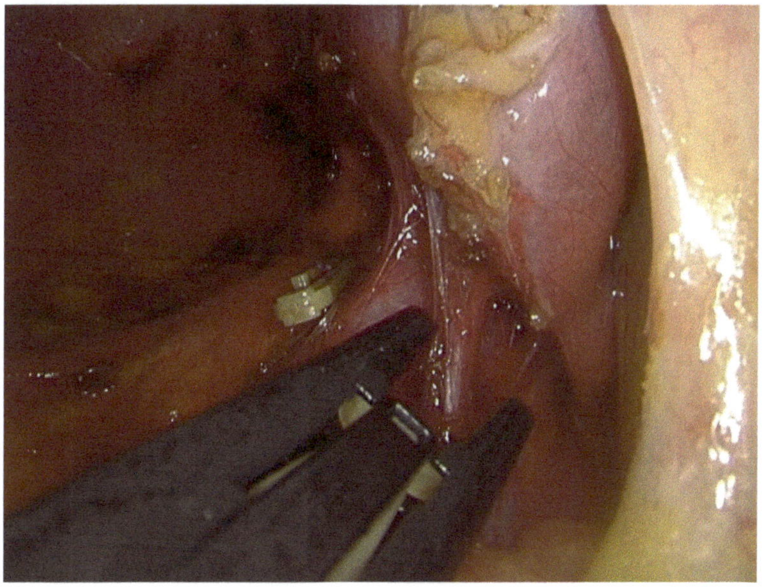

Fig. 5.14 The short hepatic vein is clamped with an absorbable clip

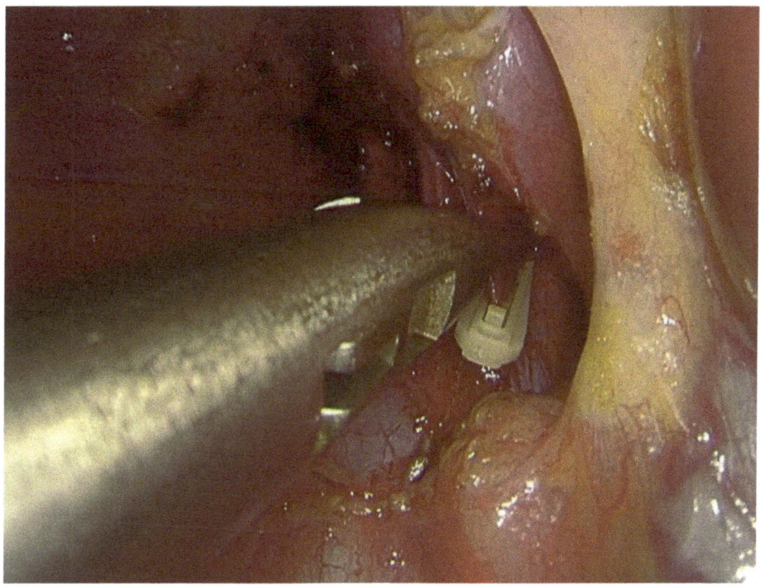

Fig. 5.15 A titanic clip is applied on the distal portion of the short hepatic vein

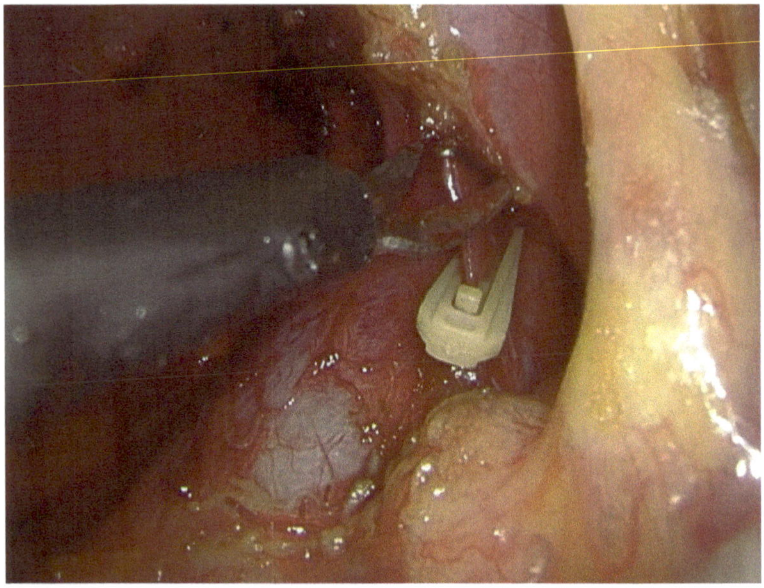

Fig. 5.16 The short hepatic vein is divided

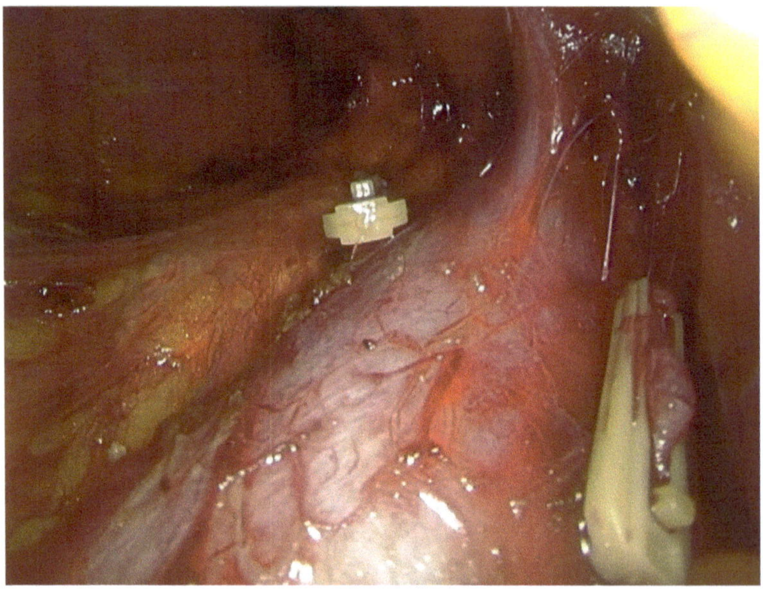

Fig. 5.17 The third short hepatic vein is visualized after the two short hepatic veins were divided

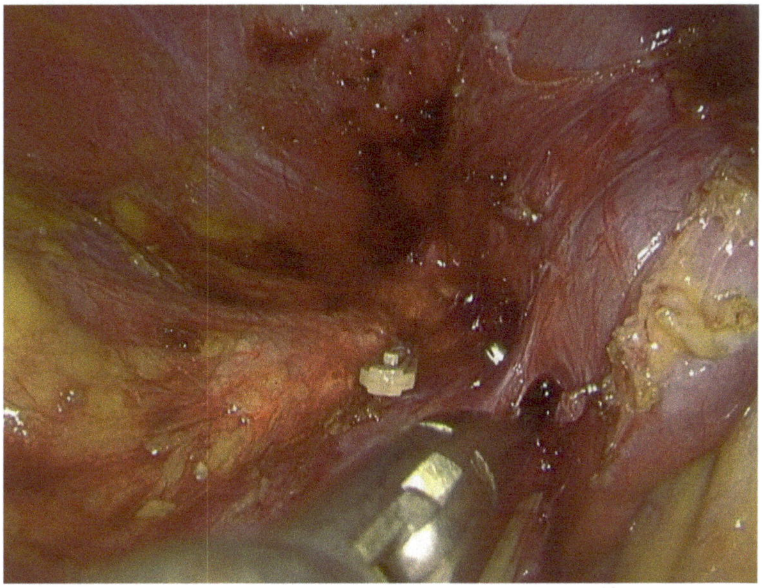

Fig. 5.18 The short hepatic vein is dissected with the forceps

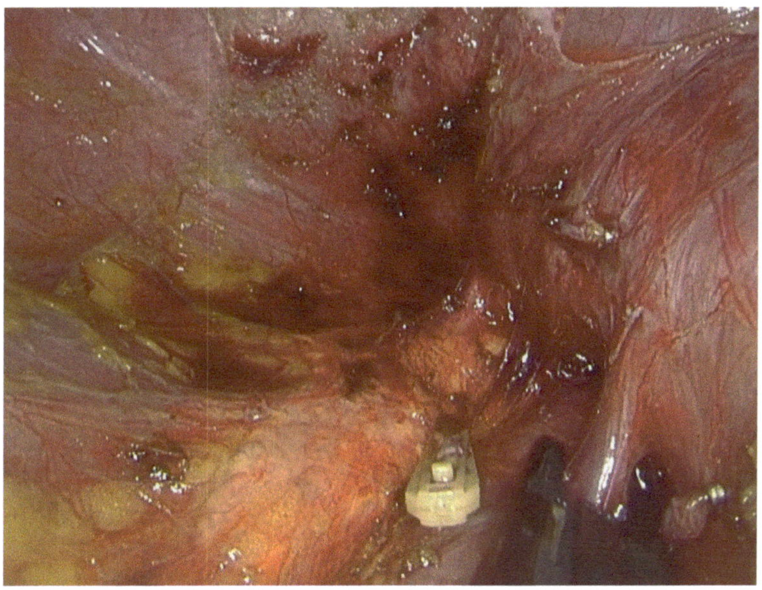

Fig. 5.19 The short hepatic vein is clamped with an absorbable clip

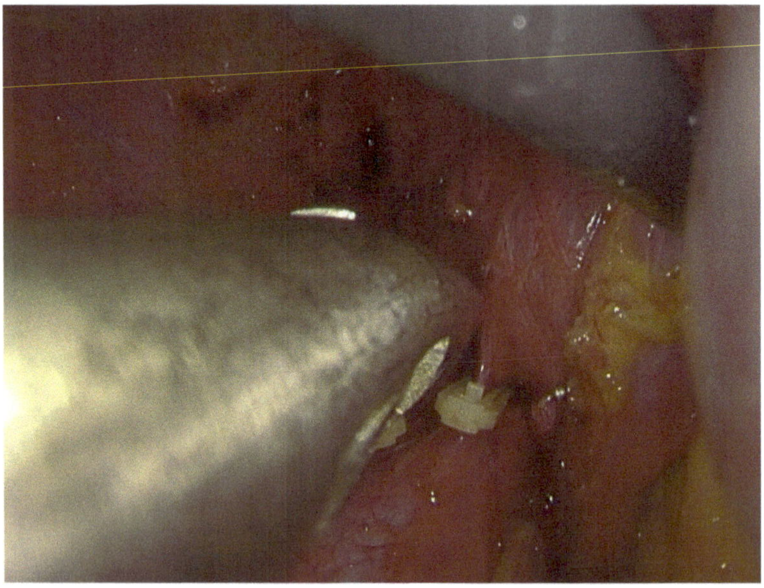

Fig. 5.20 A titanic clip is applied on the distal portion of the short hepatic vein

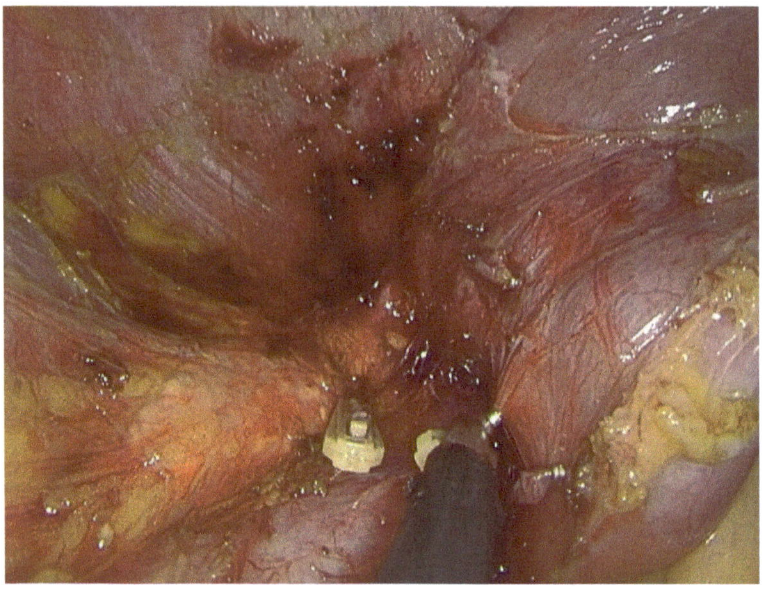

Fig. 5.21 The short hepatic vein is divided

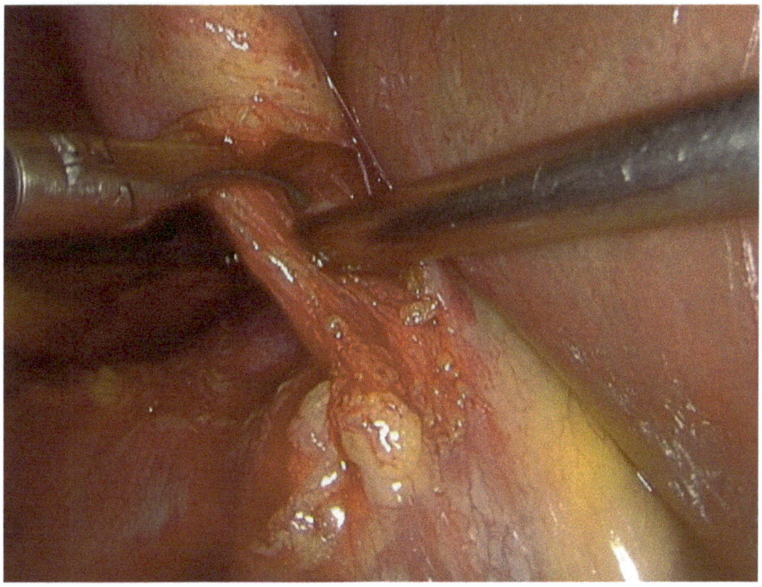

Fig. 5.22 The gallbladder is mobilized upward and the cystic duct is dissected

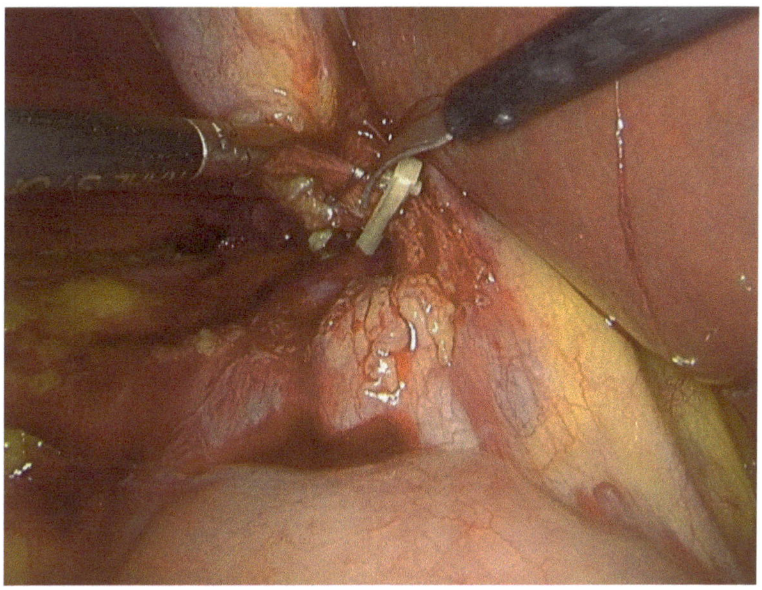

Fig. 5.23 After being clamped with clips, the cystic duct is divided

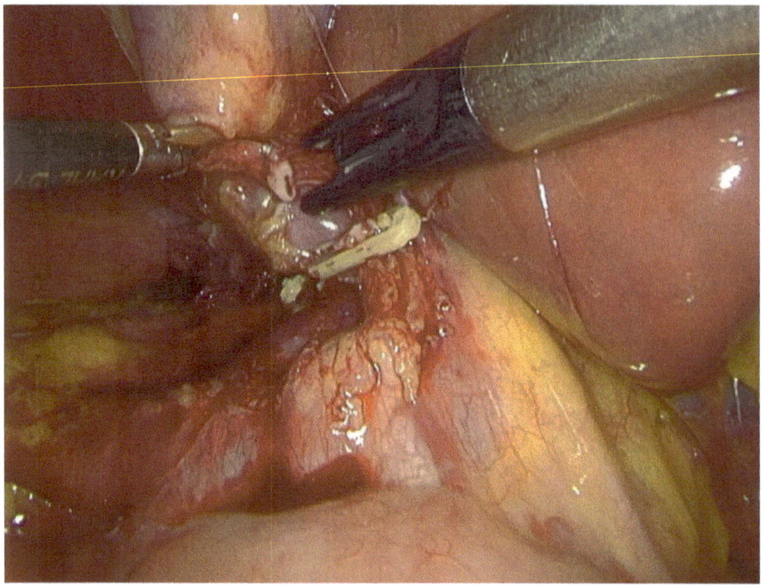

Fig. 5.24 After being dissected, the cystic artery is clamped with an absorbable clip

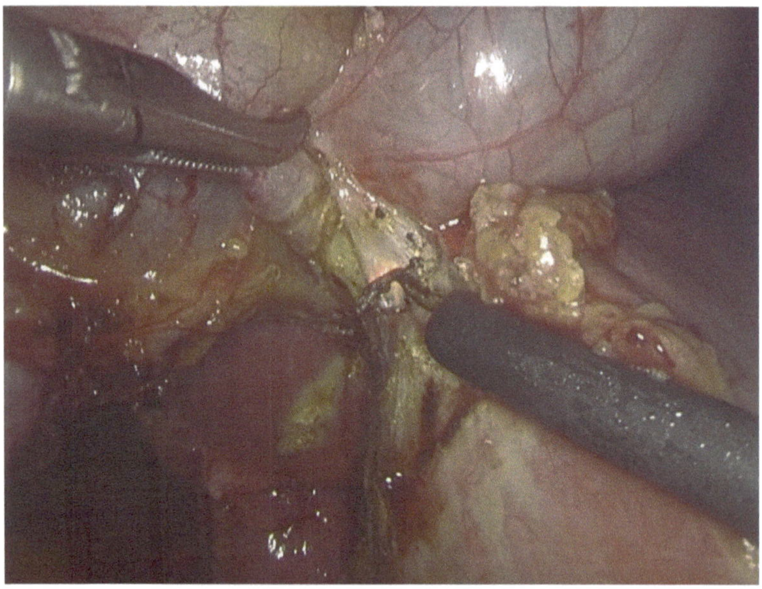

Fig. 5.25 The gallbladder is resected after the cystic artery was divided

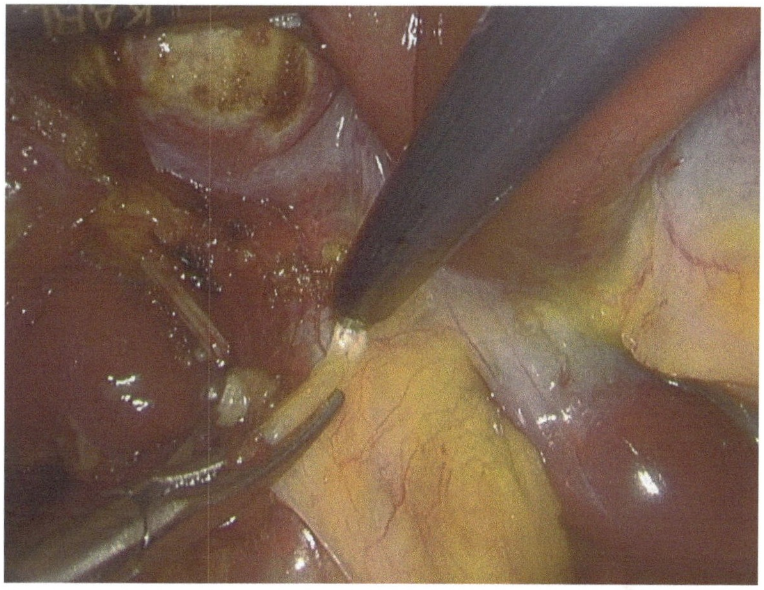

Fig. 5.26 The hepatoduodenal ligament (HDL) is dissected with LPMOD

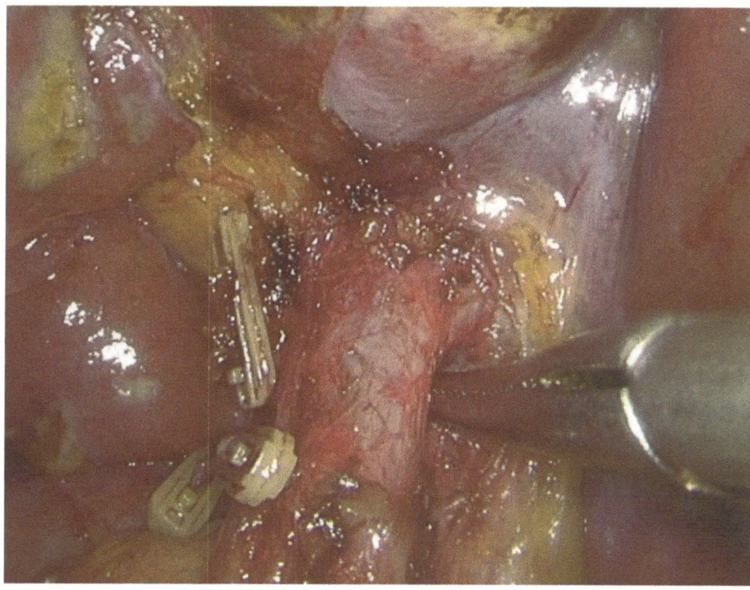

Fig. 5.27 The common bile duct is dissected

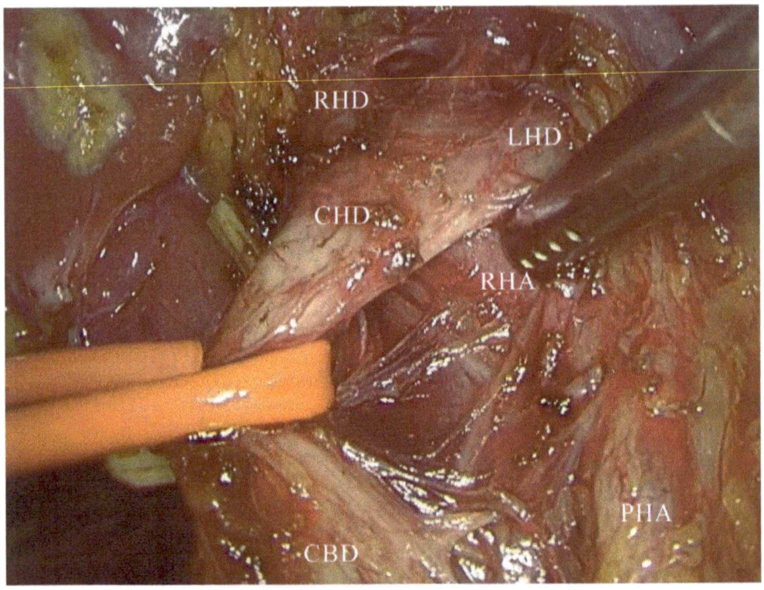

Fig. 5.28 The CBD is pulled to the right with a #8 urinary catheter, and the right hepatic artery (*RHA*) is visualized

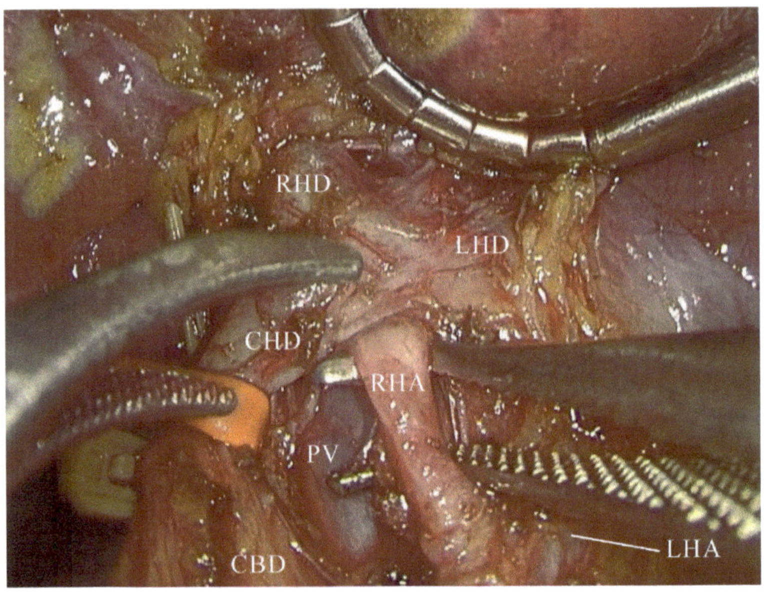

Fig. 5.29 The right hepatic artery is dissected

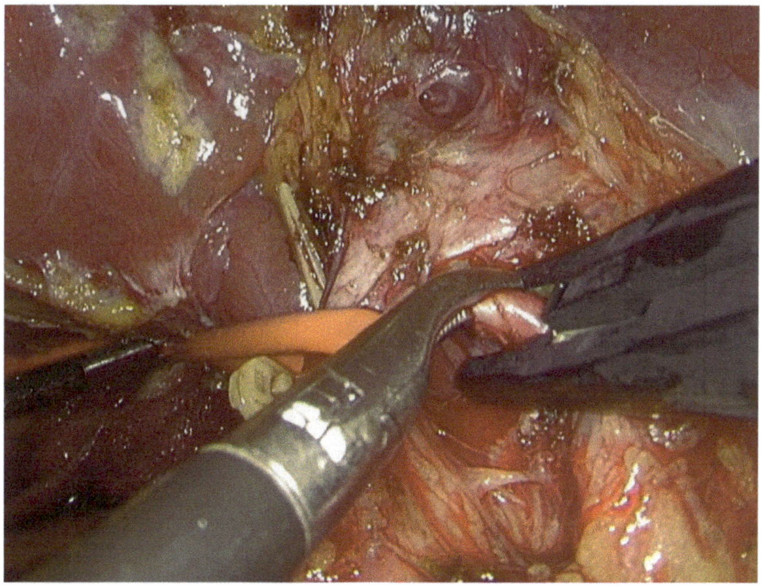

Fig. 5.30 The right hepatic artery is clamped with an absorbable clip

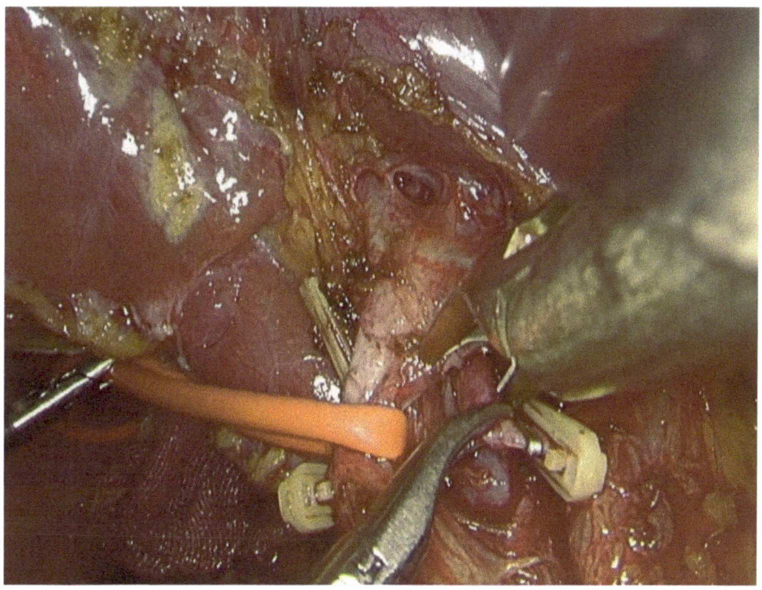

Fig. 5.31 A titanic clip is applied on the distal portion of the right hepatic artery

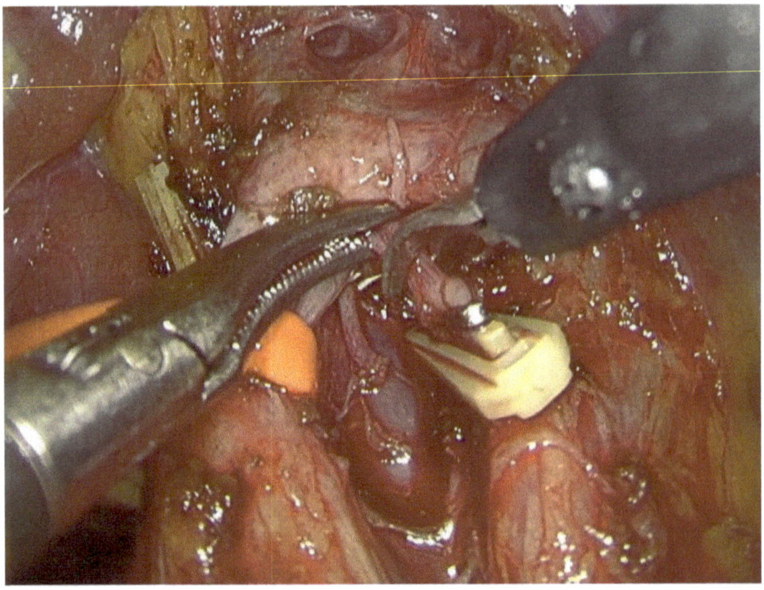

Fig. 5.32 The right hepatic artery is divided

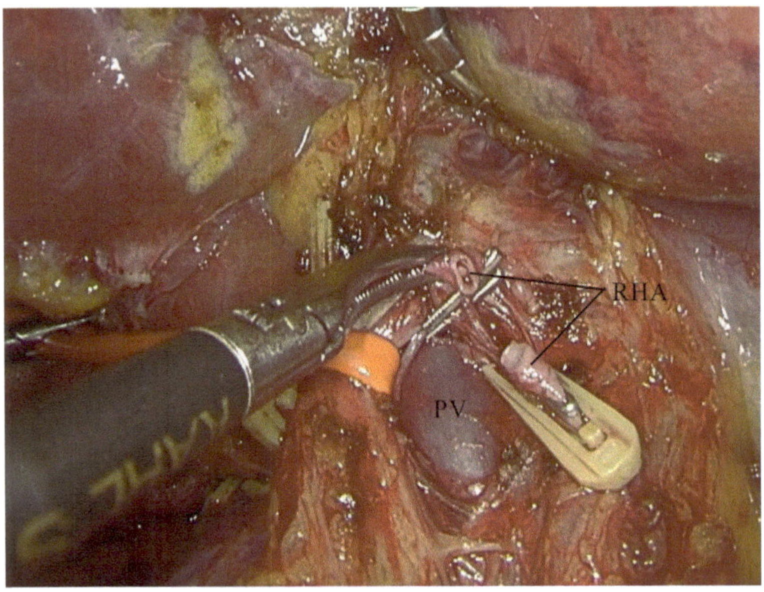

Fig. 5.33 The portal vein (*PV*) is visualized after the RHA was divided

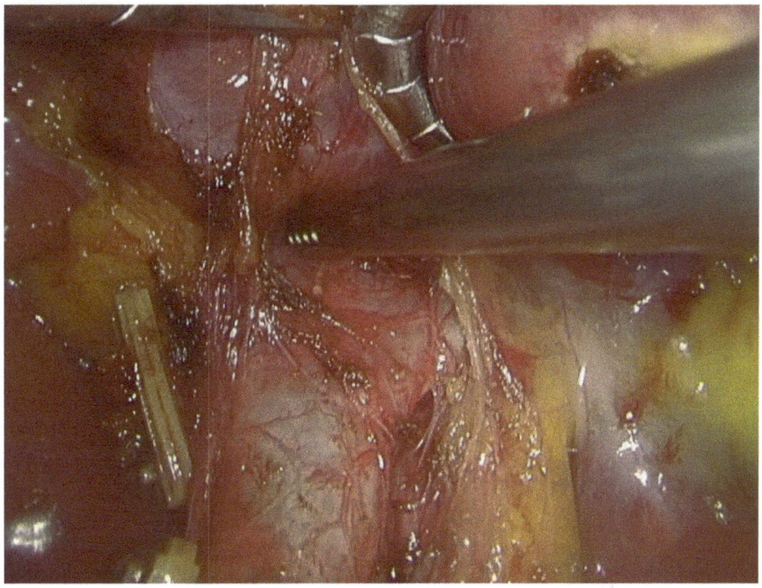

Fig. 5.34 The porta hepatis is exposed by pulling the hilar plate, and the right hepatic duct (RHD) is dissected

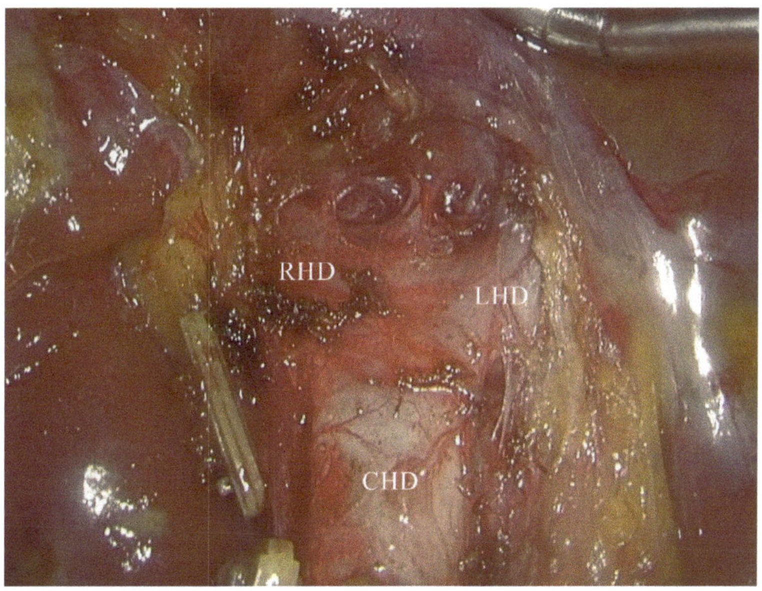

Fig. 5.35 The bifurcation of the hepatic duct (BHD) is identified

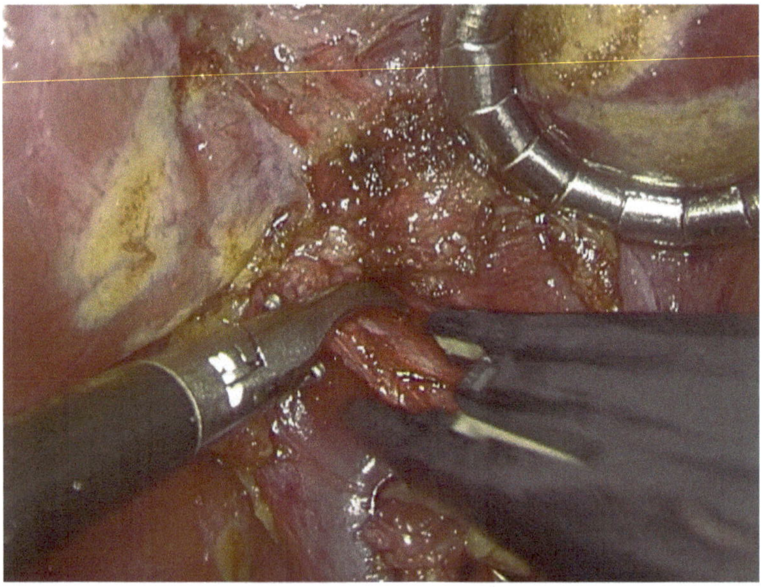

Fig. 5.36 The right hepatic duct is clamped with an absorbable clip

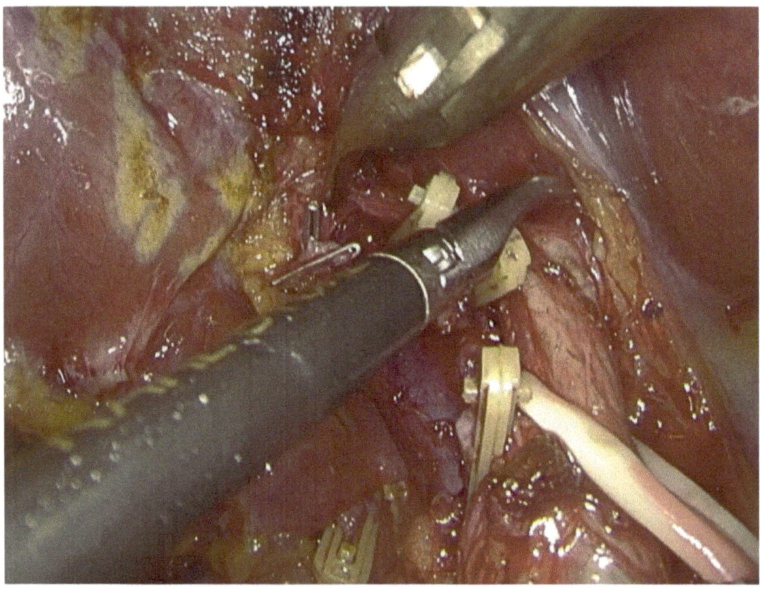

Fig. 5.37 A titanic clip is applied on the right hepatic duct

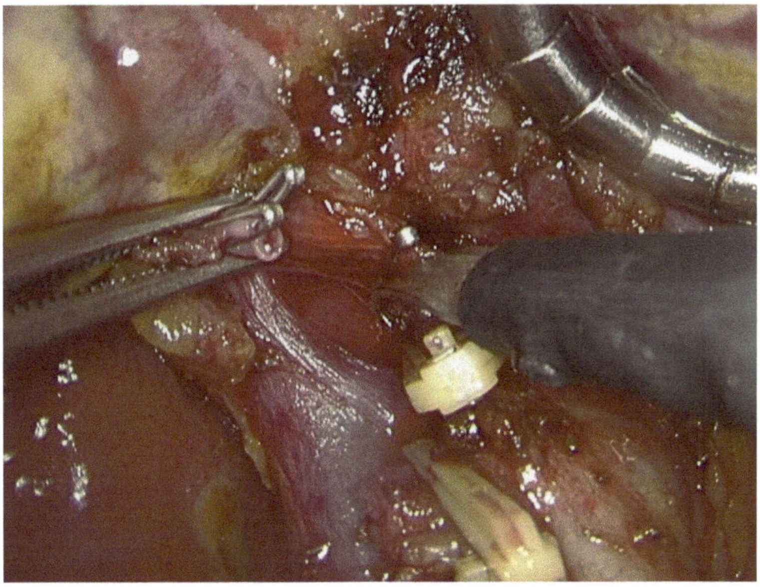

Fig. 5.38 The right hepatic duct is divided

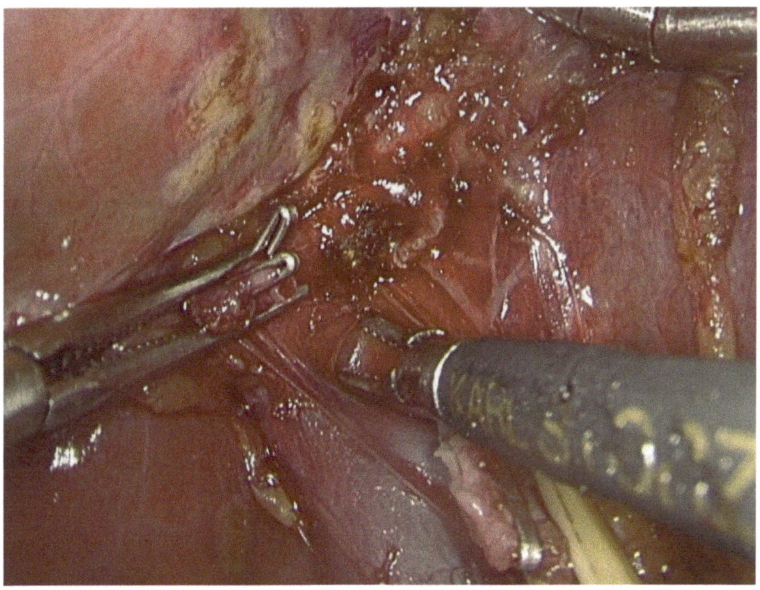

Fig. 5.39 The right branch of portal vein is dissected with a forceps

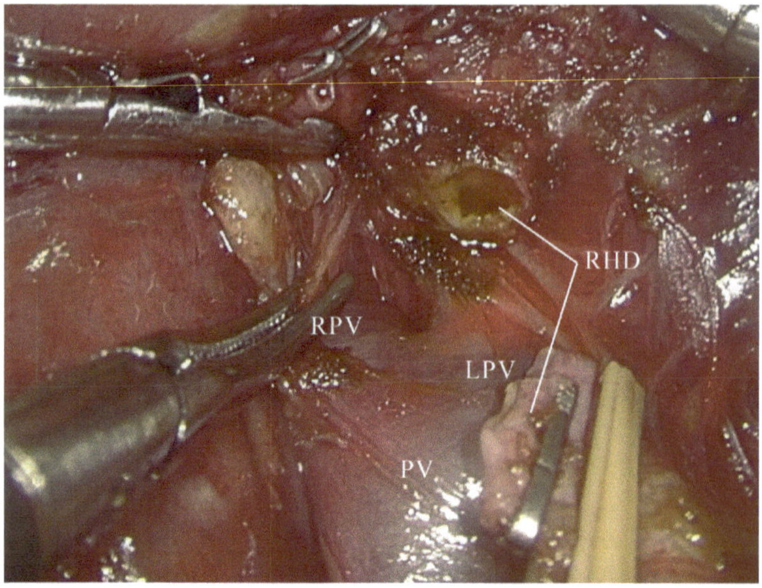

Fig. 5.40 The bifurcation of the portal vein is identified

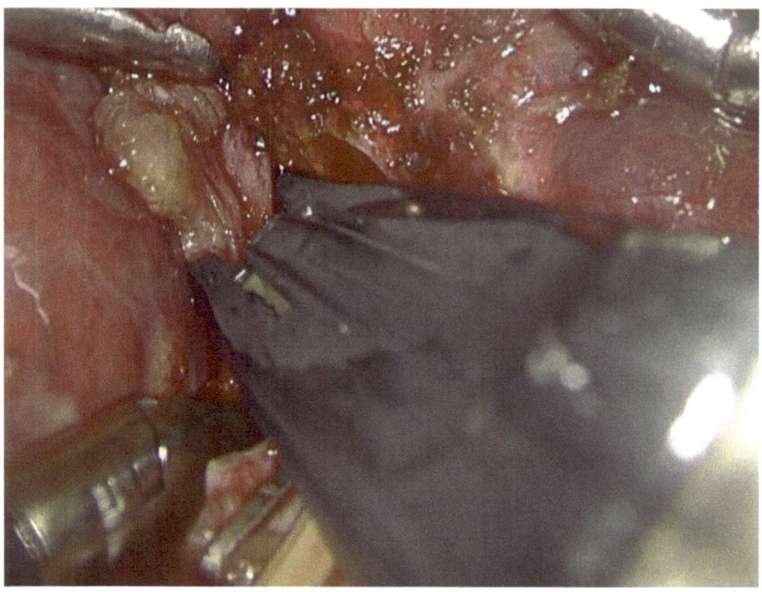

Fig. 5.41 The right branch of portal vein (RPV) is clamped with an absorbable clip

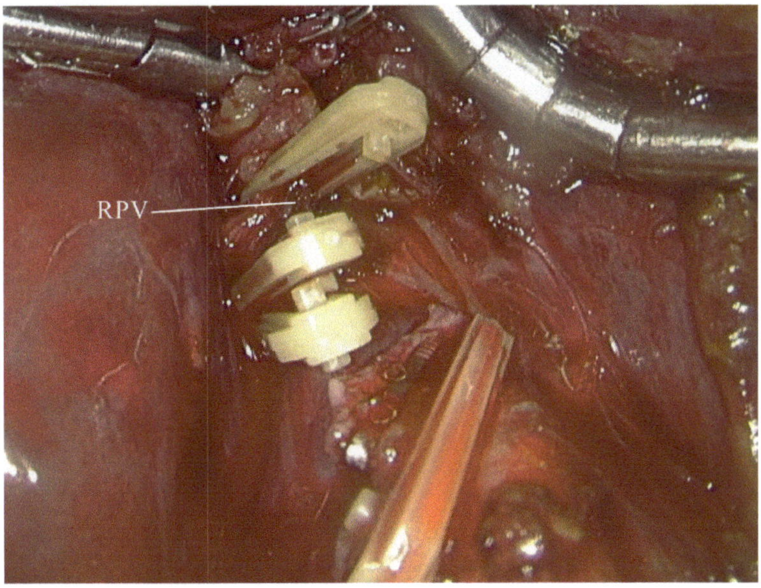

Fig. 5.42 The RPV is occluded with absorbable clips, and the selective right inflow occlusion is completed

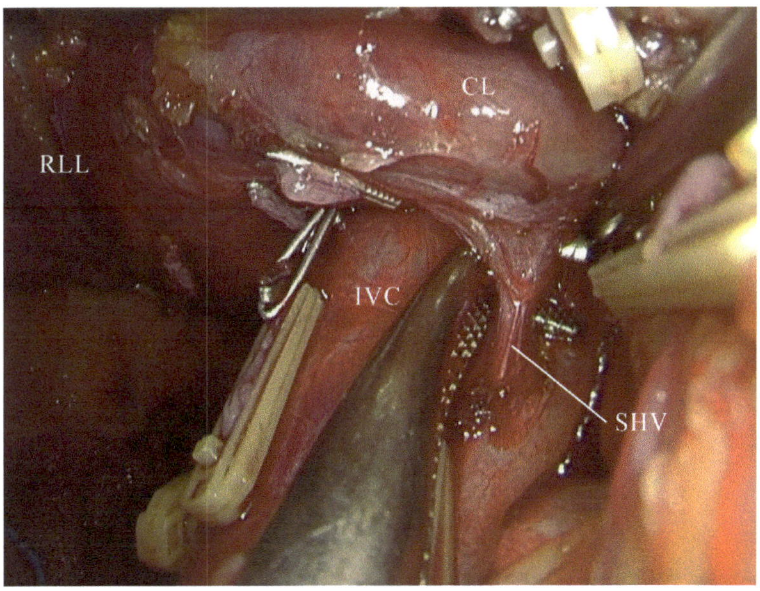

Fig. 5.43 After the right hepatic pedicle was divided, a short hepatic vein to the caudate lobe (*CL*) is exposed and is dissected

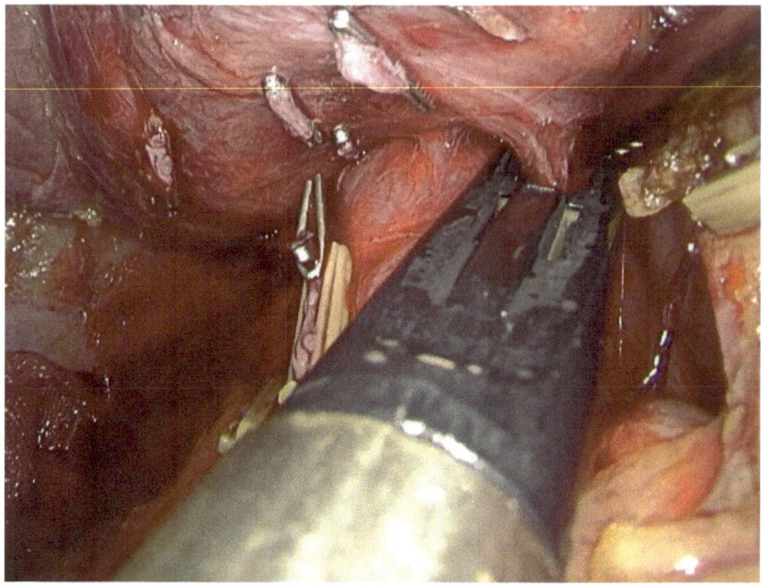

Fig. 5.44 The short hepatic vein is clamped with an absorbable clip

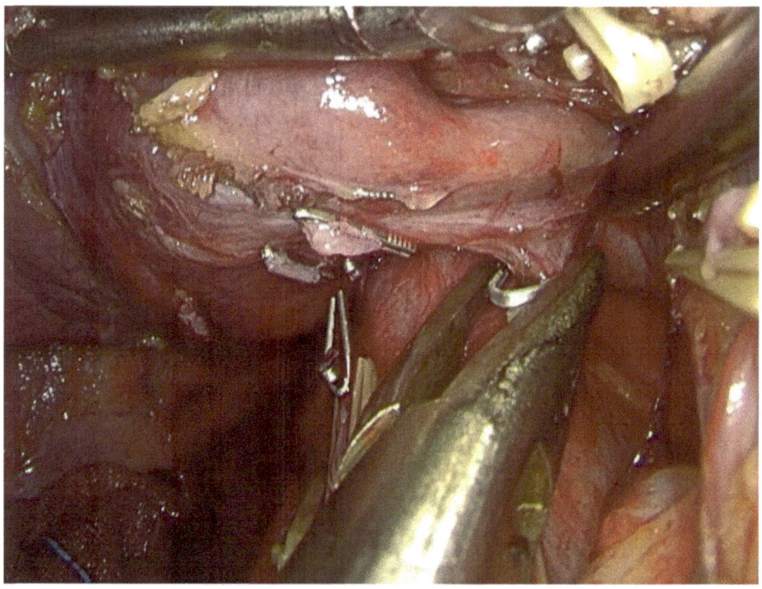

Fig. 5.45 A titanic clip is applied on the distal portion of the short hepatic vein

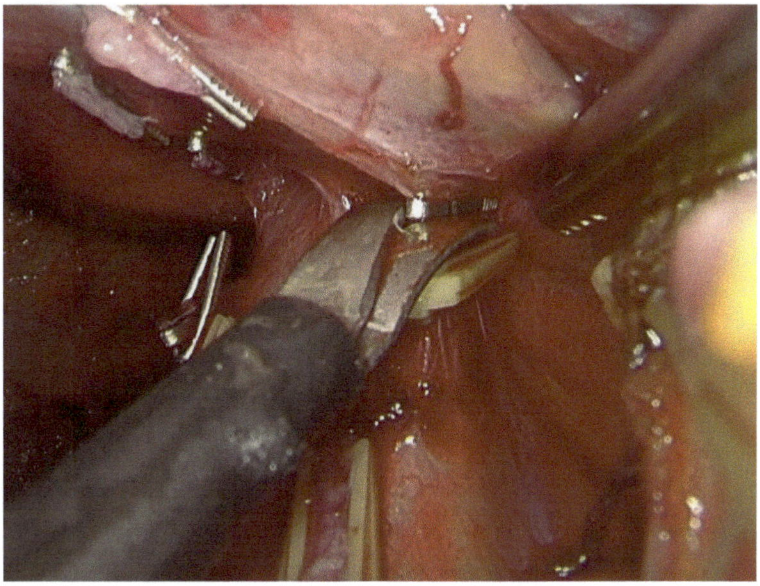

Fig. 5.46 The short hepatic vein is divided

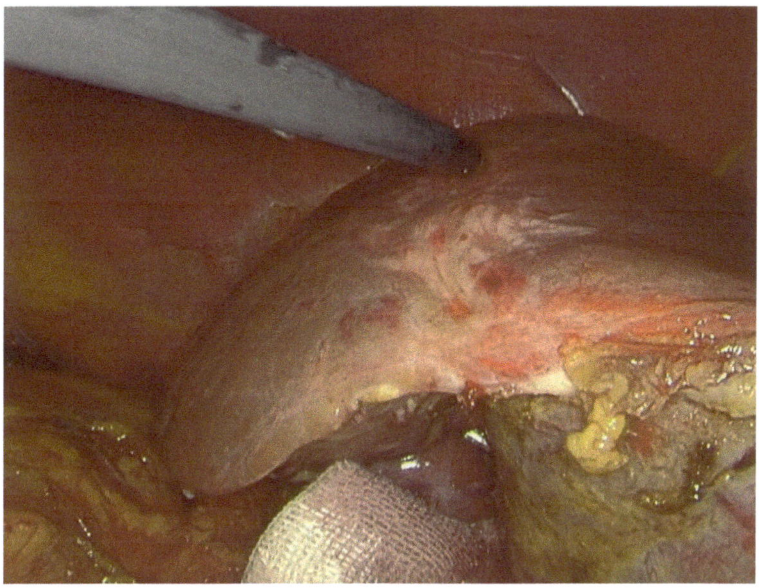

Fig. 5.47 The right lobe of the liver is completely freed

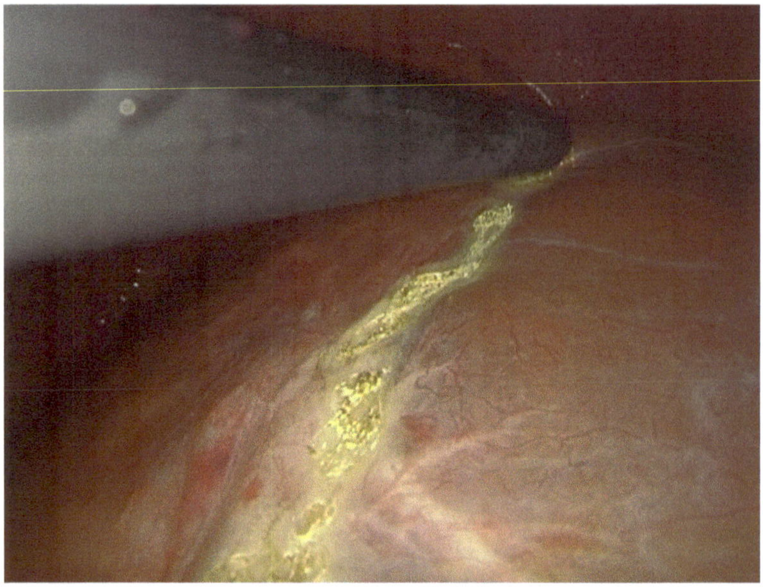

Fig. 5.48 A transection line is marked on the liver surface with LPMOD

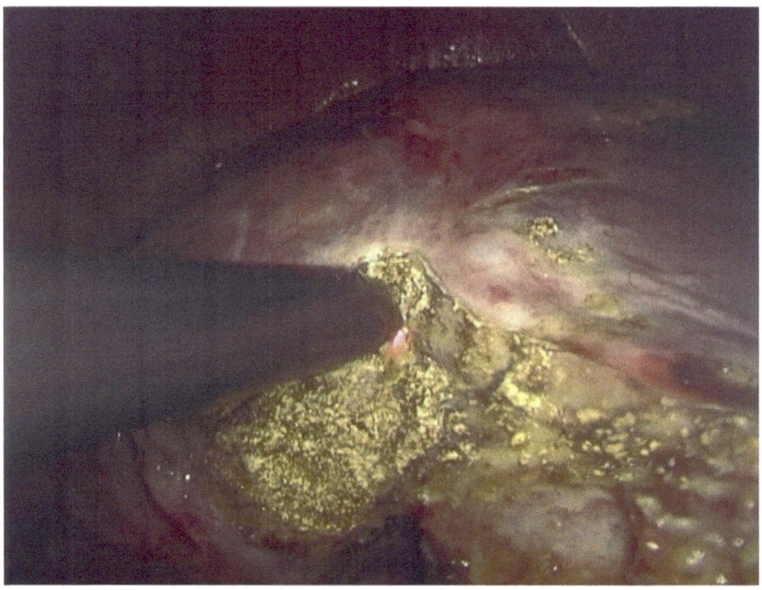

Fig. 5.49 The liver parenchyma is transected with LPMOD

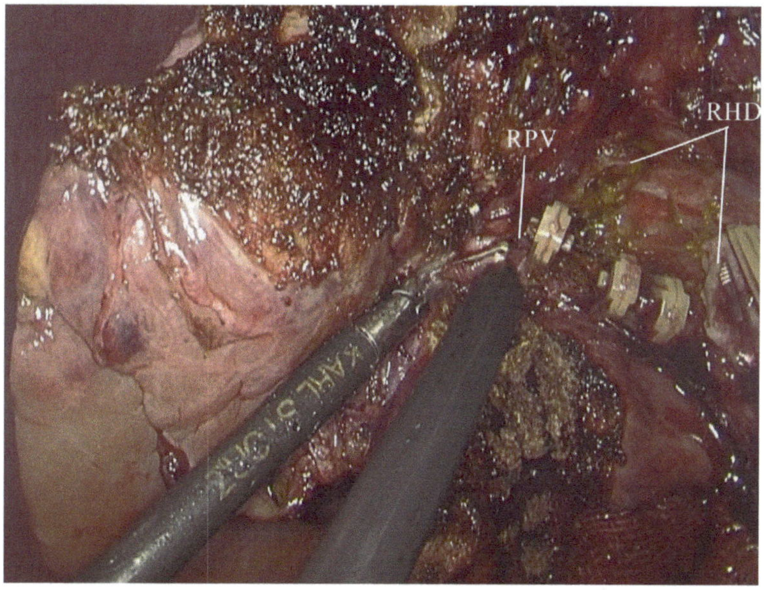

Fig. 5.50 The RPV is divided with LPMOD

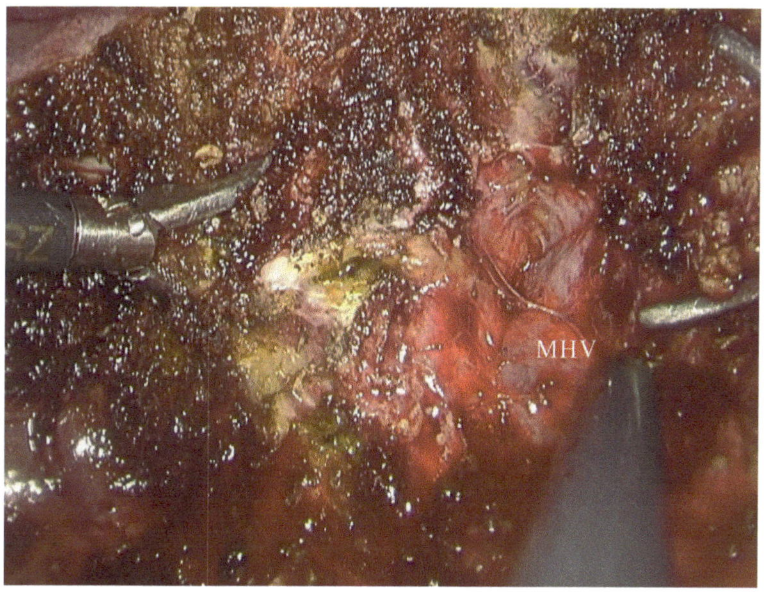

Fig. 5.51 The MHV is visualized in the transection of the liver parenchyma

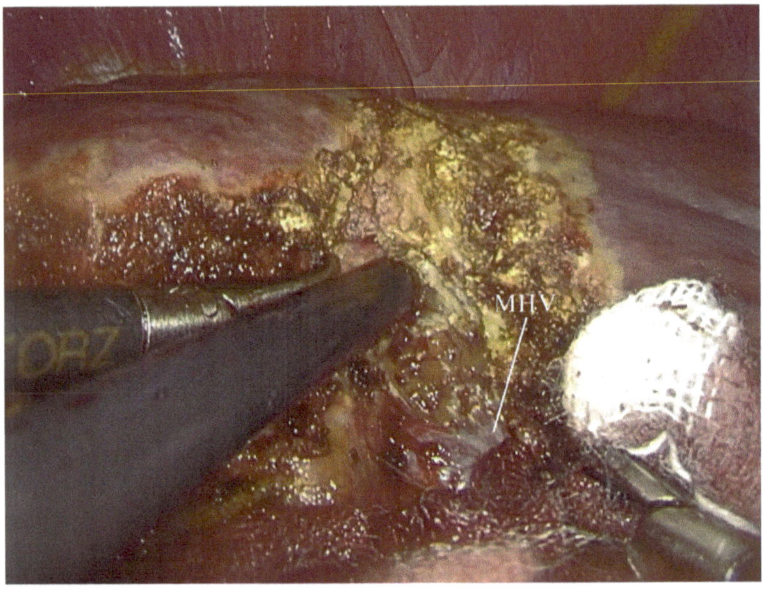

Fig. 5.52 Liver parenchyma is transected along the middle hepatic vein and a branch of middle hepatic vein is visualized

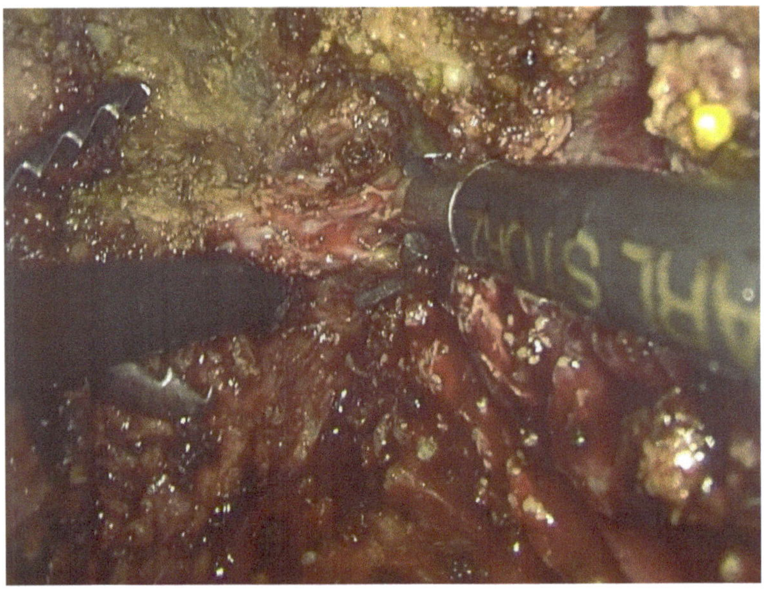

Fig. 5.53 The branch of MHV is dissected with LPMOD

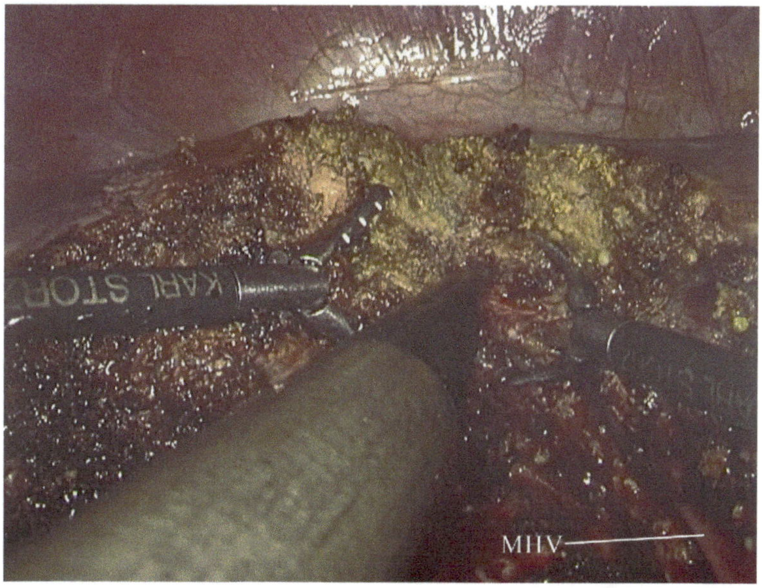

Fig. 5.54 The branch of MHV is clamped with an absorbable clip

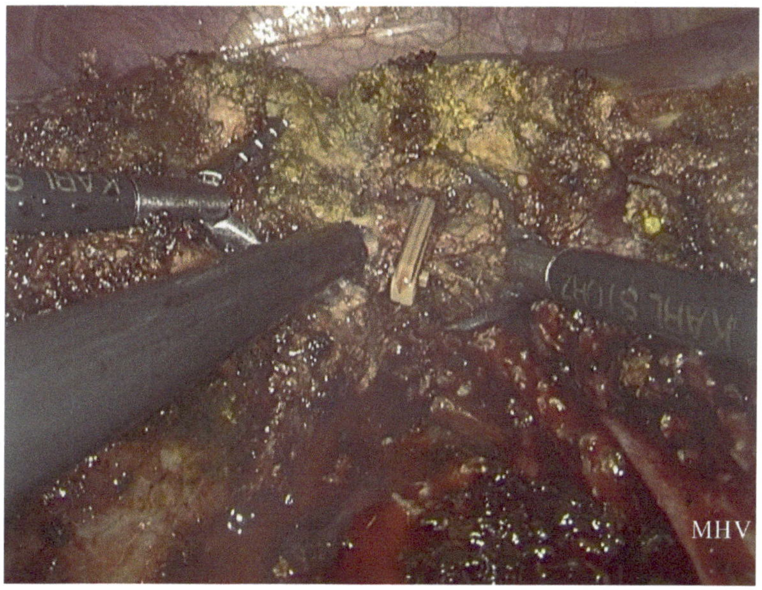

Fig. 5.55 The branch of MHV is divided with LPMOD

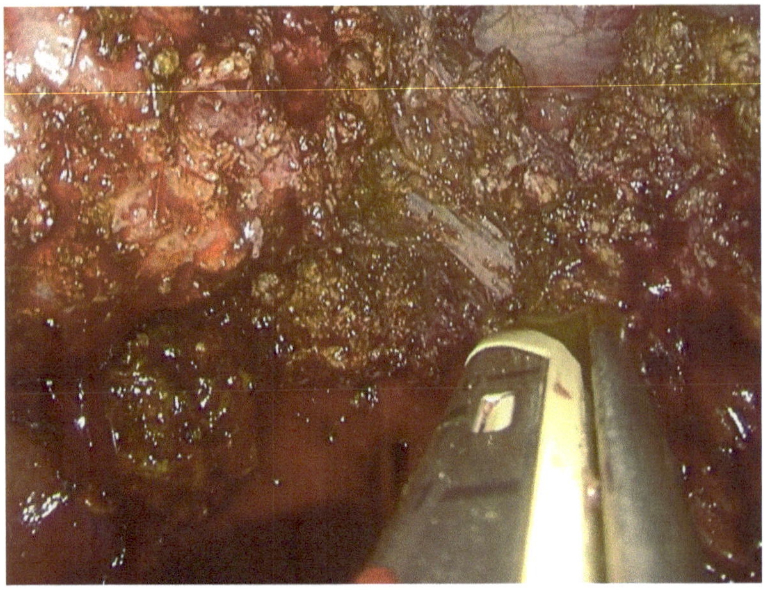

Fig. 5.56 The right hepatic vein is visualized

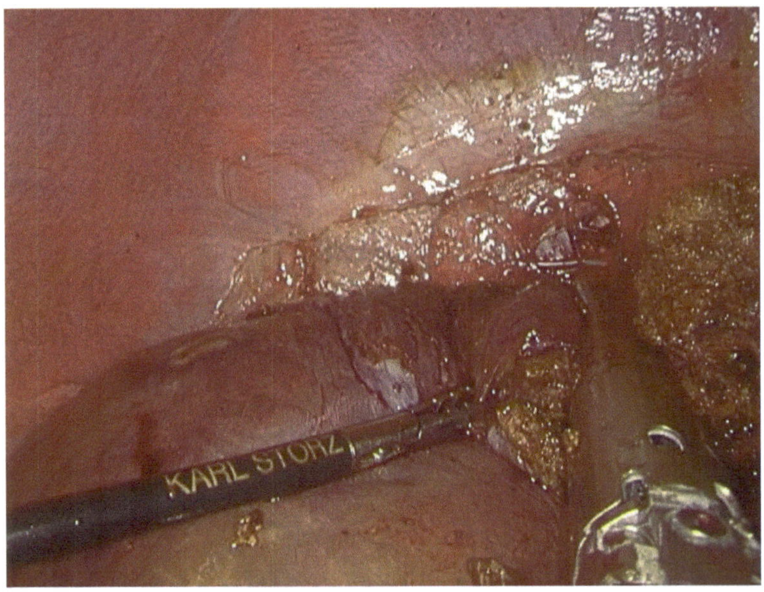

Fig. 5.57 The right hepatic vein and the remainder of the liver parenchyma are transected with linear staples

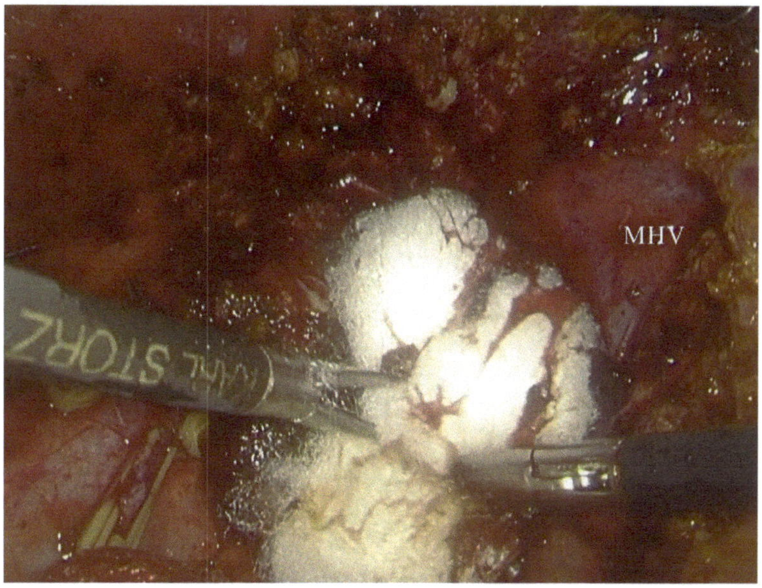

Fig. 5.58 The right lobe is removed and the MHV can be visualized on the transection plane

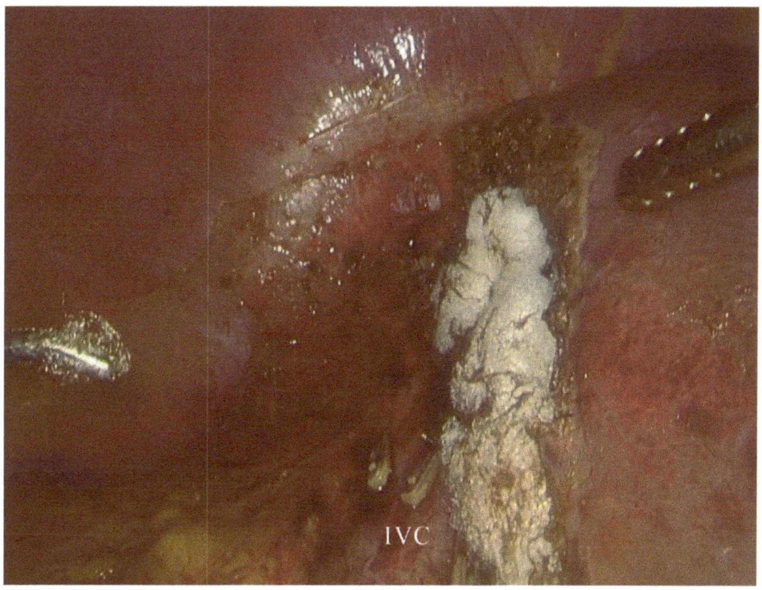

Fig. 5.59 The view of the transection plane after the right lobe was removed

References

Malassagne B, Cherqui D, Alon R, et al. Safety of selective vascular clamping for major hepatectomies. J Am Coll Surg. 1998;187:482–6.

O'Rourke N, Fielding G. Laparoscopic right hepatectomy: surgical technique. J Gastrointest Surg. 2004;8: 213–6.

Sahin M, Avsar FM, Ozel H, et al. The effects of dimethyl sulfoxide on liver damage caused by ischemia-reperfusion. Transplant Proc. 2004;36:2590–2.

Teoh NC, Farrell GC. Hepatic ischemia reperfusion injury: pathogenic mechanisms and basis for hepatoprotection. J Gastroenterol Hepatol. 2003;18: 891–902.

6 Laparoscopic Resection of the Caudate Lobe

The caudate lobe (CL) of the liver is located between the porta hepatis (PH) and the inferior vena cava (IVC). It is divided into three parts: the Spiegel process (SP) (Couinaud's Segment 1), the paracaval portion (Couinaud's Segment 9), and the caudate process (CP). The Spiegel lobe is situated behind the ligamentum venosum (LV) and lies on the left of the IVC. The paracaval portion is located in front of the IVC. The caudate process extends to the left and can be used for the traction of the caudate lobe. The caudate lobe is supplied by branches of hepatic artery and portal vein (CPV), and the bile is drained by branches of hepatic duct (HD); these vessels and ducts are called caudate portal triad (CPT). The blood of the caudate lobe usually drains directly into the IVC through the short hepatic veins (SHVs) and, in some cases, drains through the hepatic veins (Fig. 6.1). The CPT and the SHVs are important structures in the resection of the caudate, and in most cases, they can be divided before the transection of the liver parenchyma. It is difficult to define the transection line in the completely isolated caudate lobectomy. Takayama et al. (1991) suggested a counterstaining identification technique to define the surgical margin in 1991, but it was not routinely used in the resection of the caudate lobe. Normally, we performed the resection of the caudate lobe along the line from the caudate process to the tip of the caudate lobe.

Resection of the caudate lobe is one of the most difficult open liver surgeries due to the anatomic position. Proper management of the short hepatic veins is the key to this procedure. In the laparoscopic approach, due to the different vision angle and manipulation space, the short hepatic veins can be fully exposed by the proper mobilization of the caudate lobe and can be safely divided after the meticulous dissection. However, it is still a most dangerous laparoscopic surgery and should be performed by experienced laparoscopic surgeons.

Electronic supplementary material The online version of this chapter at (doi: 10.1007/978-94-017-9840-2_6) contains supplementary material, which is available to authorized users.

X. Cai, *Laparoscopic Hepatectomy: Atlas and Techniques*,
DOI 10.1007/978-94-017-9840-2_6,

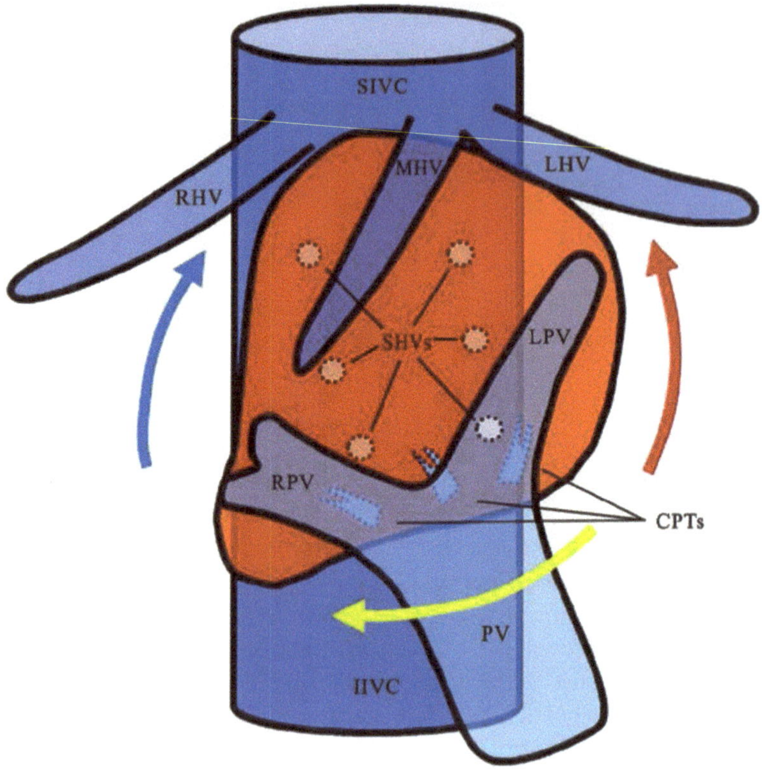

Fig. 6.1 Anatomy of the caudate lobe. *SIVC* suprahepatic inferior vena cava, *RHV* right hepatic vein, *MHV* middle hepatic vein, *LHV* left hepatic vein, *SHV* short hepatic vein, *RPV* right branch of portal vein, *LPV* left branch of portal vein, *PV* portal vein, *CPT* caudate portal triad, *IIVC* infrahepatic inferior vena cava. *The red arrow*: a left approach to raise the caudate lobe and divide the SHVs. *The yellow arrow*: the caudate portal triad is dissected and divided, close to the base of the umbilical fissure. *The blue arrow*: the caudate lobe is transected from the caudate process to the tip of the caudate lobe (From the RPV to the LHV)

6.1 Indications and Contraindications

The indications include benign liver tumors or intrahepatic bile duct stones with irreversible diseases (biliary stricture, severe parenchymal fibrosis or atrophy) requiring isolated or combined resection of the caudate lobe and liver function of Child A to B classification. Contraindications include extrahepatic bile duct stricture and acute suppurative cholangitis or history of biliary surgeries such as exploration of the common bile duct (CBD), or cholangiojejunostomy (cholecystectomy is not regarded as a contraindication).

6.2 Patient Position and Trocars' Position

Patients are placed in the supine position under general anesthesia. Three surgeons are needed in the operation. The senior surgeon stands on the left side of the patient, one assistant surgeon stands on the right side of the senior surgeon controlling the aspiration device, and the other assistant surgeon stands on the right side of the patient. Four entries are made. A supraumbilical 10-mm trocar is inserted as the observation port. A 12-mm trocar below the left costal margin is inserted as the main manipulation port. And two 5-mm trocars are inserted at the right flank area as assistant manipulation ports (Fig. 6.2).

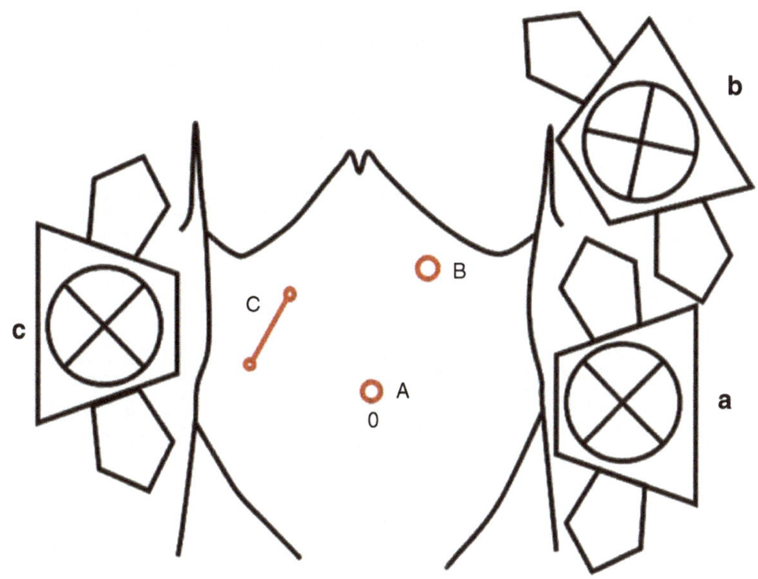

Fig. 6.2 Trocars' position and surgeons' position. (*A*) Observation port; (*B*) Main manipulation port; (*C*) Two assistant ports and the incision for removing specimen; (**a**) The senior surgeon stands on the left side of the patient; (**b**) One assistant stands on the right side of the senior surgeon controlling the aspiration device; (**c**) The other assistant surgeon stands on the right side of the patient

6.3 Laparoscopic Isolated Resection of the Caudate Lobe

See Figs. 6.3, 6.4, 6.5, 6.6, 6.7, 6.8, 6.9, 6.10, 6.11, 6.12, 6.13, and Video 6.1.

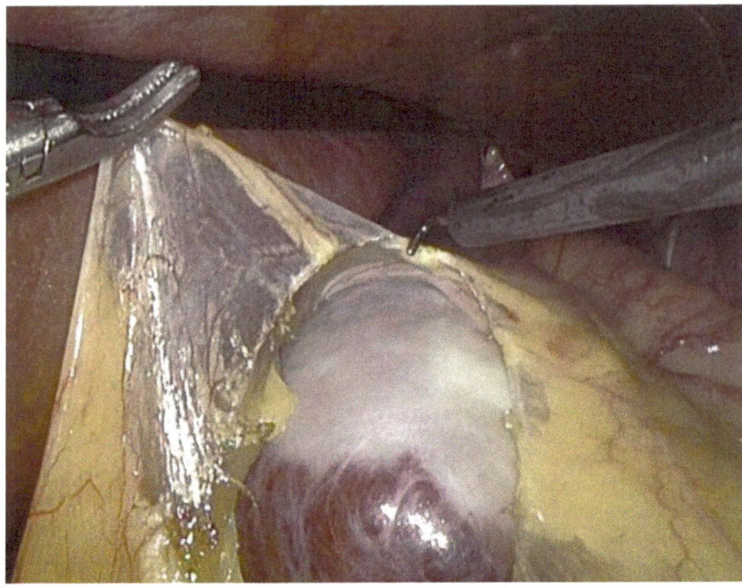

Fig. 6.3 The left lobe (LL) of the liver is elevated with a laparoscopic grasping forceps, and the lesser omentum (LO) is divided

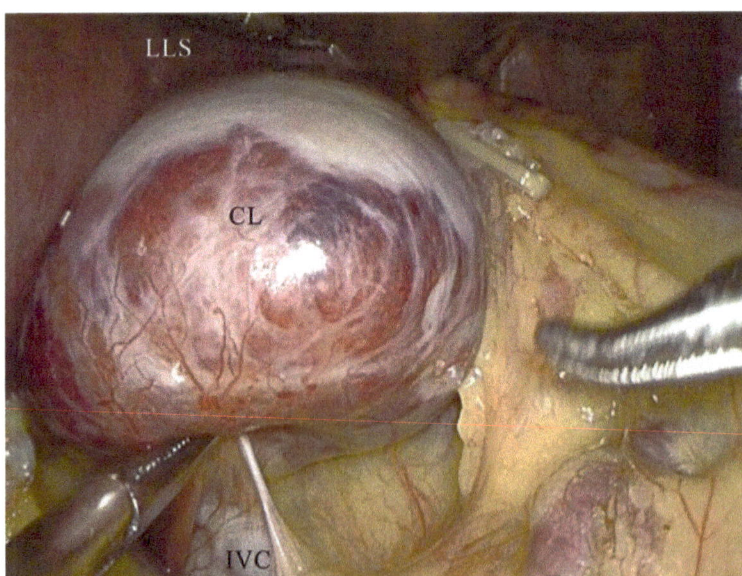

Fig. 6.4 The CL of the liver (a hemangioma) is elevated and the IVC is visualized

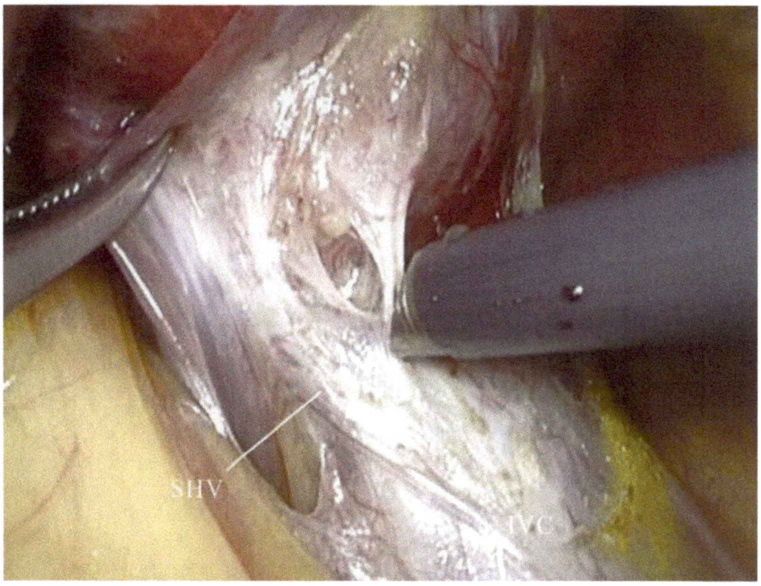

Fig. 6.5 A SHV is visualized in the dissection

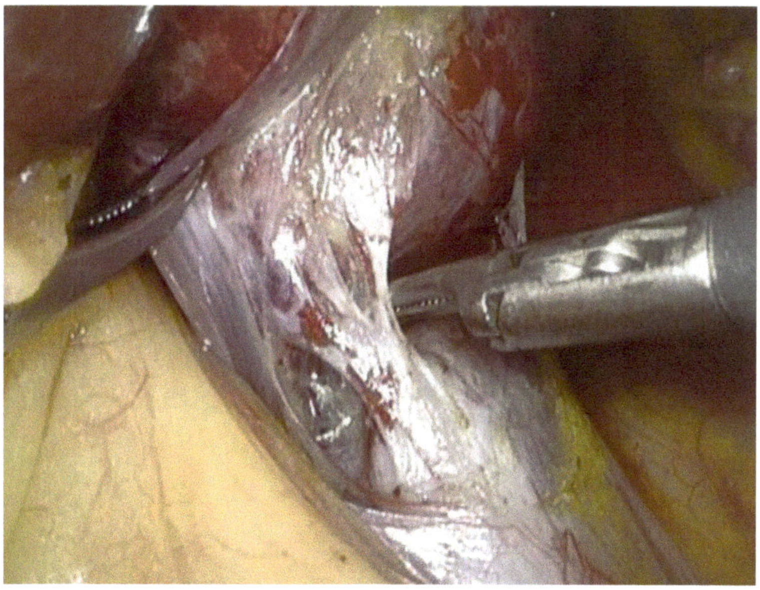

Fig. 6.6 The SHV is dissected and is freed with a curved dissecting forceps

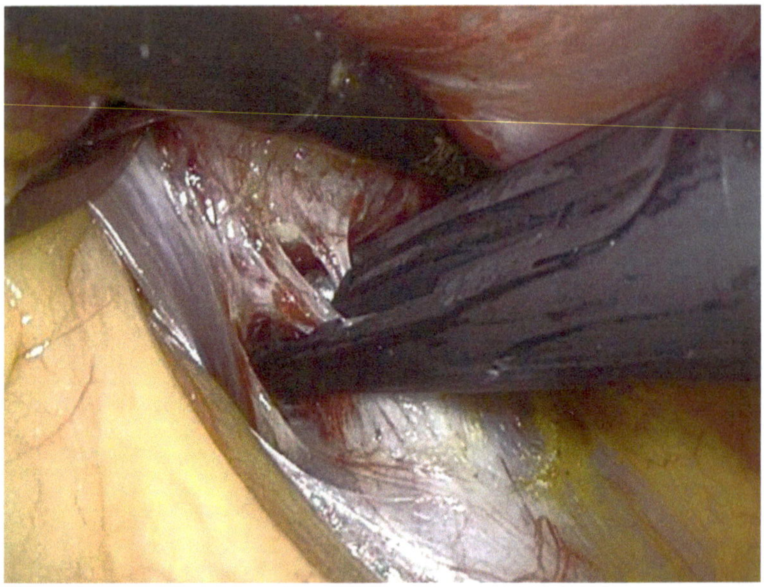

Fig. 6.7 The SHV is clamped with an absorbable clip

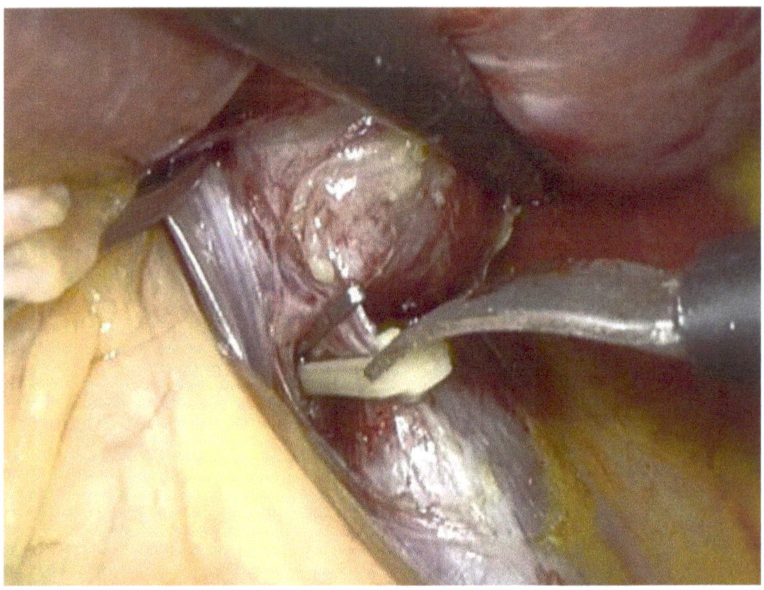

Fig. 6.8 The SHV is divided

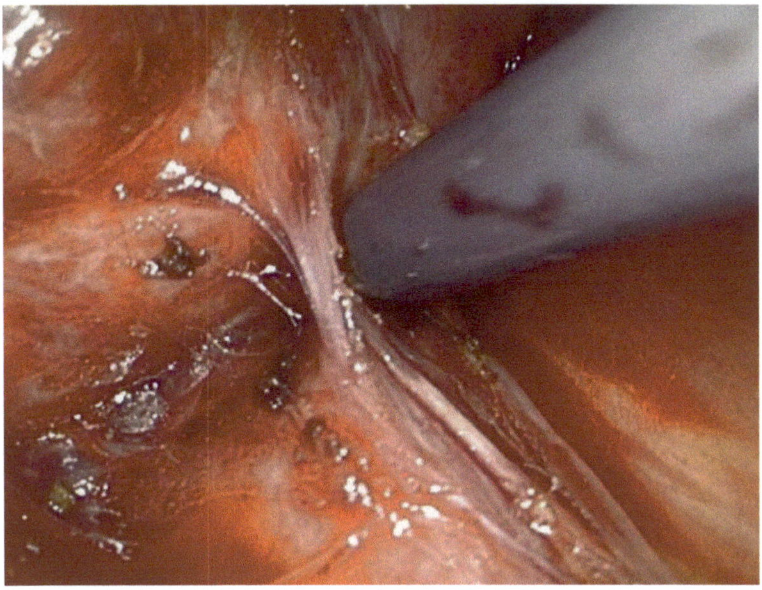

Fig. 6.9 Another SHV is dissected with LPMOD

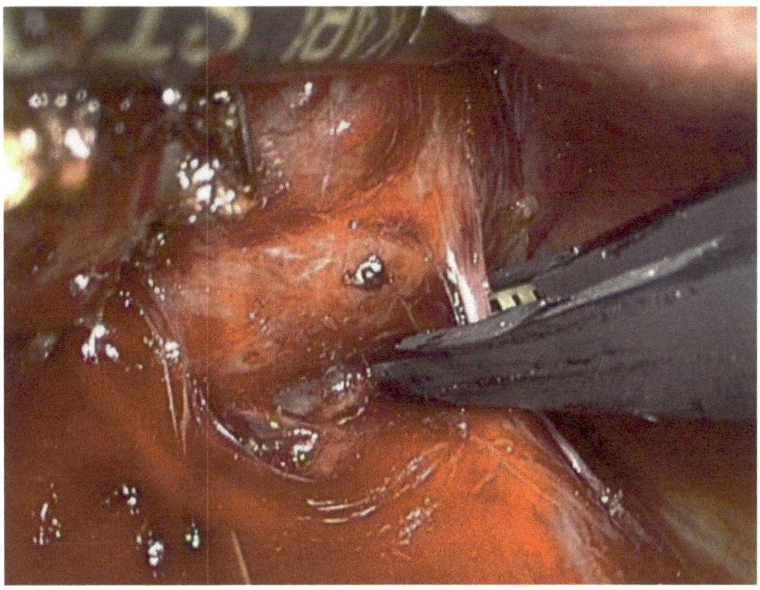

Fig. 6.10 The SHV is clamped with an absorbable clip

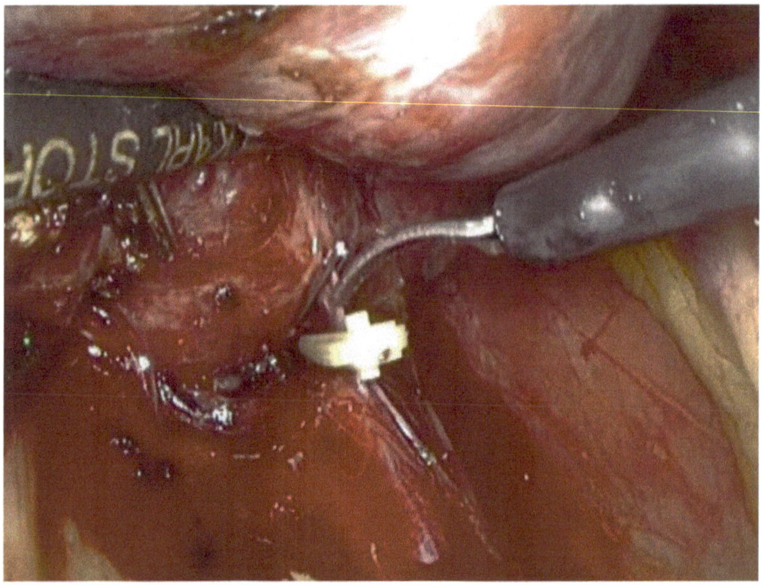

Fig. 6.11 The SHV is divided

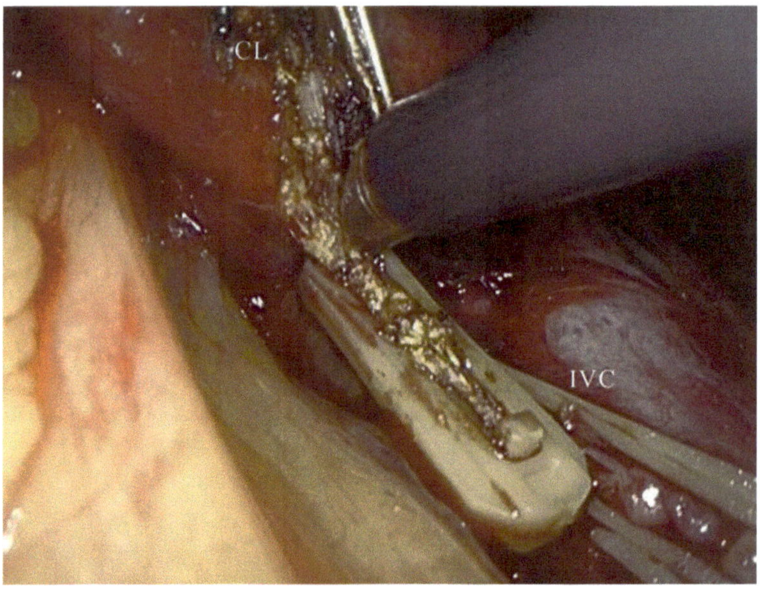

Fig. 6.12 After being clamped with an absorbable clip, liver parenchyma and the caudate portal triad are transected with LPMOD

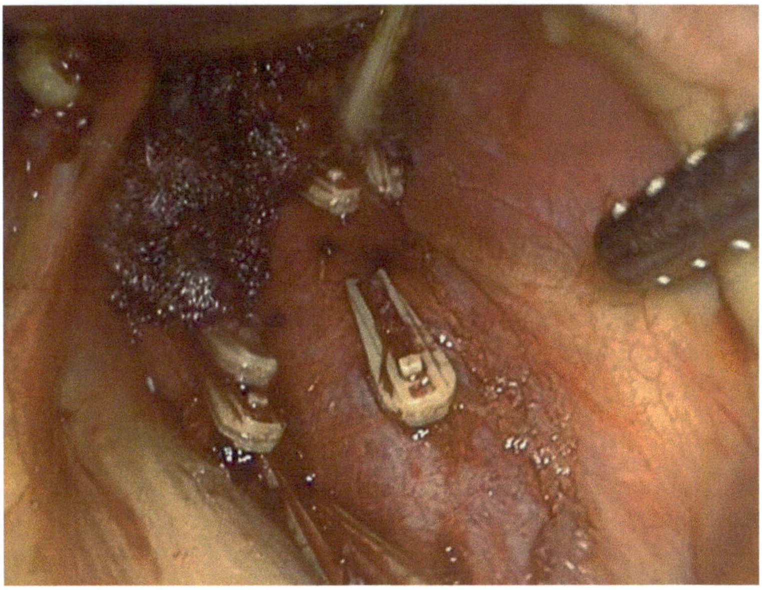

Fig. 6.13 The inferior vena cava is visualized after the resection of caudate lobe

6.4 Laparoscopic Combined Resection of the Caudate Lobe: Laparoscopic Left Lateral Segmentectomy and Resection of the Caudate Lobe

See Figs. 6.14, 6.15, 6.16, 6.17, 6.18, 6.19, 6.20, 6.21, 6.22, 6.23, 6.24, 6.25, 6.26, 6.27, 6.28, 6.29, 6.30, 6.31, 6.32, 6.33, 6.34, 6.35, 6.36, 6.37, 6.38, 6.39, 6.40, 6.41, 6.42, 6.43, 6.44, 6.45, 6.46, 6.47, 6.48, 6.49, 6.50, 6.51, 6.52, 6.53, 6.54, and Video 6.2.

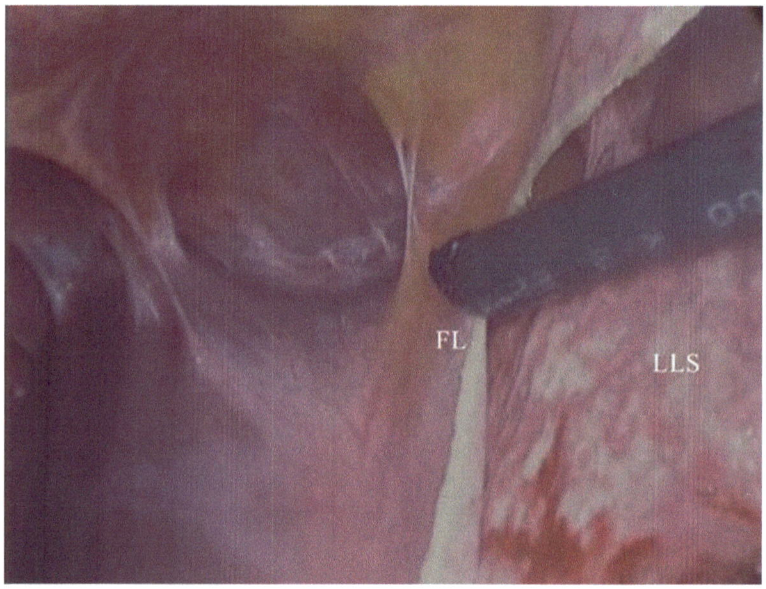

Fig. 6.14 The round ligament (RL), the falciform ligament (FL), and the adhesion are divided with LPMOD

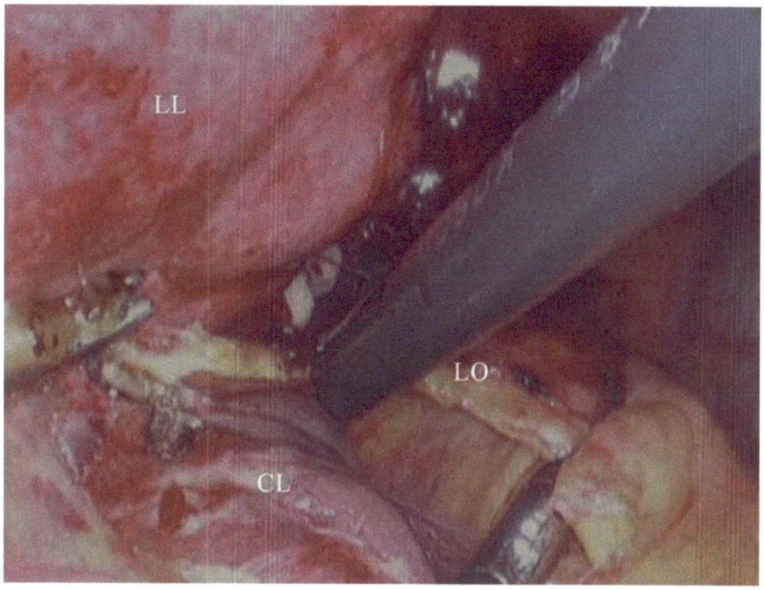

Fig. 6.15 The LO is divided with LPMOD

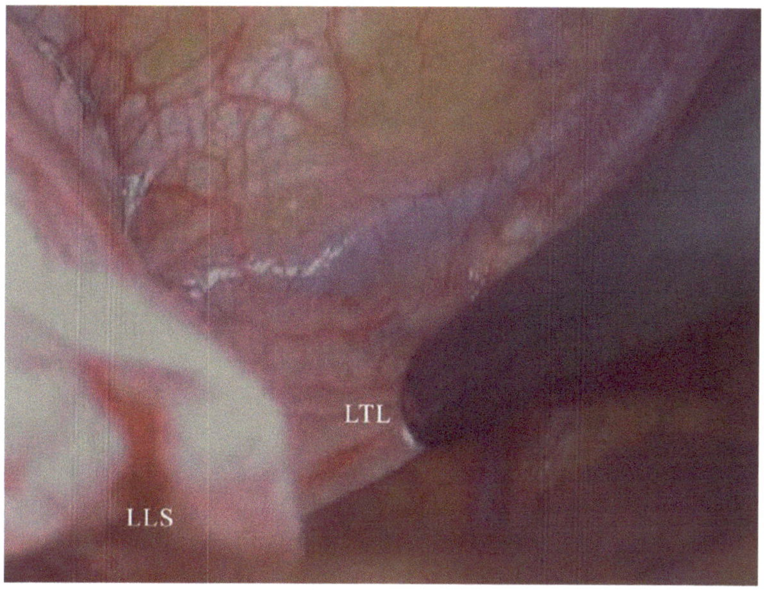

Fig. 6.16 The LL of the liver is mobilized to the right, and the LTL is divided with LPMOD

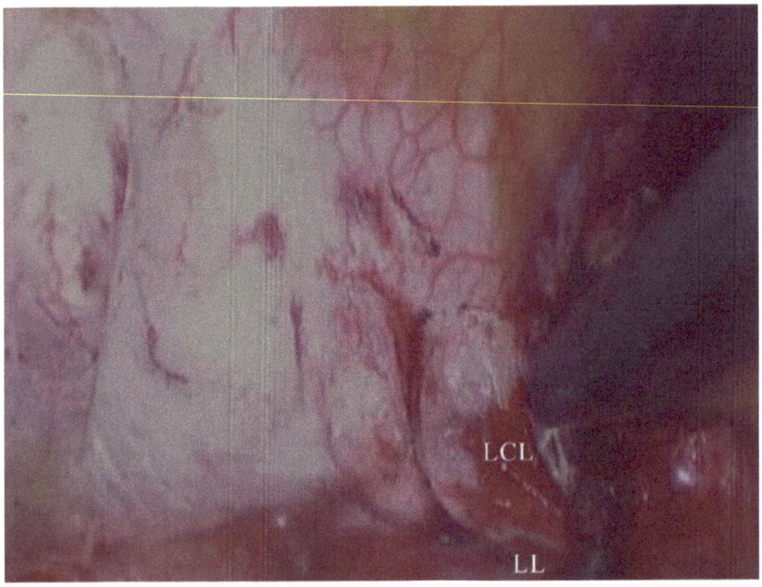

Fig. 6.17 The LL of the liver is pressed downward, and the left coronary ligament (*LCL*) is divided with LPMOD

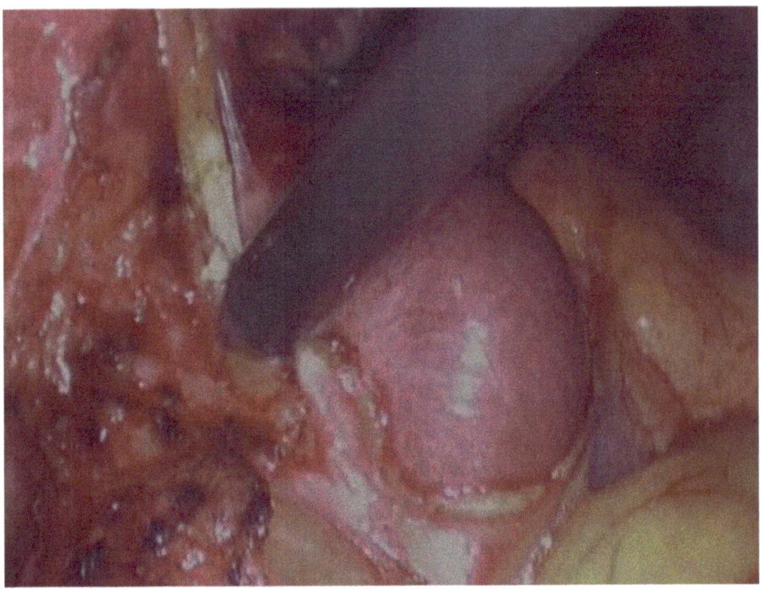

Fig. 6.18 The CL of the liver is fully visualized after the division of ligaments

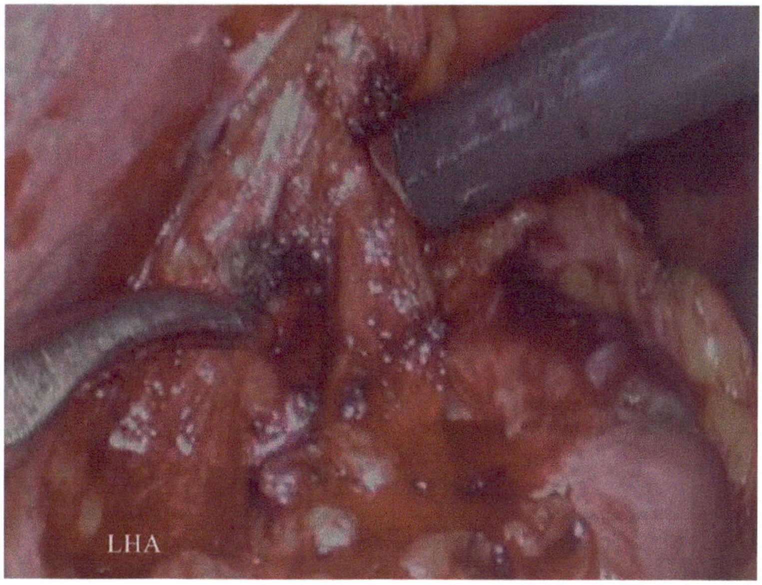

Fig. 6.19 The branch of LHA is dissected with LPMOD

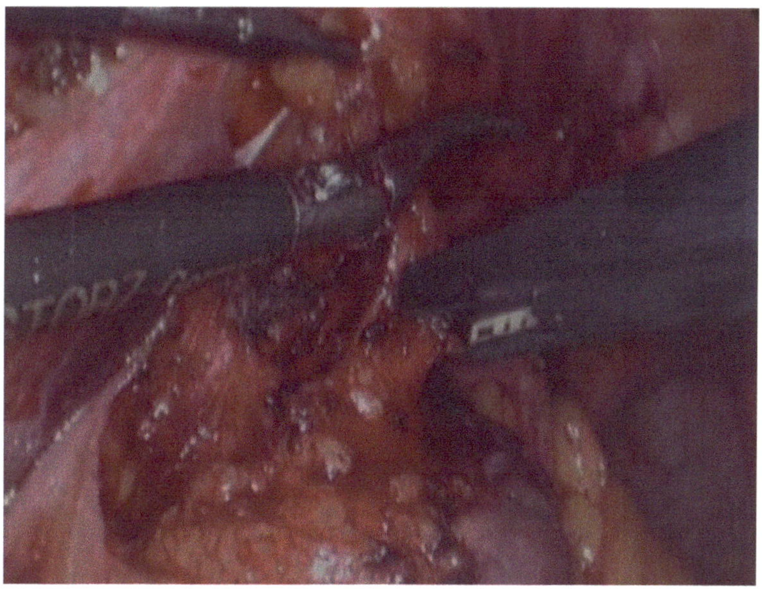

Fig. 6.20 The branch of LHA is clamped with an absorbable clip

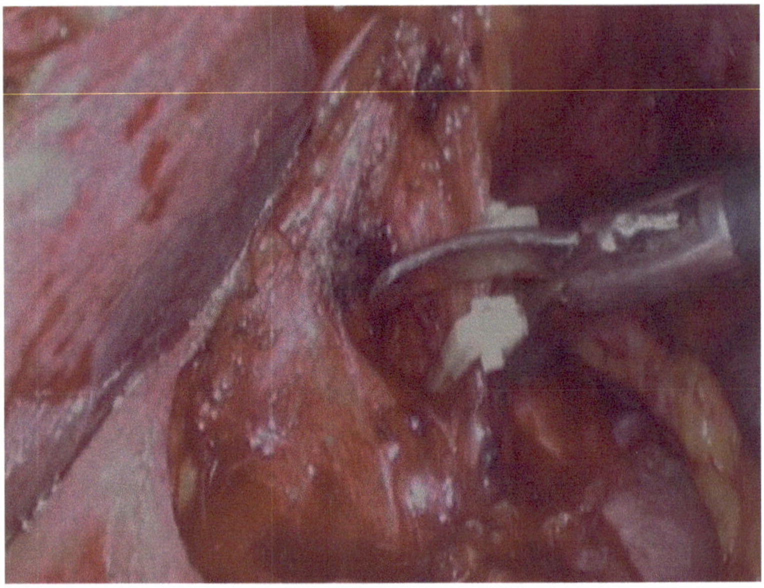

Fig. 6.21 The branch of LHA is divided

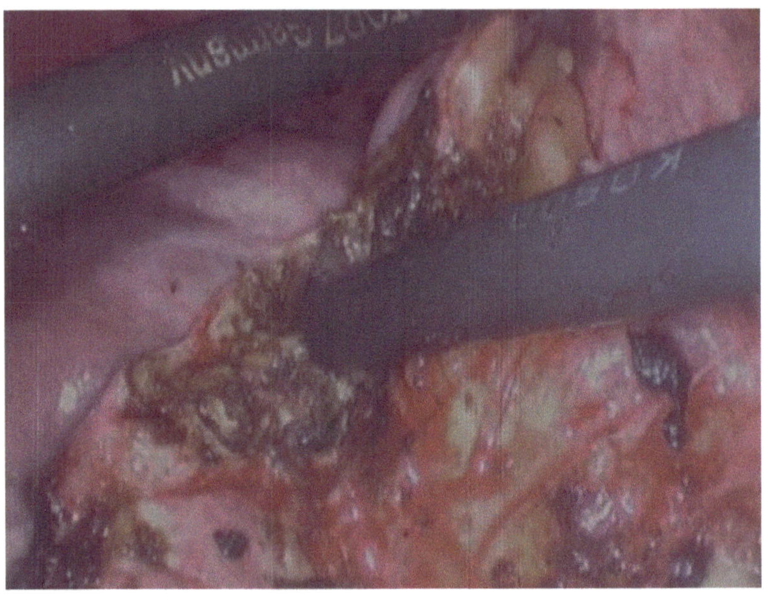

Fig. 6.22 Liver parenchyma is transected with LPMOD along the falciform ligament

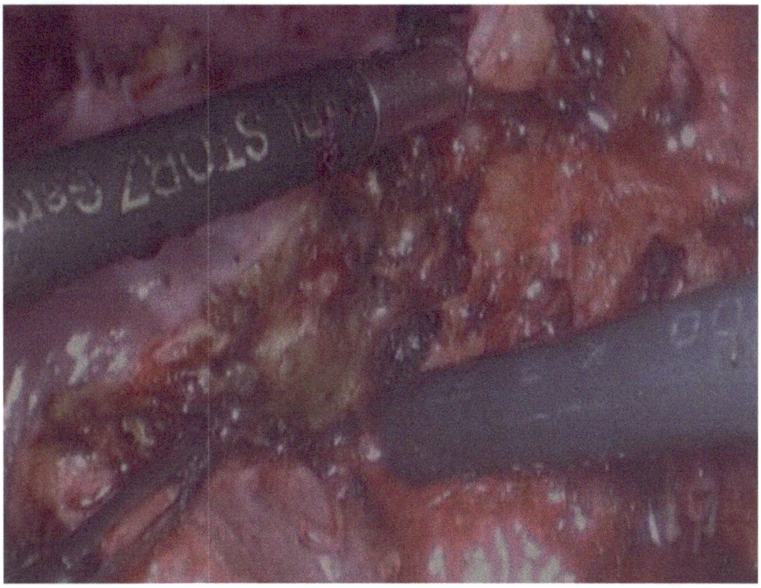

Fig. 6.23 The branch of bile duct to the left lateral segment is transected and the bile can be visualized

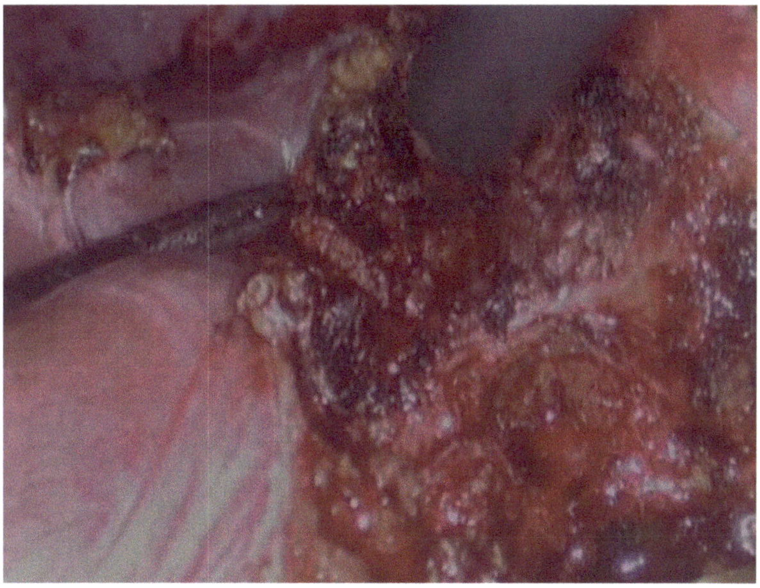

Fig. 6.24 A small artery is dissected with LPMOD in the transection of liver parenchyma

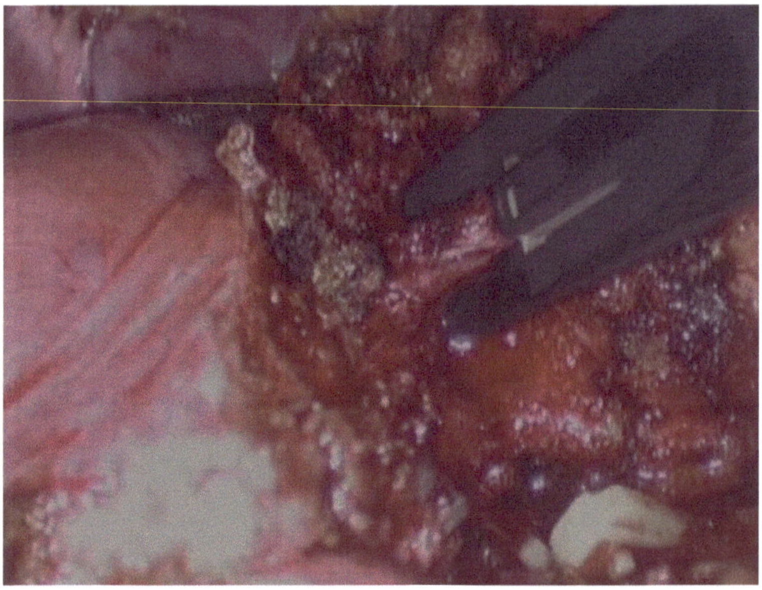

Fig. 6.25 The small artery is clamped with an absorbable clip

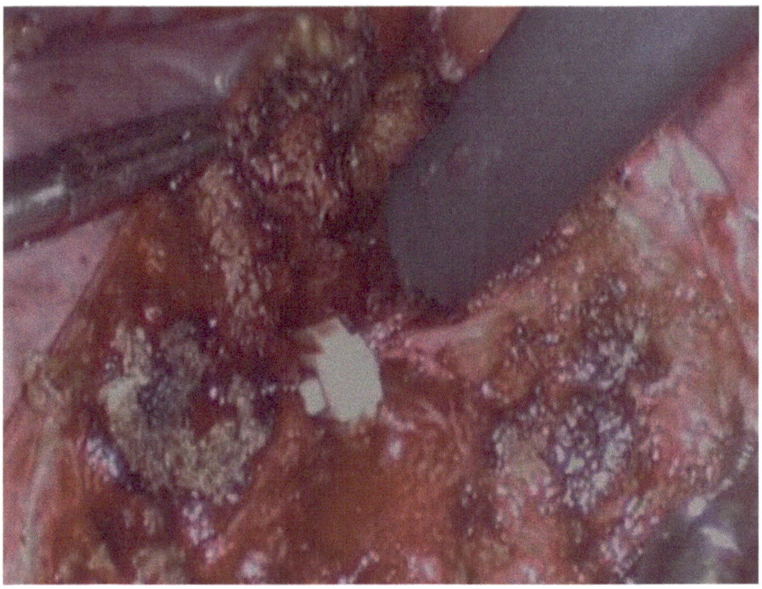

Fig. 6.26 The small artery is transected with LPMOD

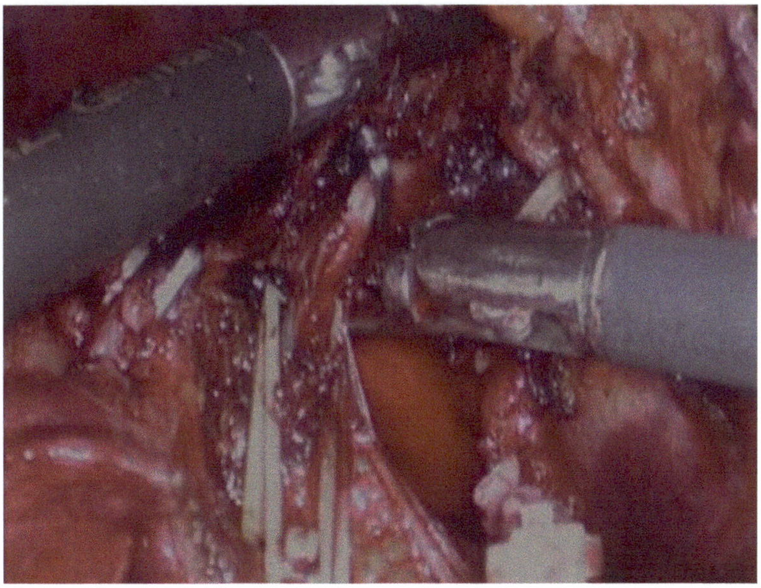

Fig. 6.27 The branch of left portal vein to the left lateral segment (LLS) is visualized in the transection of liver parenchyma and is dissected with a curved dissecting forceps

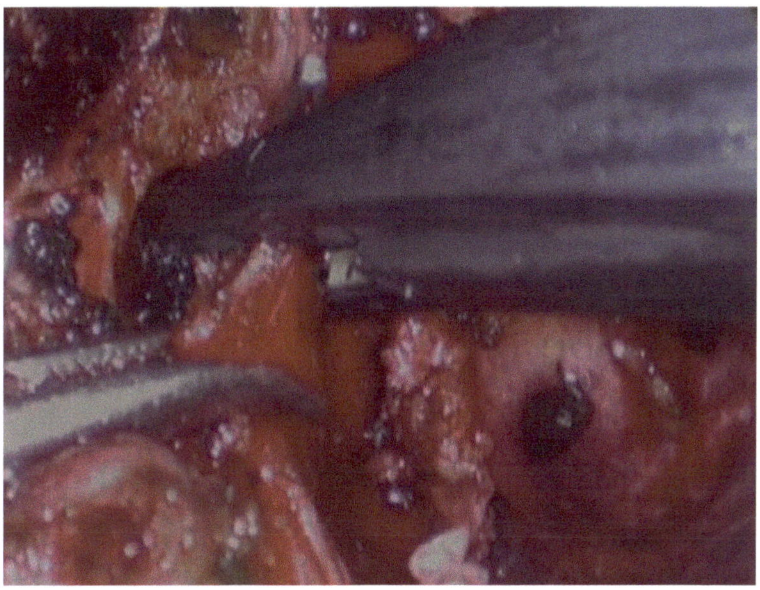

Fig. 6.28 The branch of left portal vein is clamped with an absorbable clip

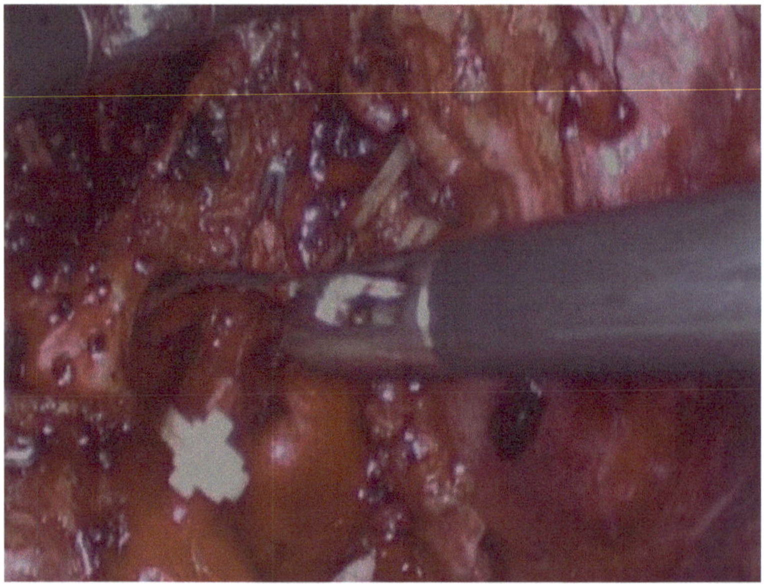

Fig. 6.29 The branch of left portal vein is divided

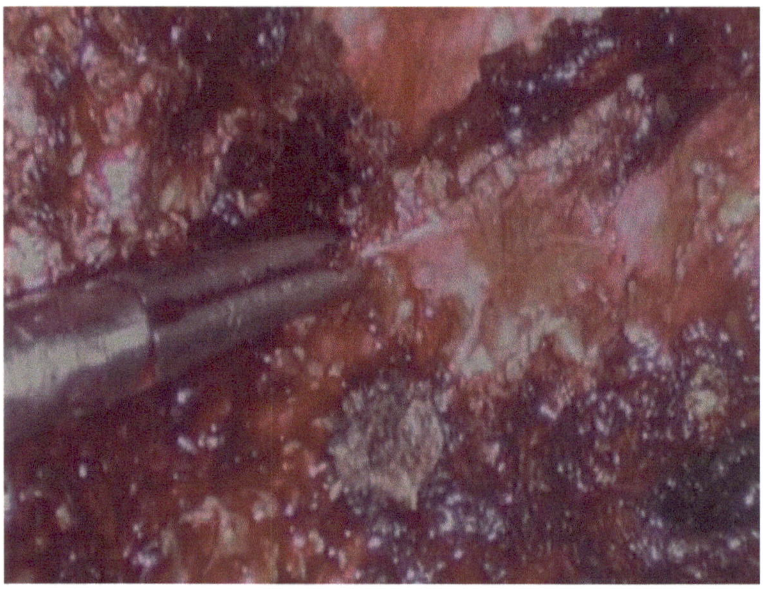

Fig. 6.30 A small vessel is visualized in the transection of liver parenchyma

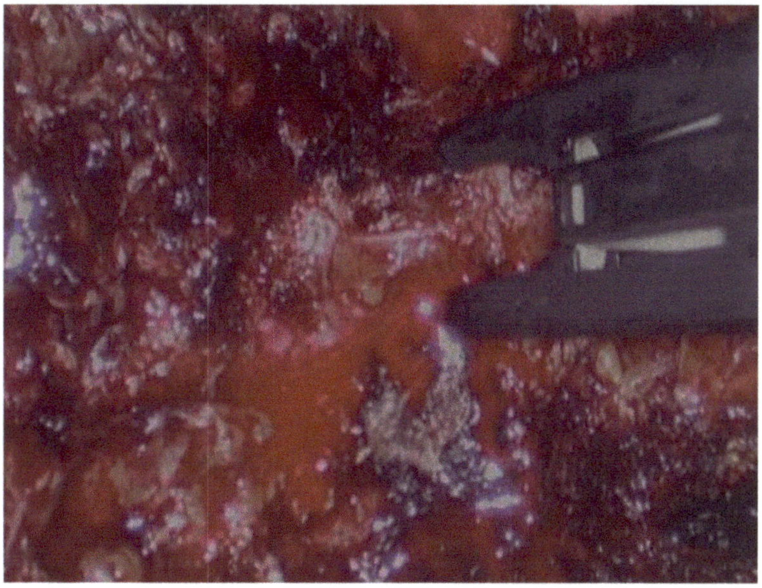

Fig. 6.31 The small vessel is clamped with an absorbable clip

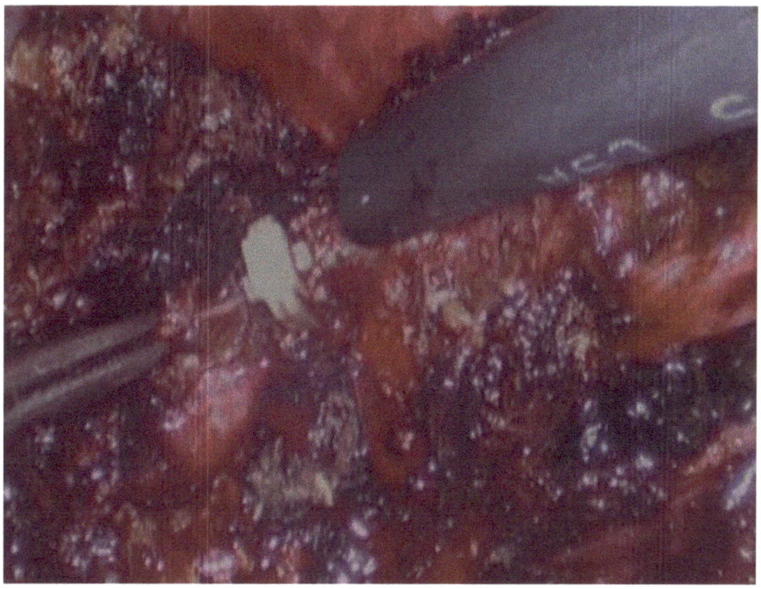

Fig. 6.32 The small vessel is divided with LPMOD

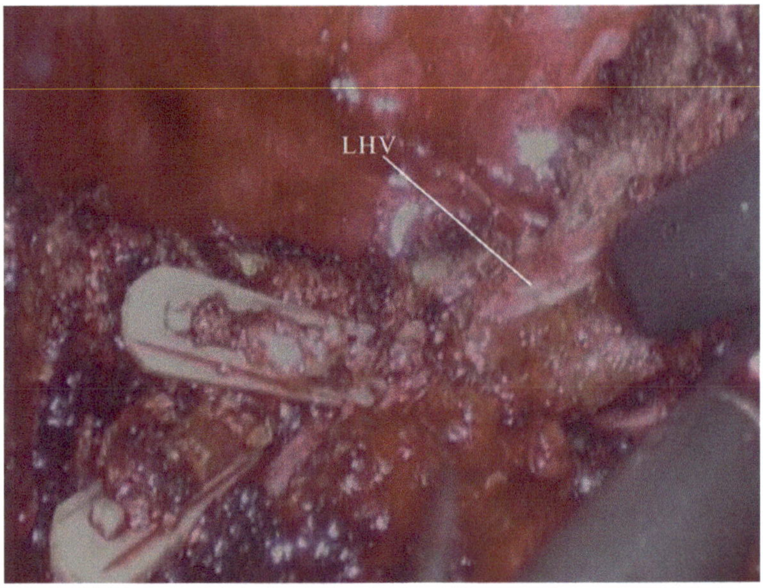

Fig. 6.33 The LHV is dissected with LPMOD

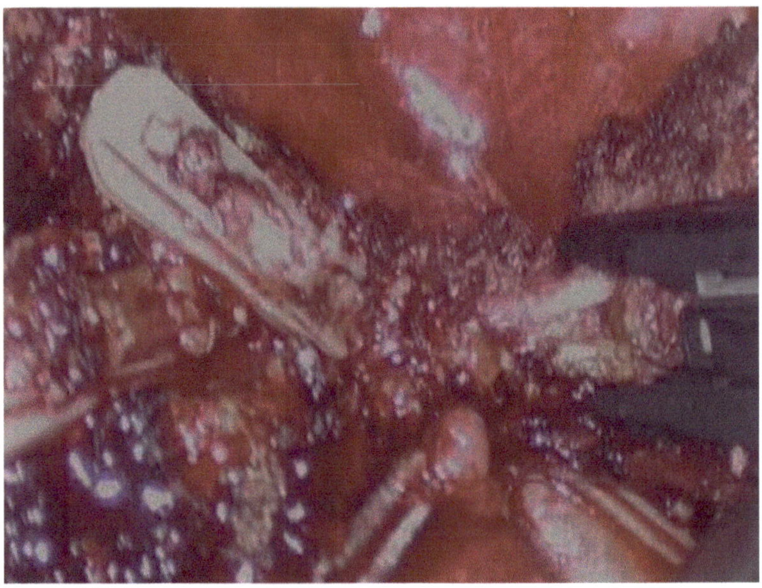

Fig. 6.34 The LHV is clamped with an absorbable clip

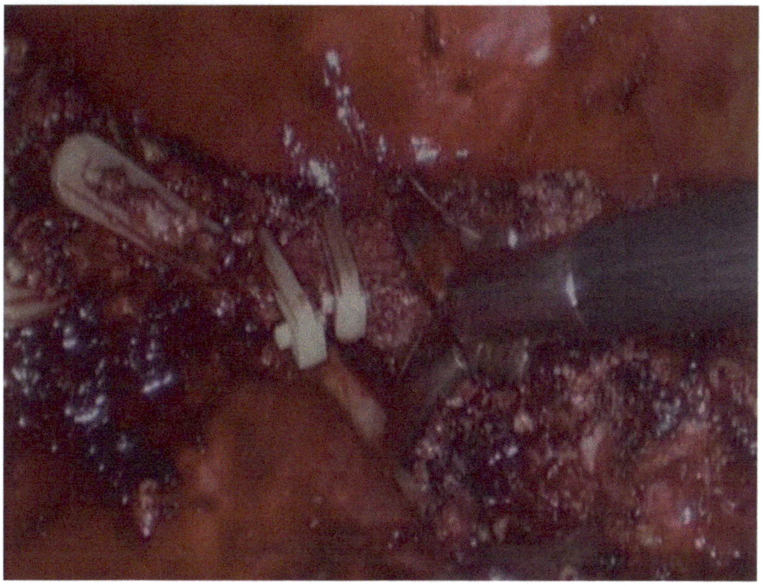

Fig. 6.35 The LHV is divided

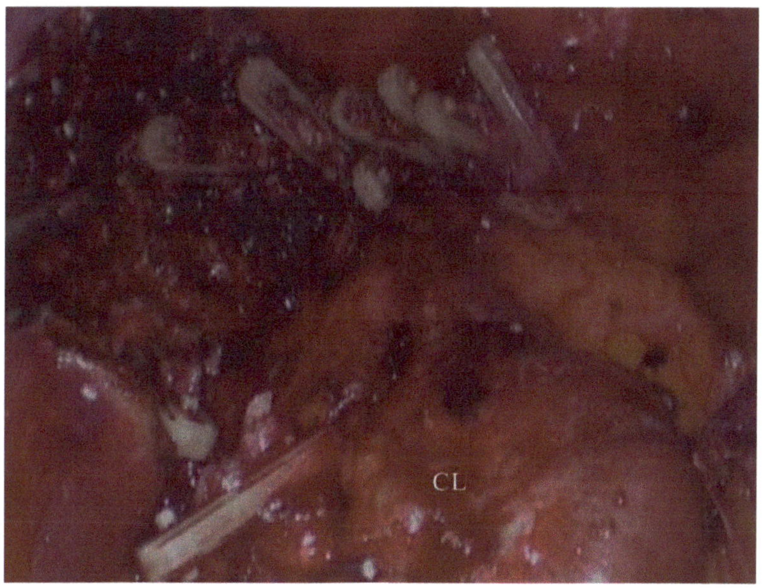

Fig. 6.36 After the left lateral segment was removed, the CL of the liver is visualized clearly

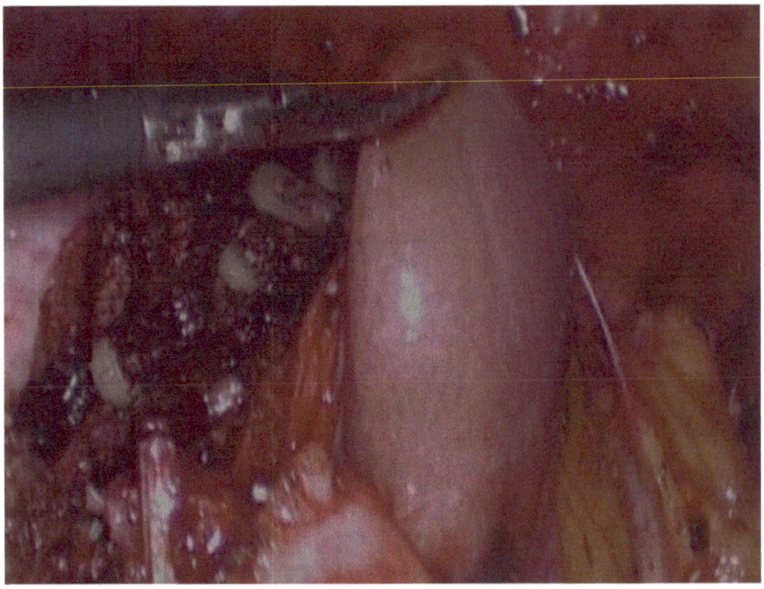

Fig. 6.37 The CL is lifted with a curved dissecting forceps

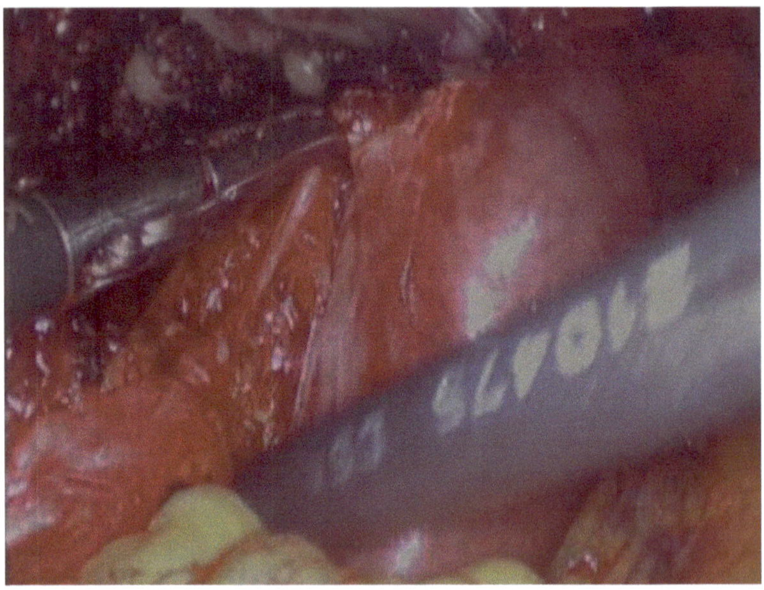

Fig. 6.38 The branch of hepatic artery is dissected with LPMOD

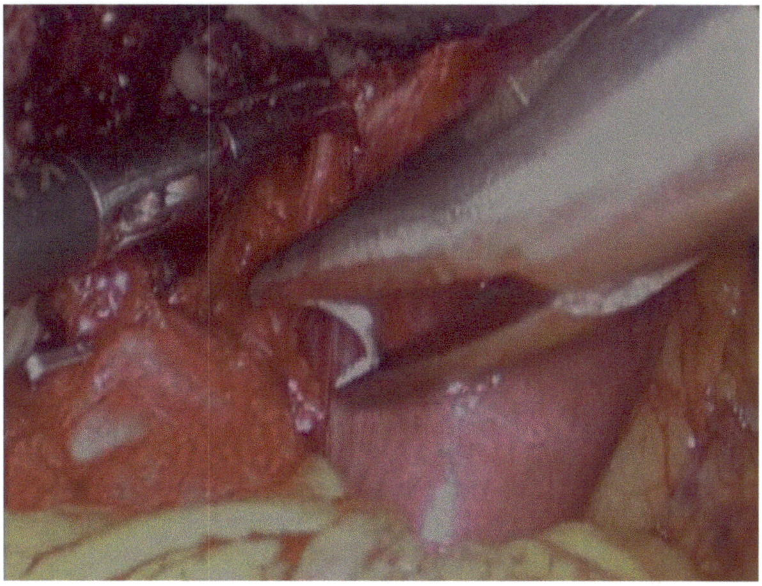

Fig. 6.39 The branch of hepatic artery is clamped with a titanic clip

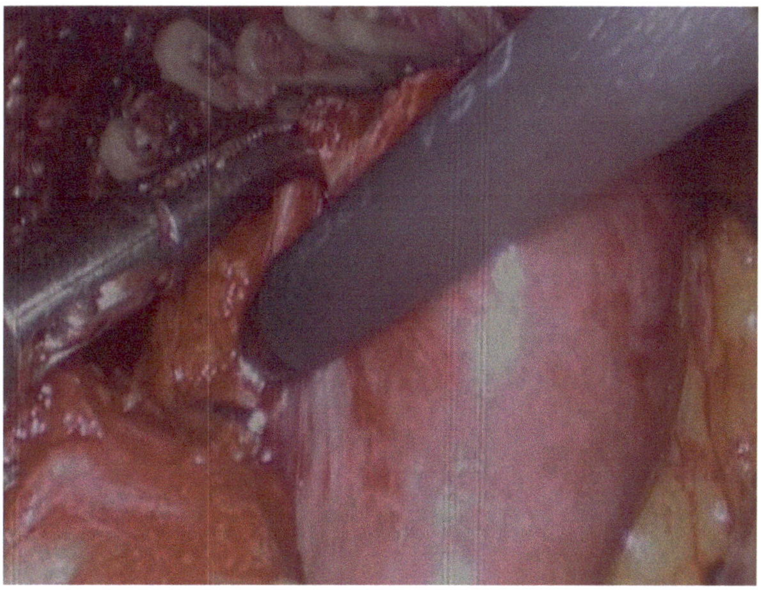

Fig. 6.40 The branch of hepatic artery is divided with LPMOD

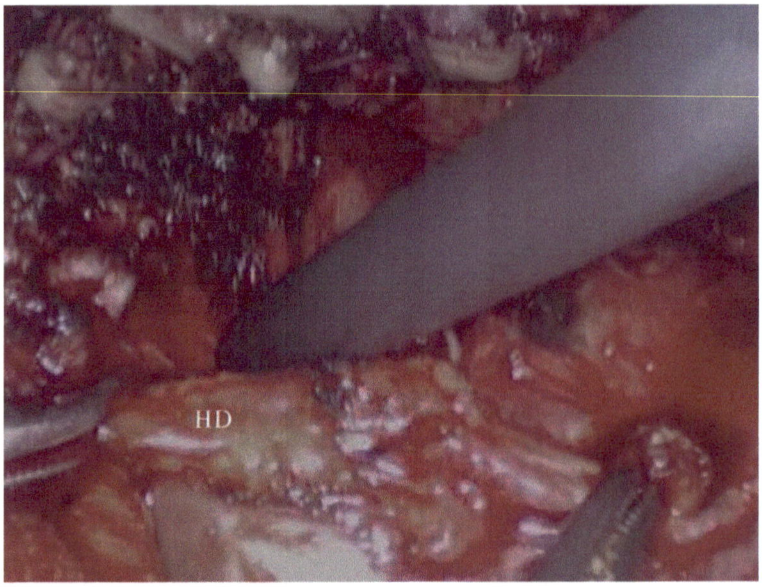

Fig. 6.41 An HD is dissected with LPMOD

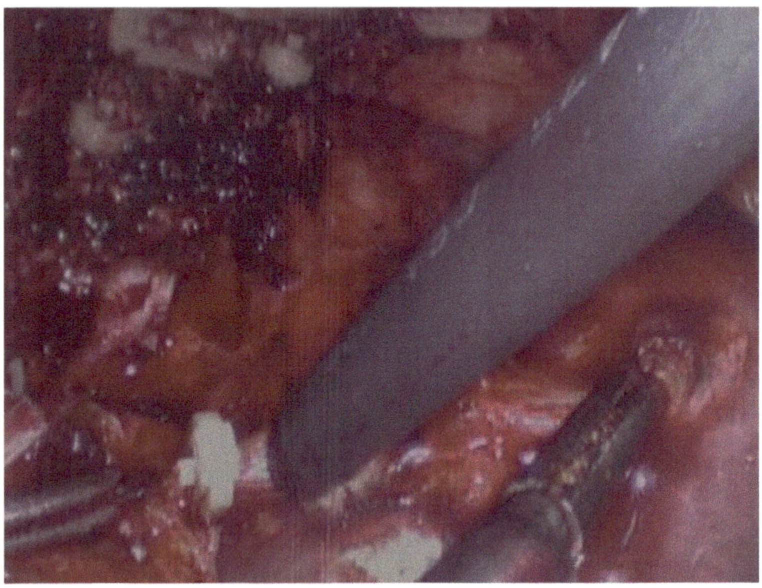

Fig. 6.42 After being clamped with an absorbable clip, the HD is divided with LPMOD

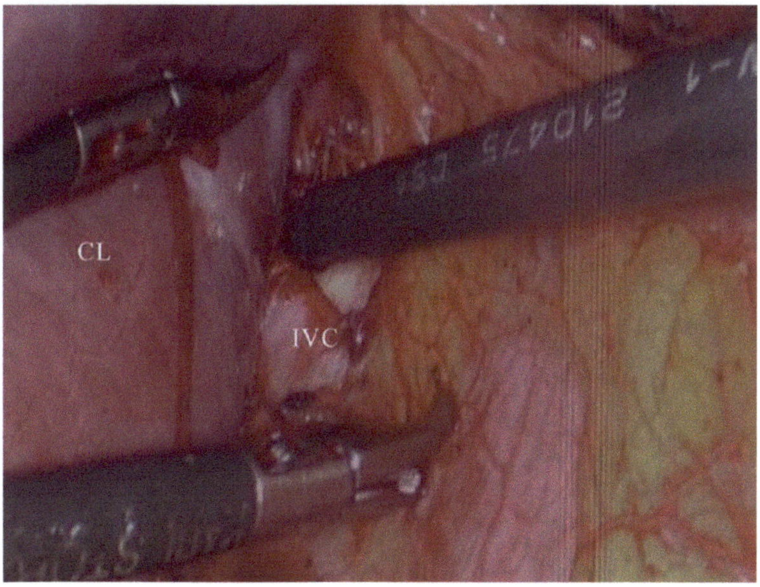

Fig. 6.43 The left wall of the IVC is visualized in the dissection

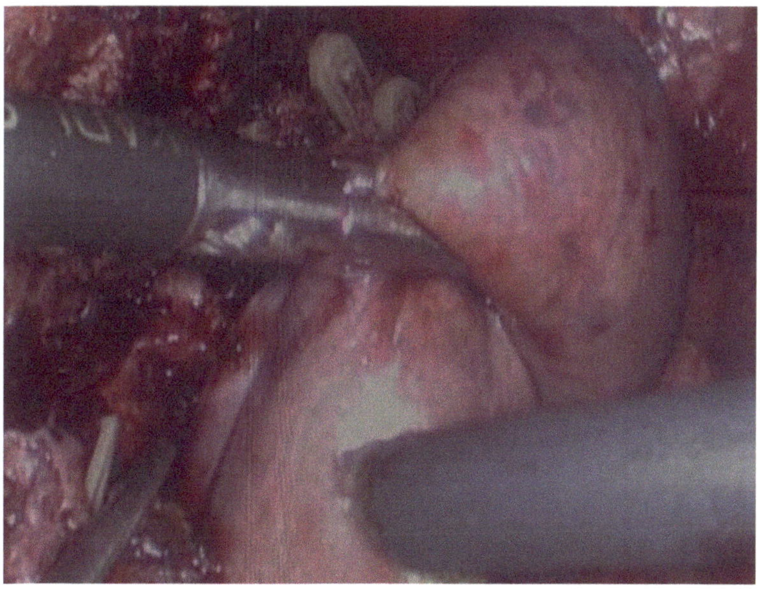

Fig. 6.44 The caudate lobe is transected with LPMOD

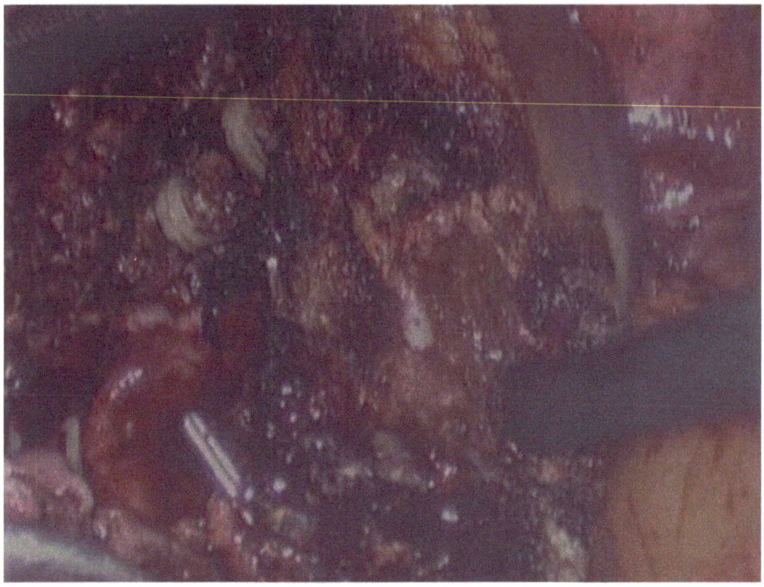

Fig. 6.45 A branch of the portal vein is visualized in the transection of liver parenchyma

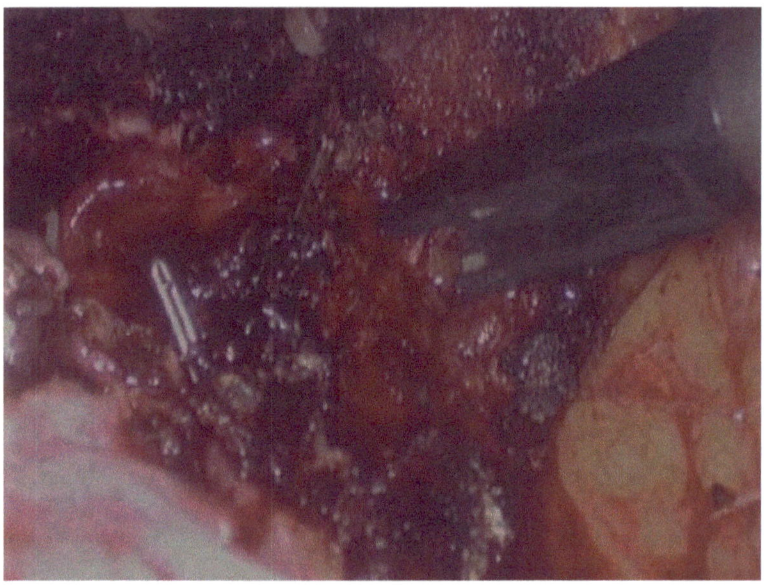

Fig. 6.46 The branch of the portal vein is clamped with an absorbable clip

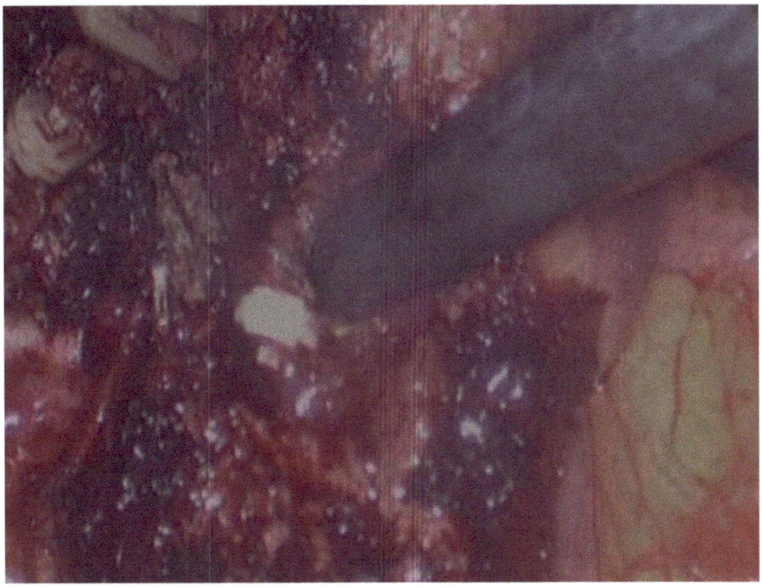

Fig. 6.47 The branch of the portal vein is divided with LPMOD

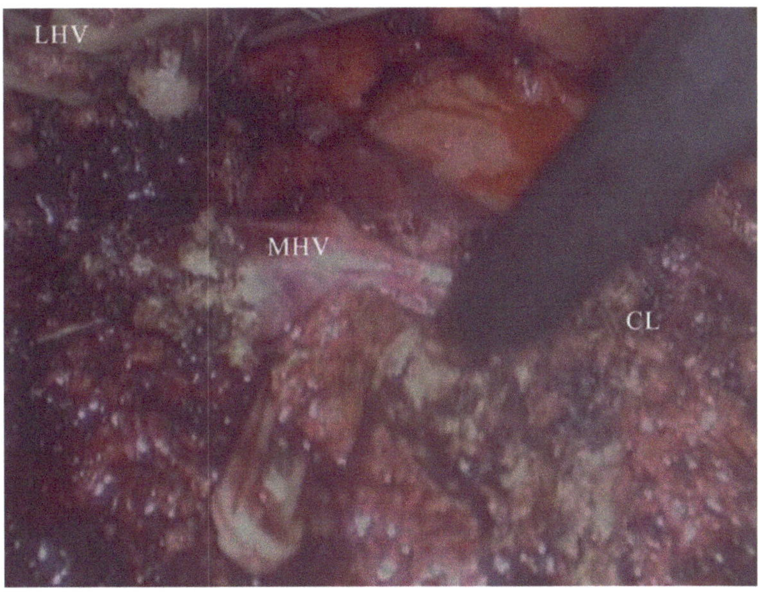

Fig. 6.48 A branch of MHV is dissected with LPMOD

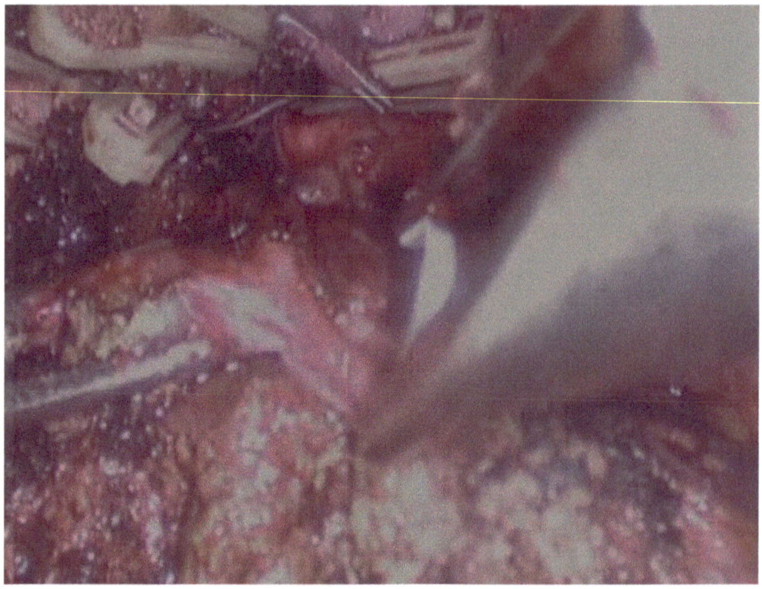

Fig. 6.49 The branch of MHV is clamped with a titanic clip

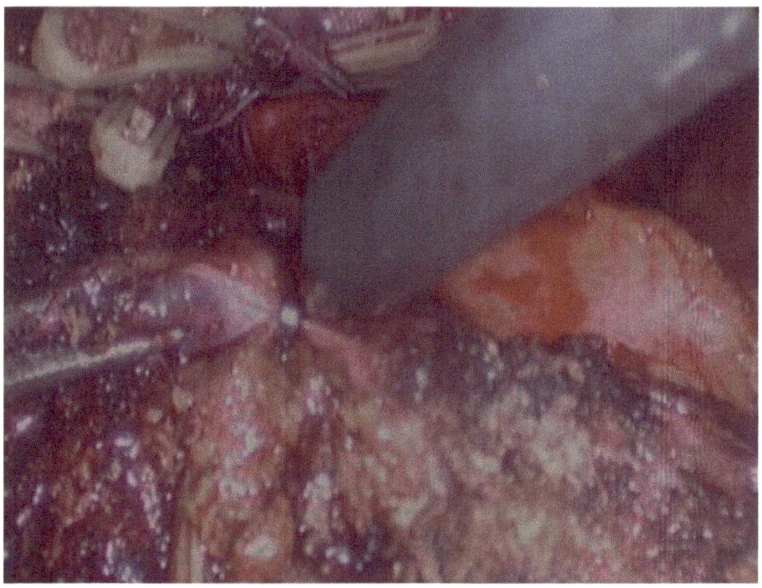

Fig. 6.50 The branch of MHV is divided

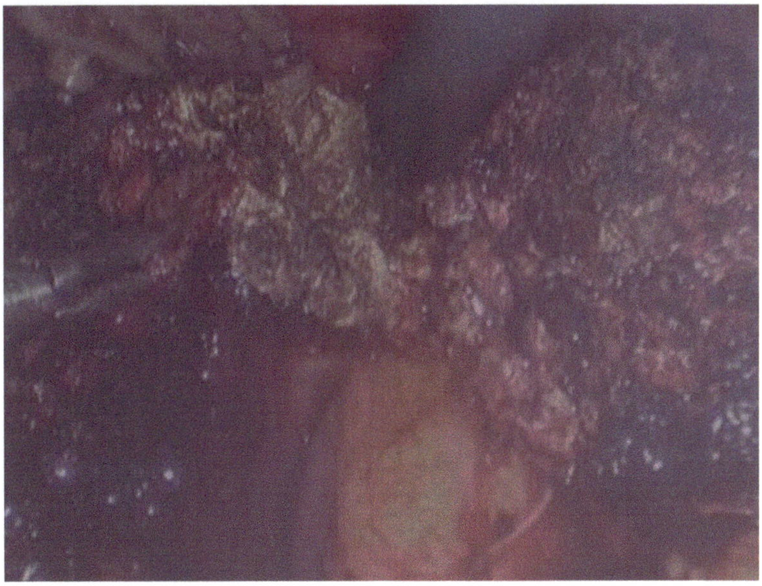

Fig. 6.51 The caudate lobe is transected with LPMOD

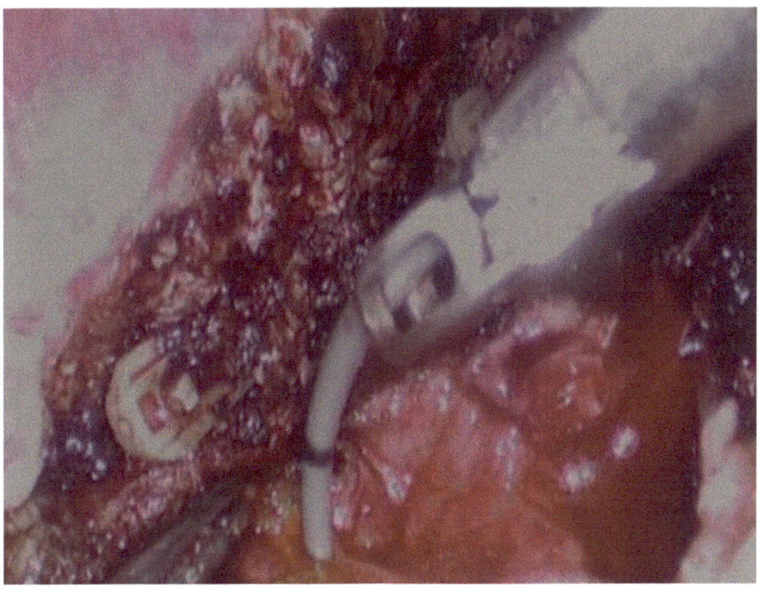

Fig. 6.52 Cholangiography is performed through the stump of the left hepatic duct (LHD) to rule out residual stones

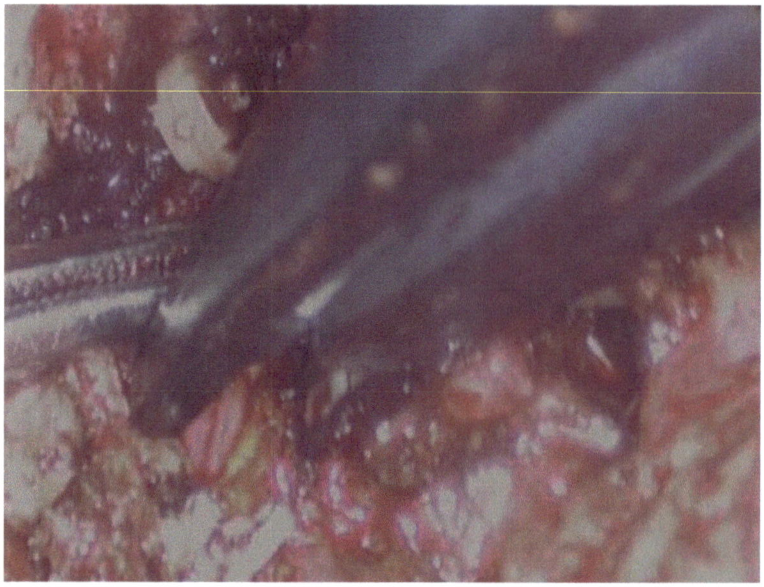

Fig. 6.53 The stump of the left hepatic duct is closed by applying an absorbable clip

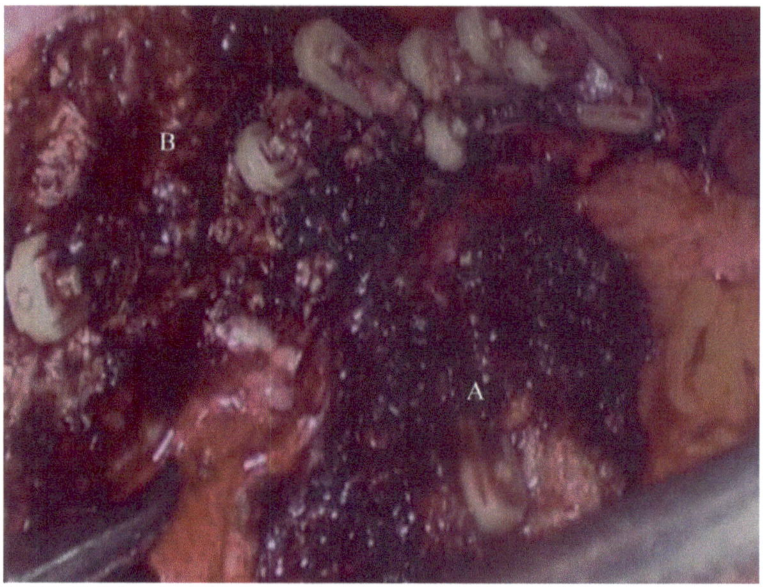

Fig. 6.54 The left caudate lobe and the left lateral segment are removed. (*A*) Raw surface of the caudate lobe; (*B*) Raw surface of the left lateral segment

6.5 Laparoscopic Combined Resection of Caudate Lobe: Laparoscopic Left Hemihepatectomy and Resection of Caudate Lobe

See Figs. 6.55, 6.56, 6.57, 6.58, 6.59, 6.60, 6.61, 6.62, 6.63, 6.64, 6.65, 6.66, 6.67, 6.68, 6.69, 6.70, 6.71, 6.72, 6.73, 6.74, 6.75, 6.76, 6.77, 6.78, 6.79, 6.80, 6.81, 6.82, 6.83, 6.84, 6.85, 6.86, 6.87, 6.88, 6.89, 6.90, 6.91, 6.92, 6.93, 6.94, and Video 6.3.

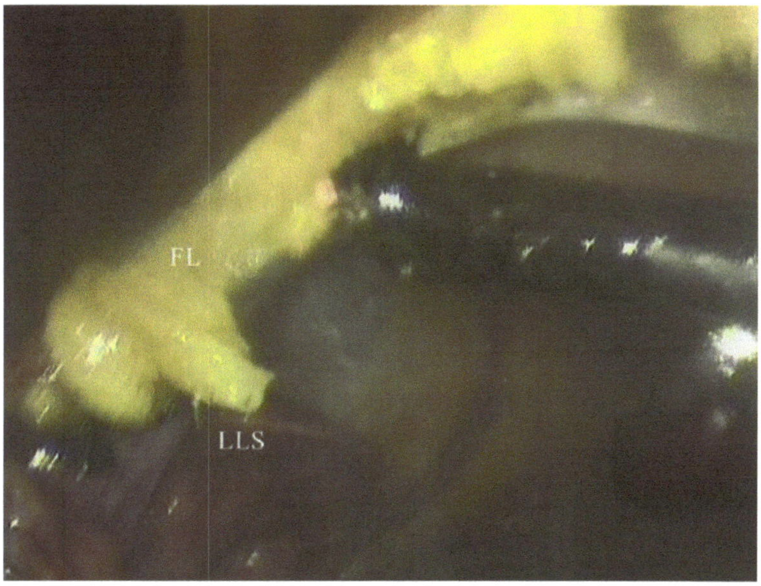

Fig. 6.55 The round ligament and FL are divided with LPMOD

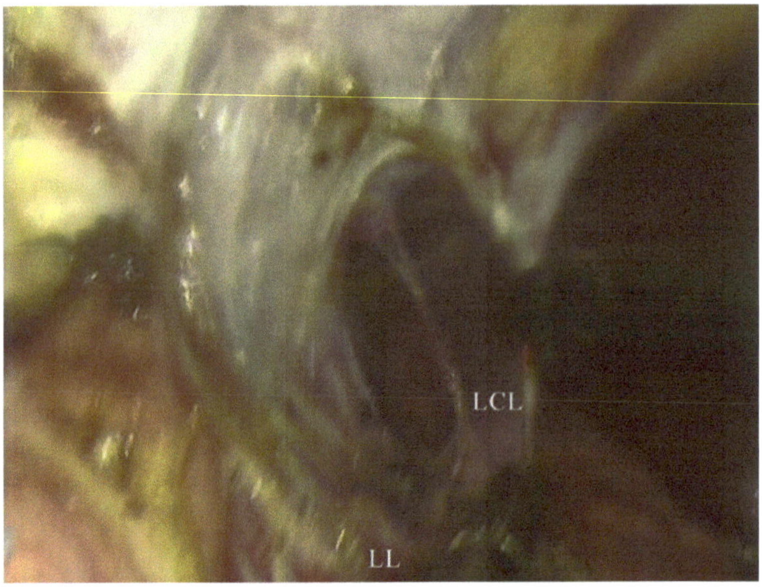

Fig. 6.56 The LCL is divided with LPMOD

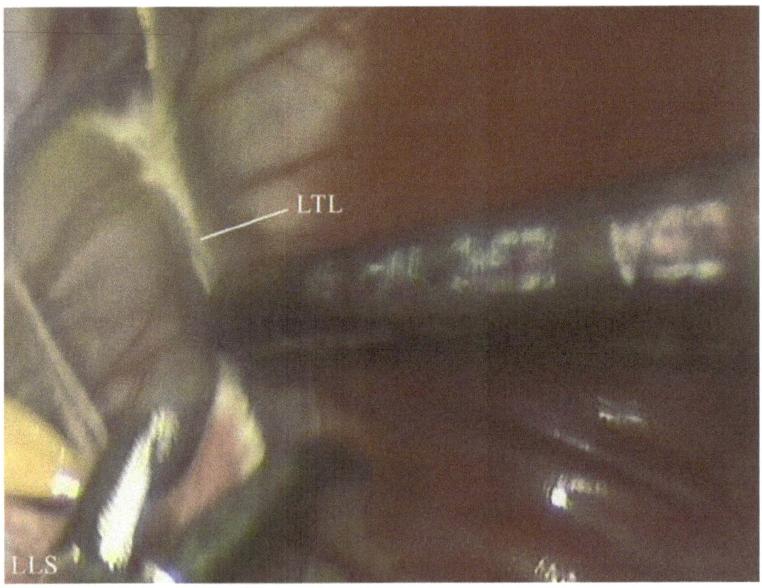

Fig. 6.57 The LTL is divided with LPMOD

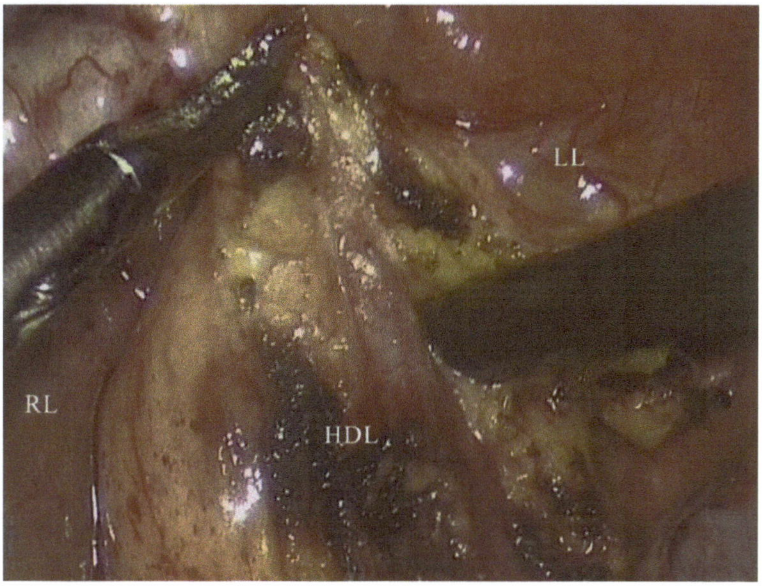

Fig. 6.58 The hepatoduodenal ligament (*HDL*) is dissected with LPMOD

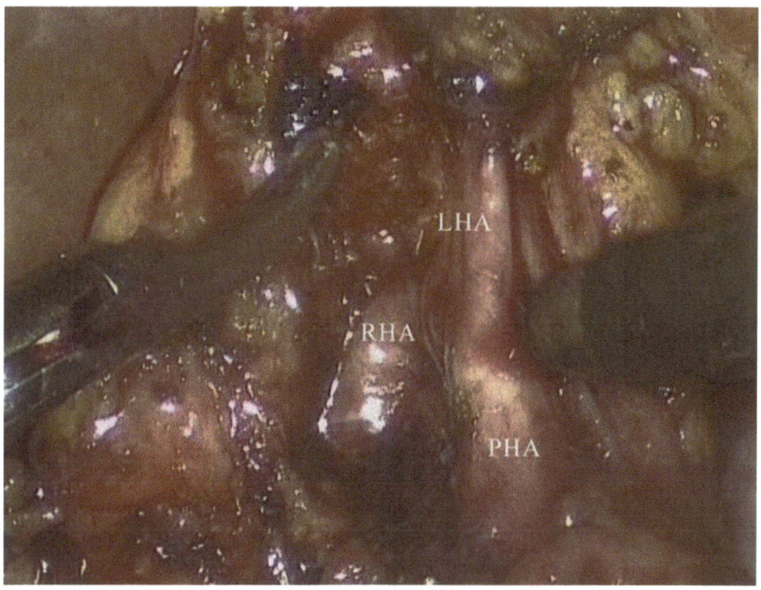

Fig. 6.59 The LHA is dissected with LPMOD

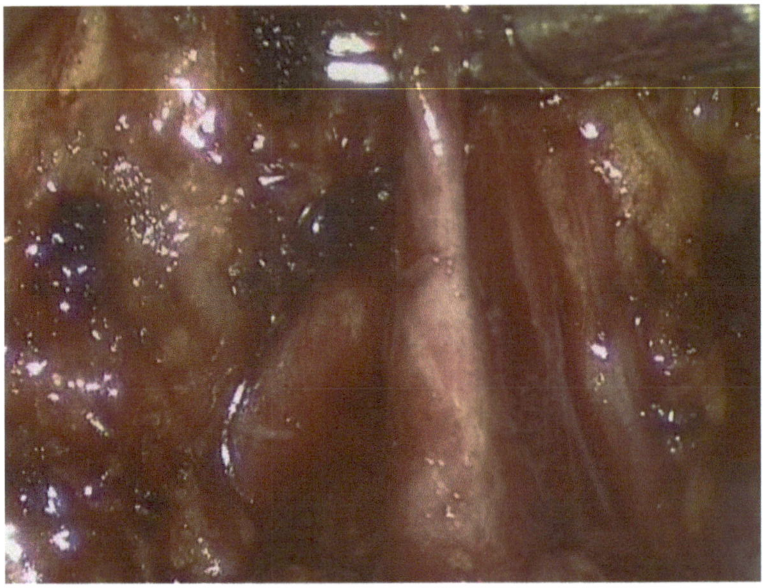

Fig. 6.60 The LHA is freed

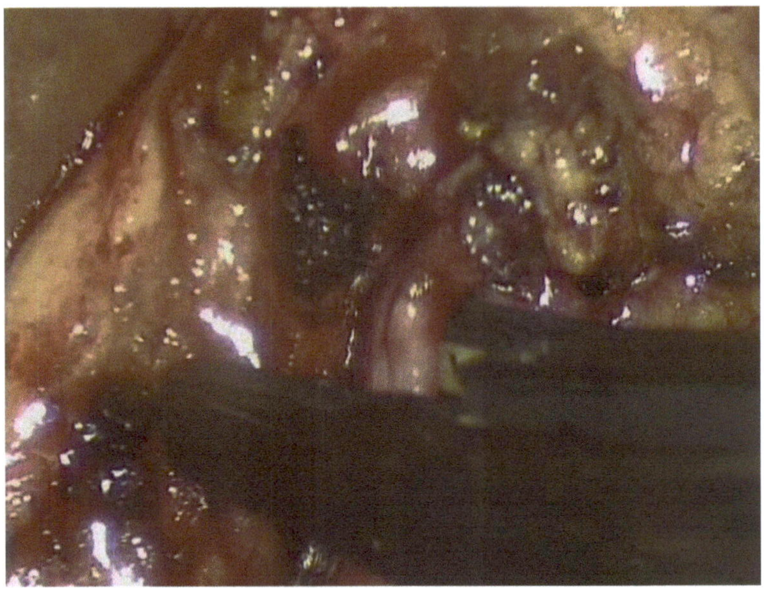

Fig. 6.61 The LHA is clamped with an absorbable clip

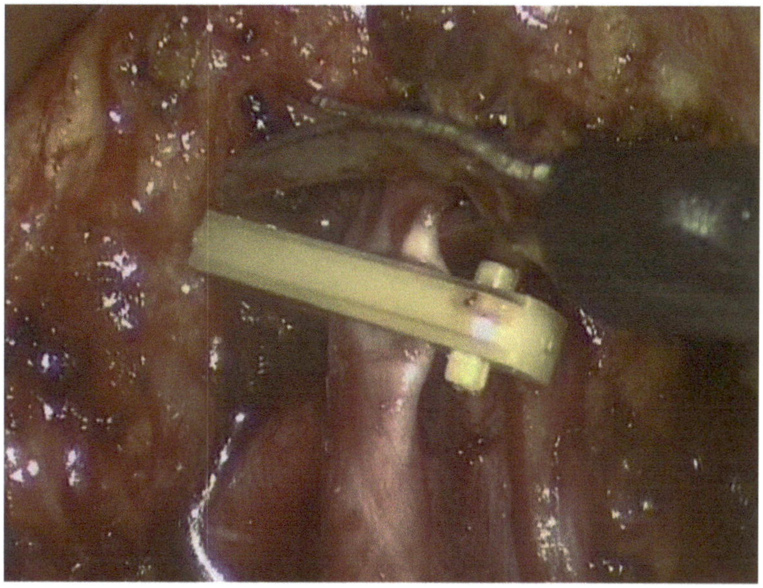

Fig. 6.62 The LHA is divided

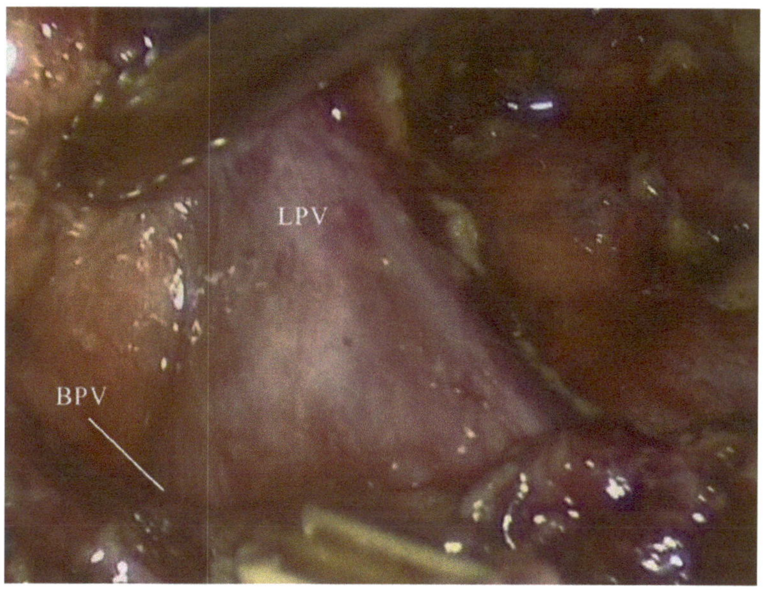

Fig. 6.63 The LPV is dissected and the BPV is visualized

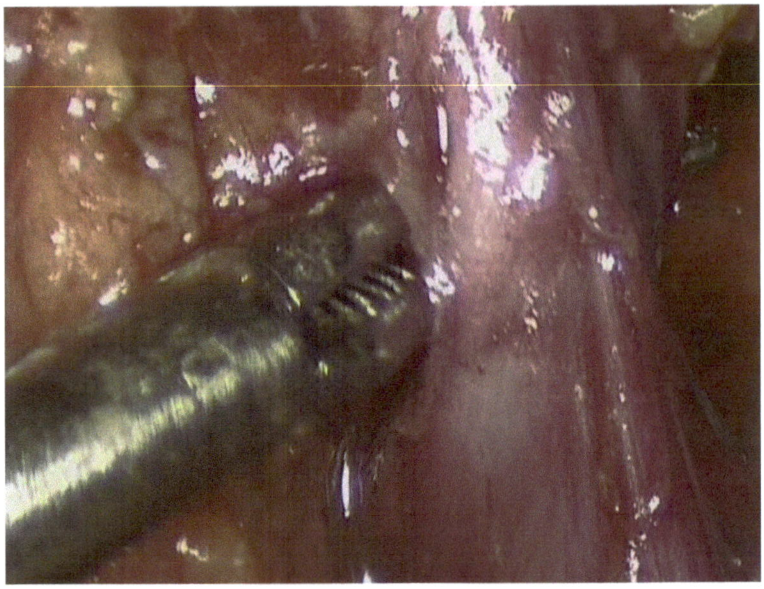

Fig. 6.64 The LPV is freed

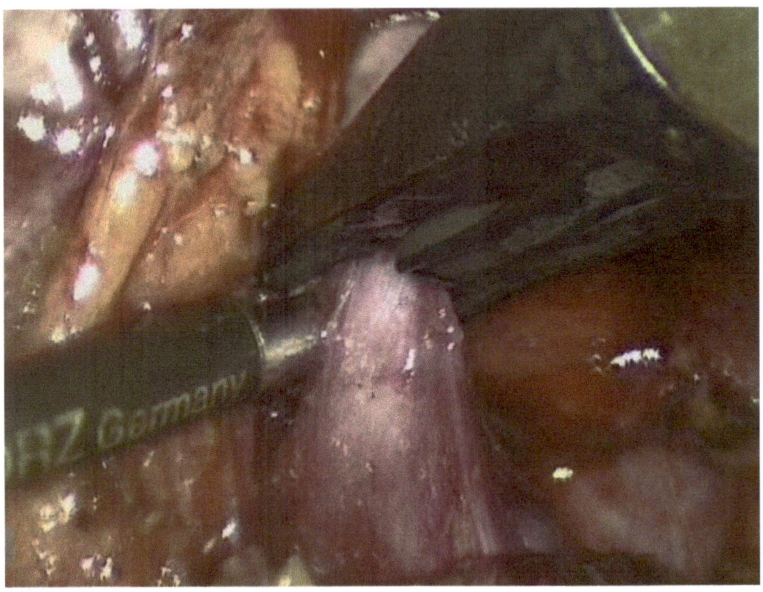

Fig. 6.65 The LPV is occluded by applying an absorbable clip

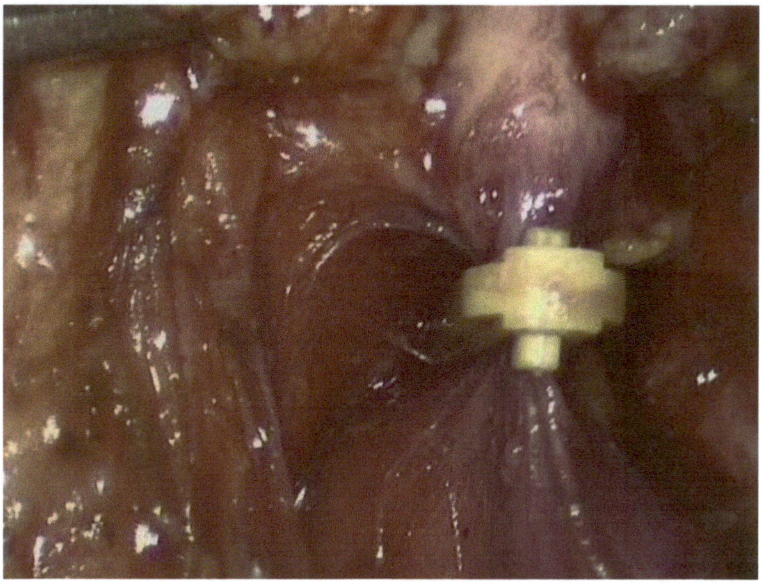

Fig. 6.66 The view of the LPV after being occluded

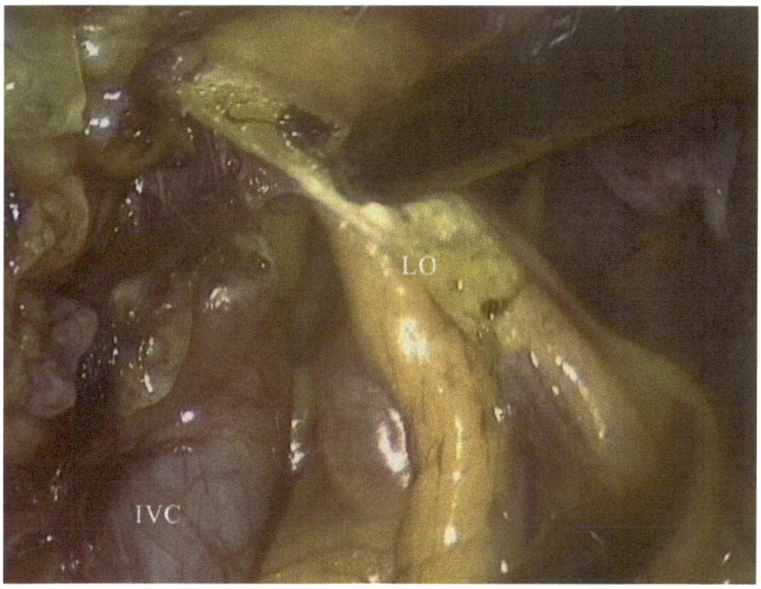

Fig. 6.67 The LO is divided with LPMOD

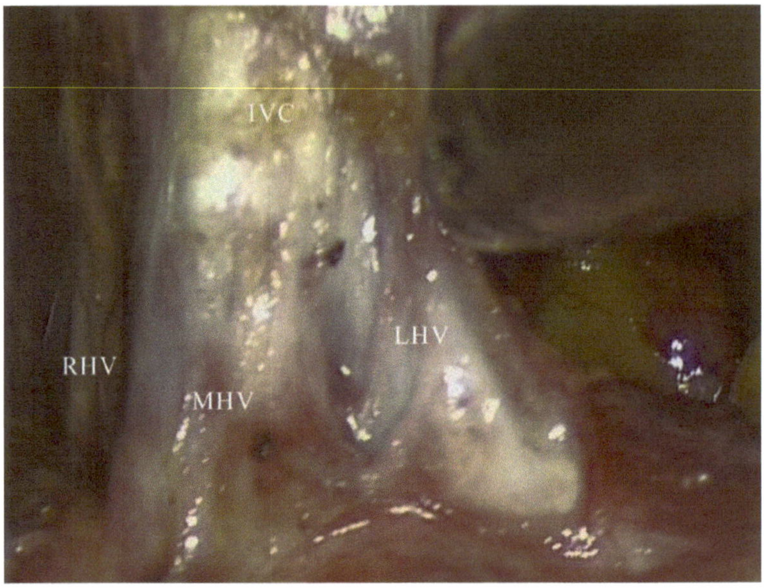

Fig. 6.68 The LHV is dissected with LPMOD

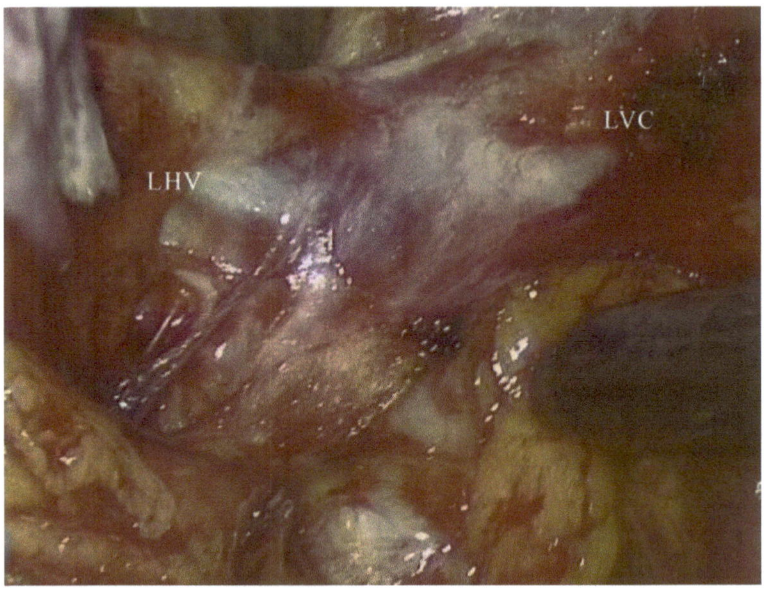

Fig. 6.69 The left lobe of the liver is mobilized to the right and the LHV is dissected with LPMOD

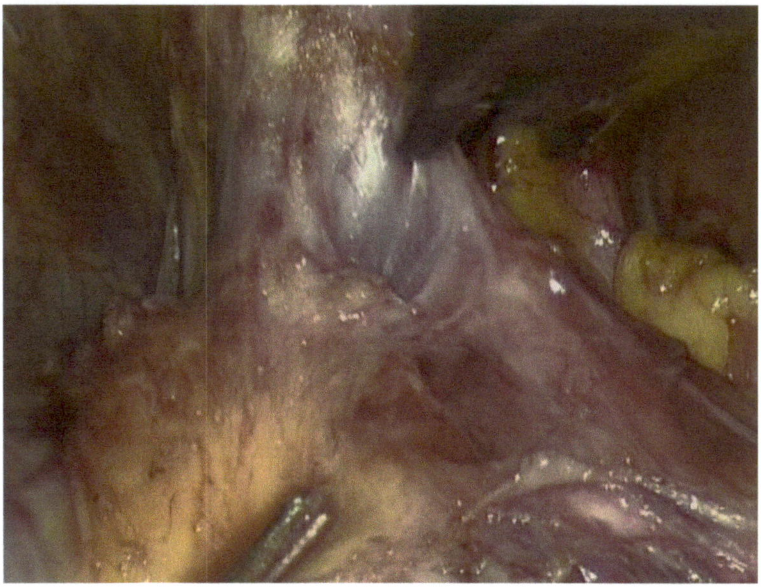

Fig. 6.70 The LHV is occluded by applying an absorbable clip on it

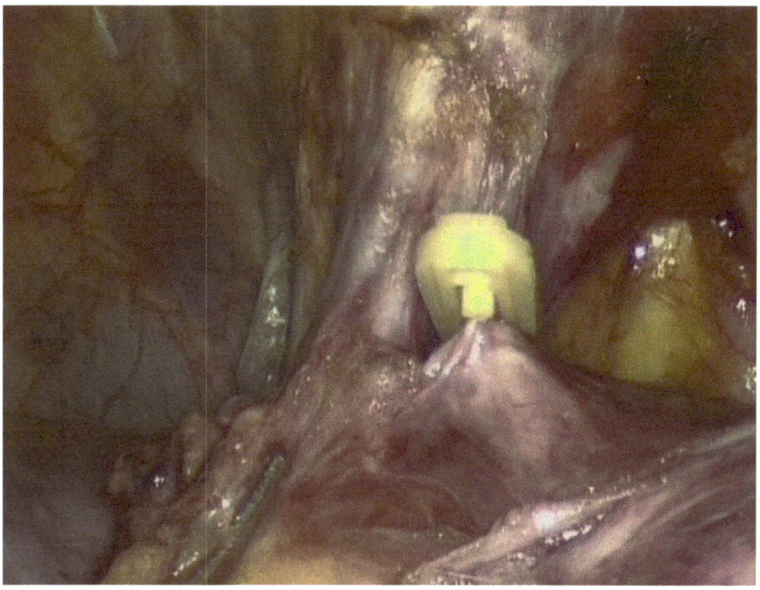

Fig. 6.71 The view of the LHV after being occluded

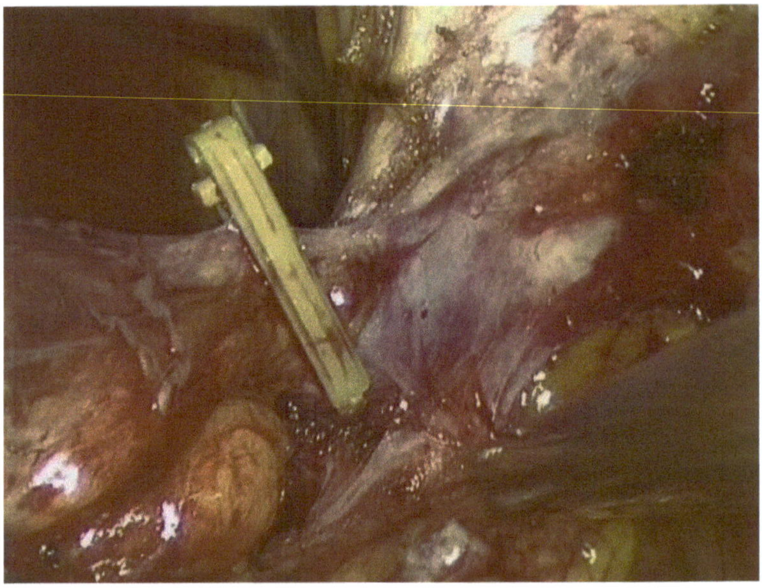

Fig. 6.72 The left lobe of the liver is mobilized to the right and the occlusion of LHV is viewed

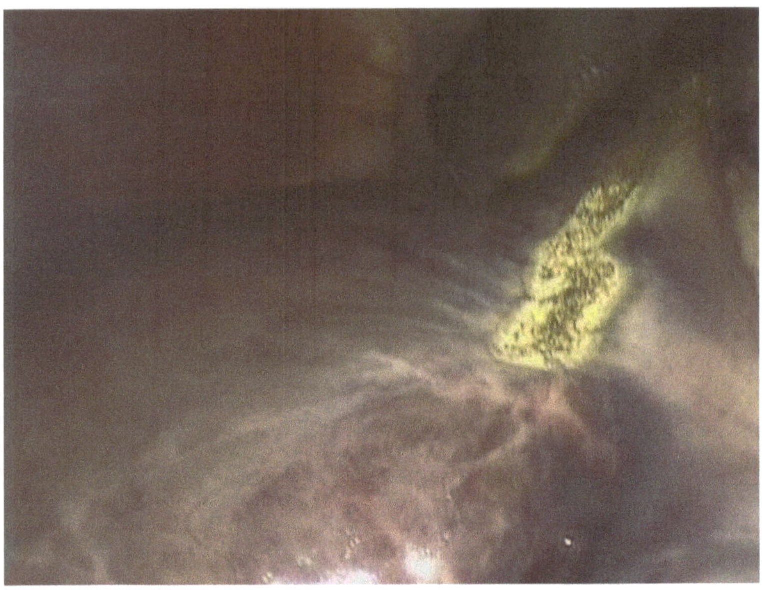

Fig. 6.73 A transection line is marked on the liver surface with LPMOD

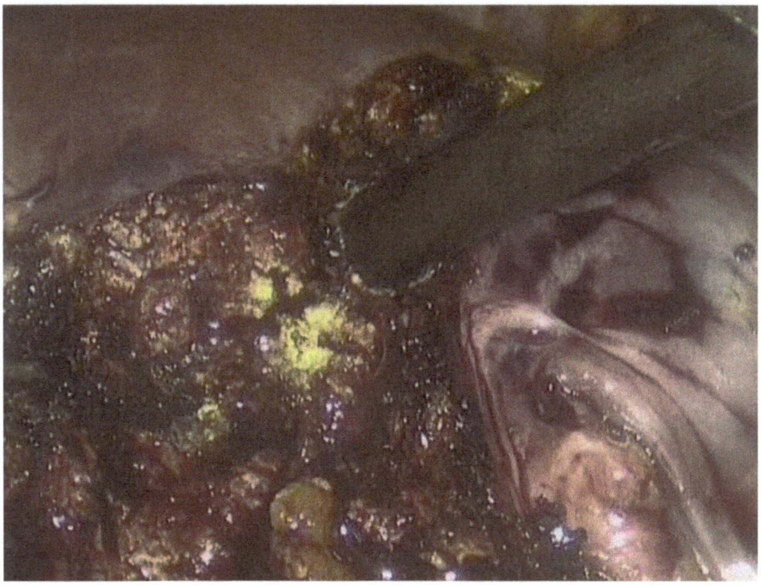

Fig. 6.74 Liver parenchyma is transected with LPMOD

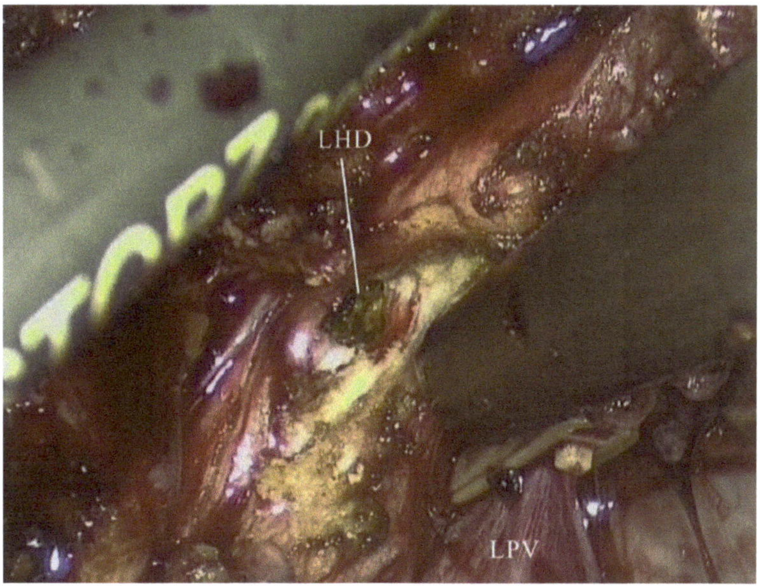

Fig. 6.75 The LHD is transected with LPMOD

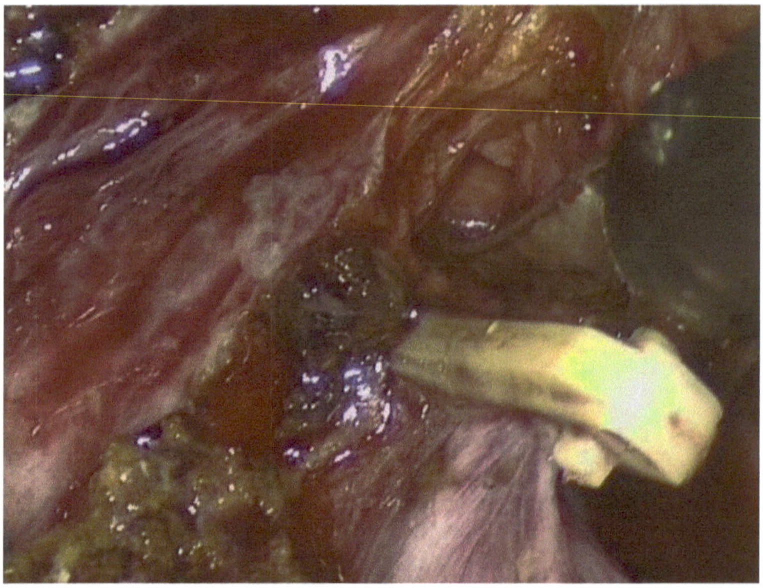

Fig. 6.76 The LPV which was occluded before liver transection is divided

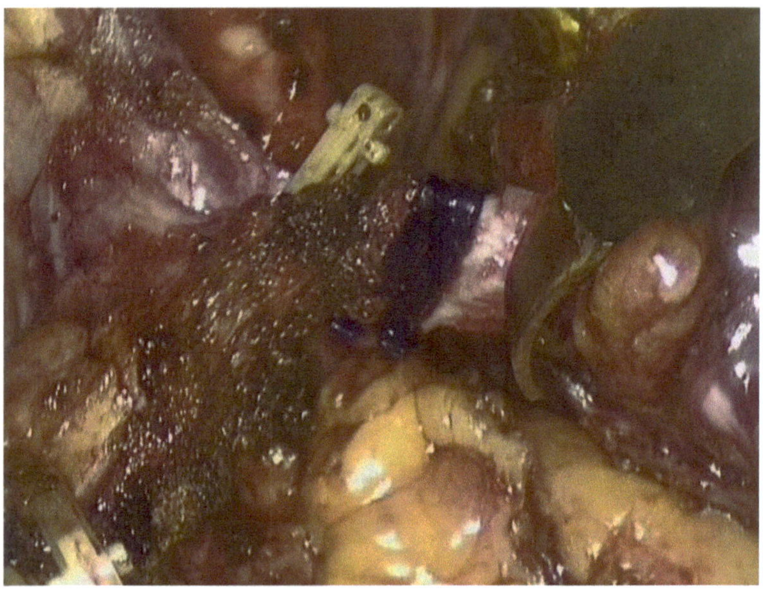

Fig. 6.77 The LHV which was occluded before the liver transection is divided, after being secured by applying two additional nonabsorbable polymer clips on it

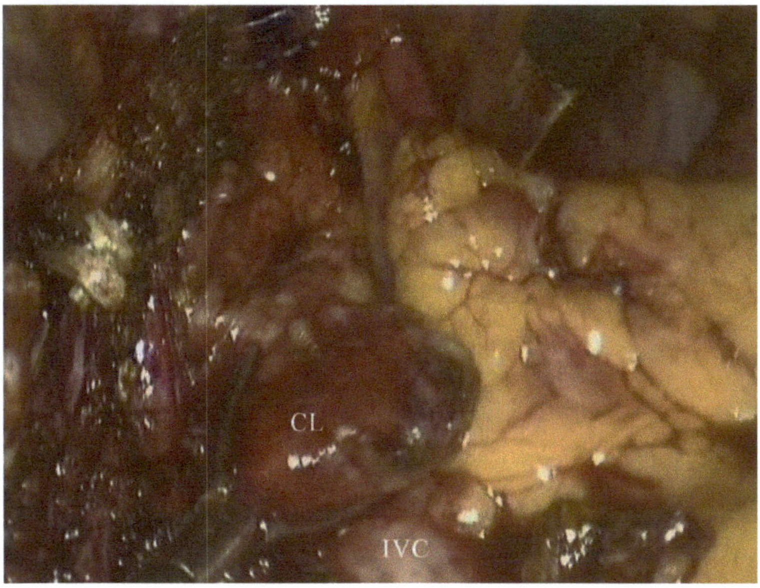

Fig. 6.78 The CL is visualized after the LL of the liver was removed

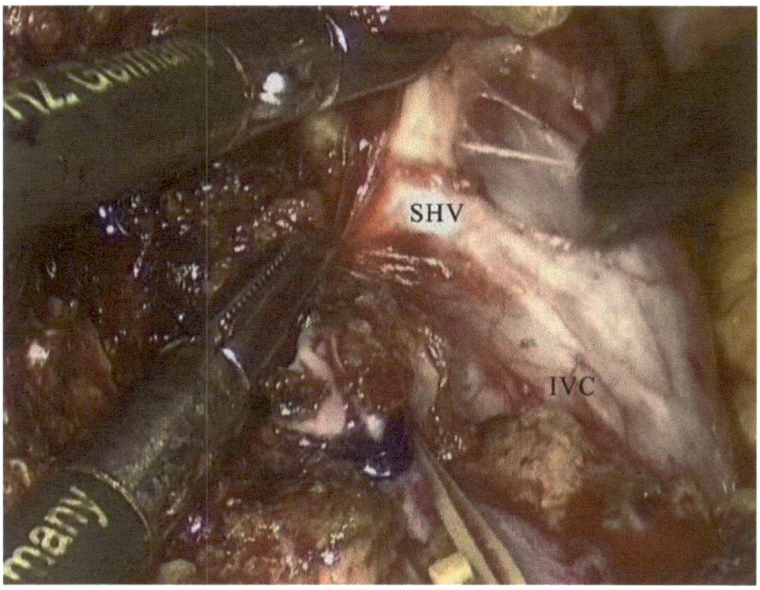

Fig. 6.79 The caudate lobe is elevated, and the SHV is visualized and is dissected with LPMOD

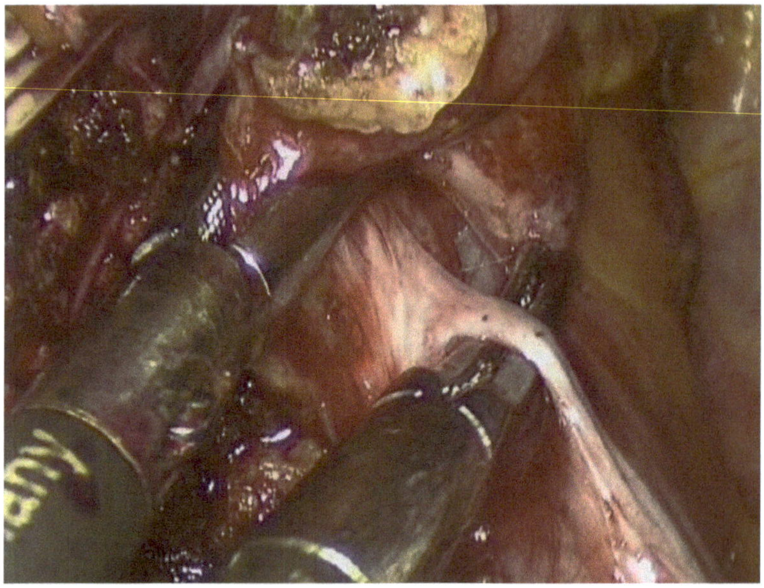

Fig. 6.80 The SHV is freed

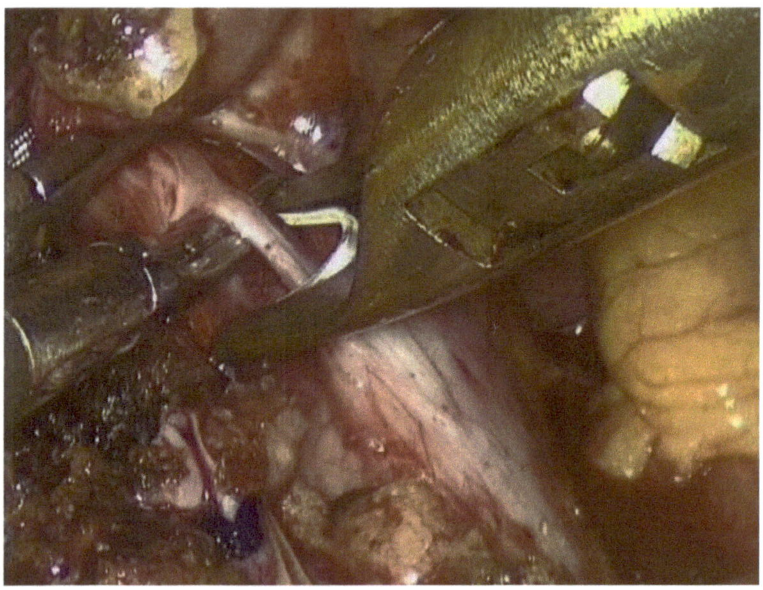

Fig. 6.81 The SHV is clamped with a titanic clip

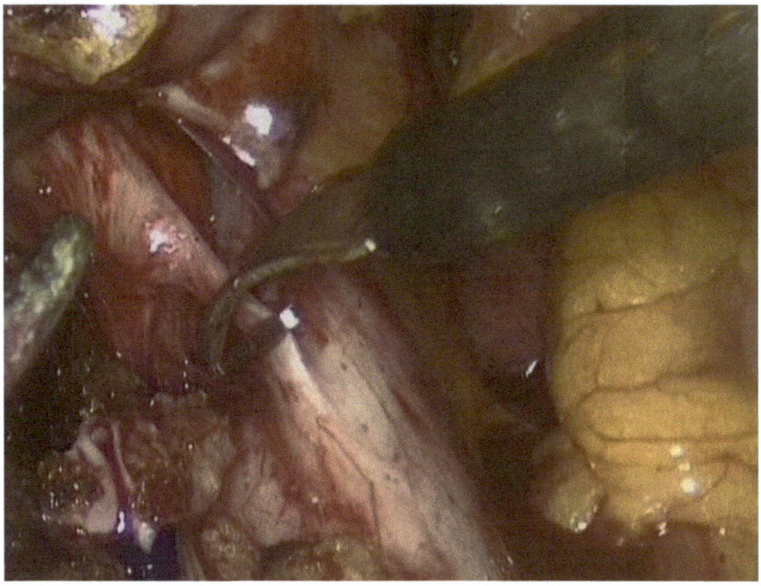

Fig. 6.82 The SHV is divided

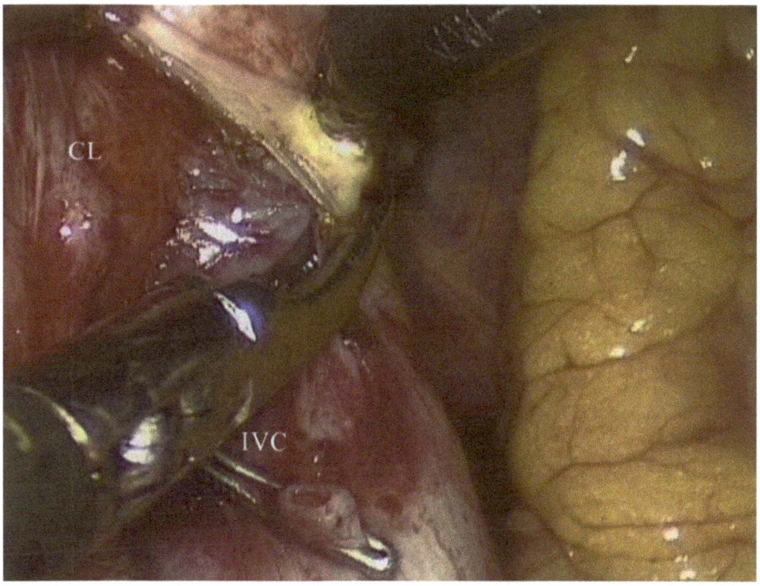

Fig. 6.83 The CL is dissected from the IVC with LPMOD

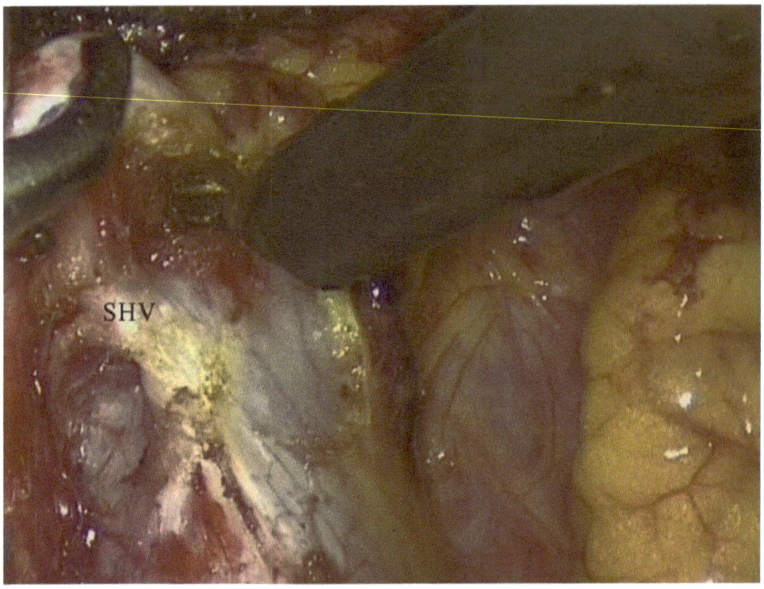

Fig. 6.84 Another SHV is dissected with LPMOD

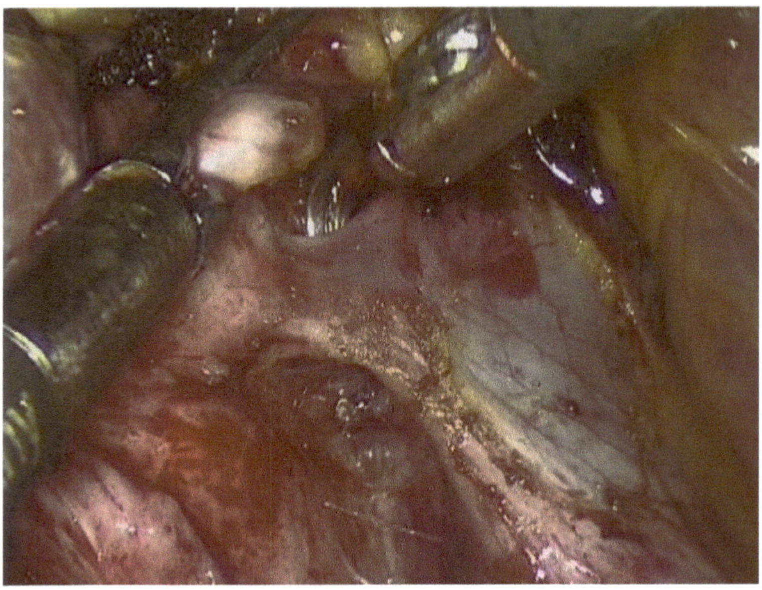

Fig. 6.85 The SHV is freed

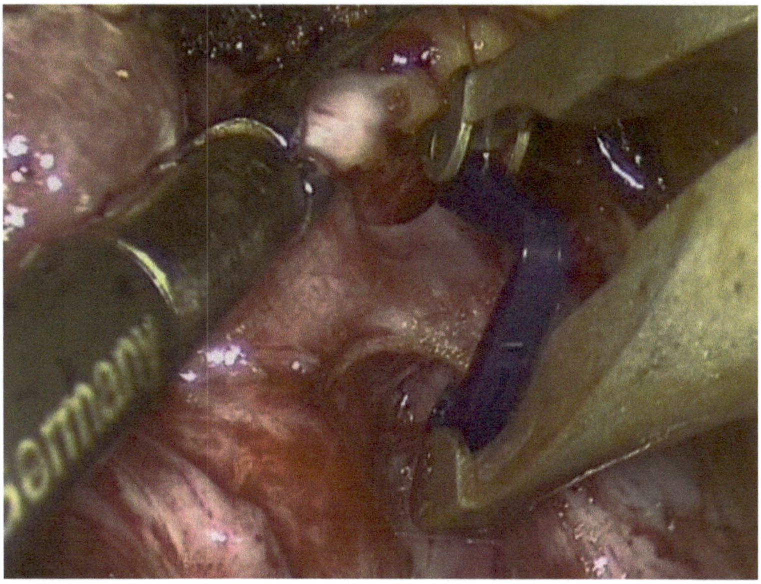

Fig. 6.86 The SHV is clamped with a nonabsorbable polymer clip

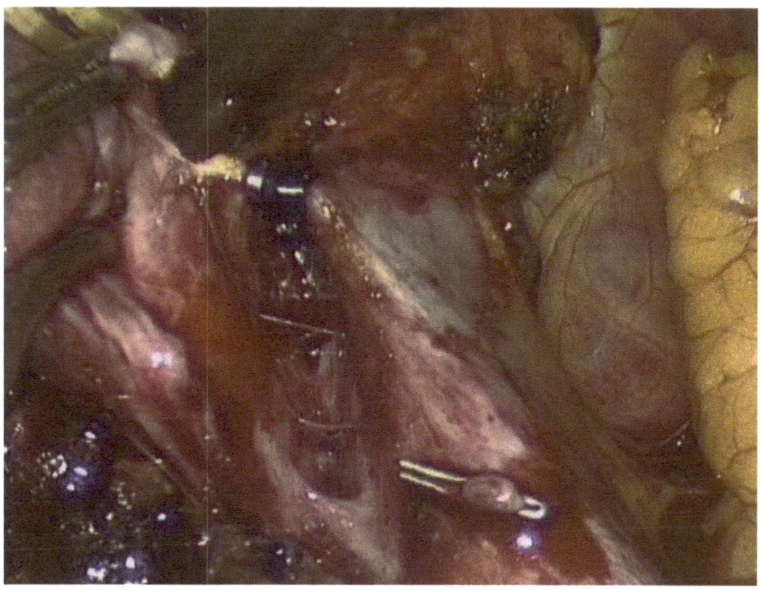

Fig. 6.87 The SHV is divided

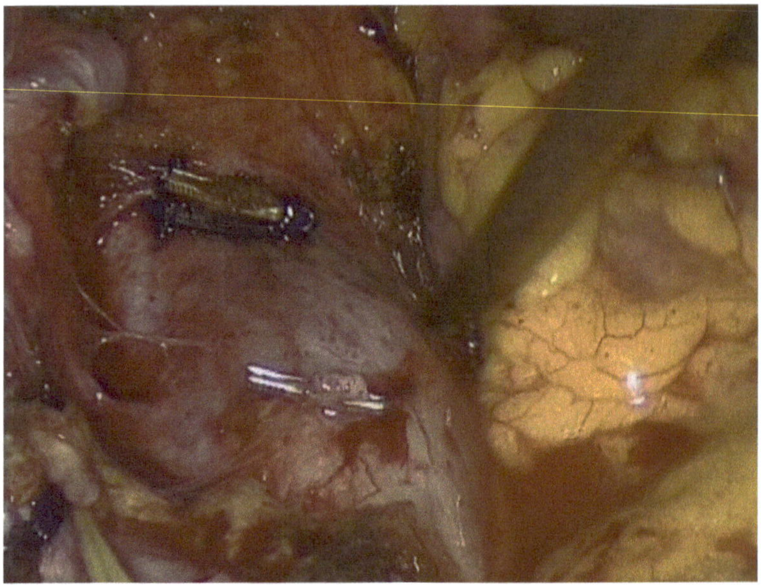

Fig. 6.88 After SHVs were divided, the CL is mobilized to the right, and the anterior wall of the inferior vena cava is visualized

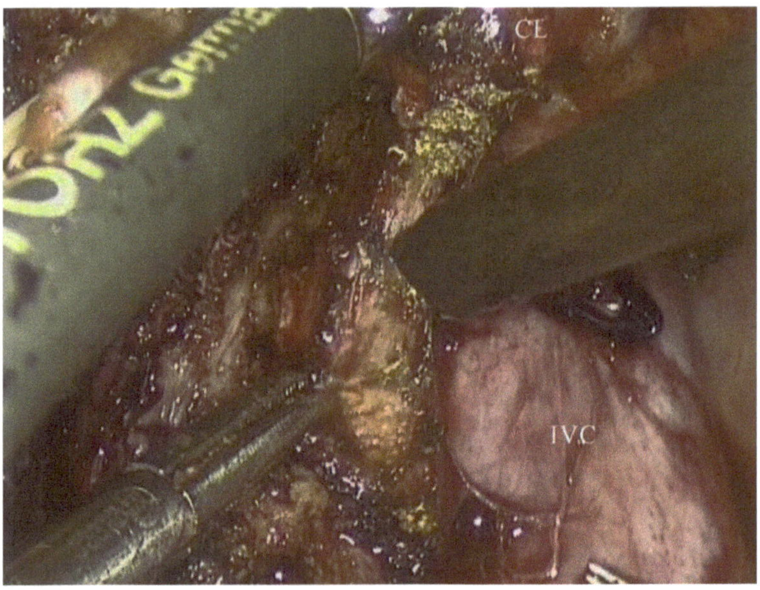

Fig. 6.89 The CL is lifted and is transected with LPMOD

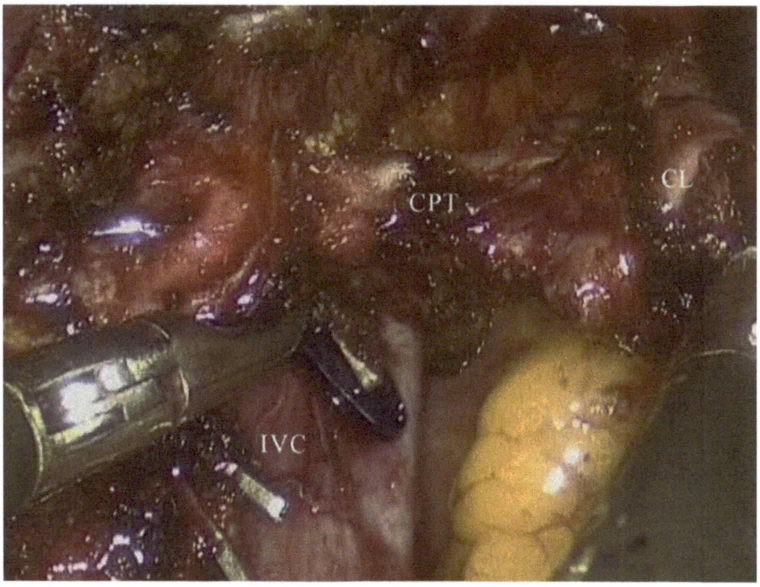

Fig. 6.90 The CL is mobilized to the left and the CPT is dissected

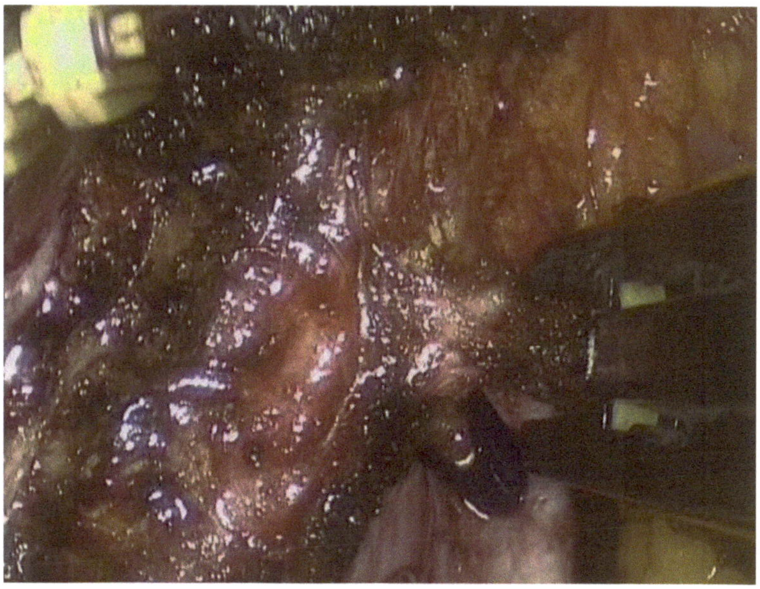

Fig. 6.91 The CPT is clamped with an absorbable clip

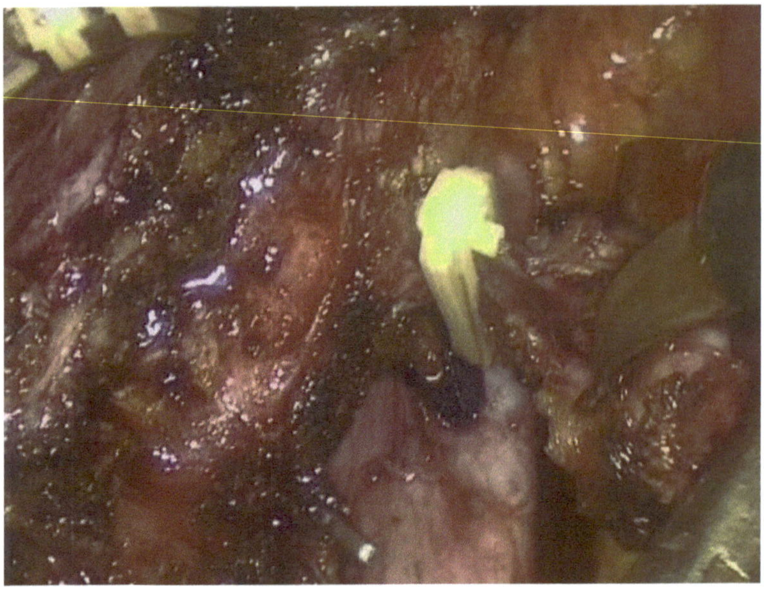

Fig. 6.92 The CPT is divided

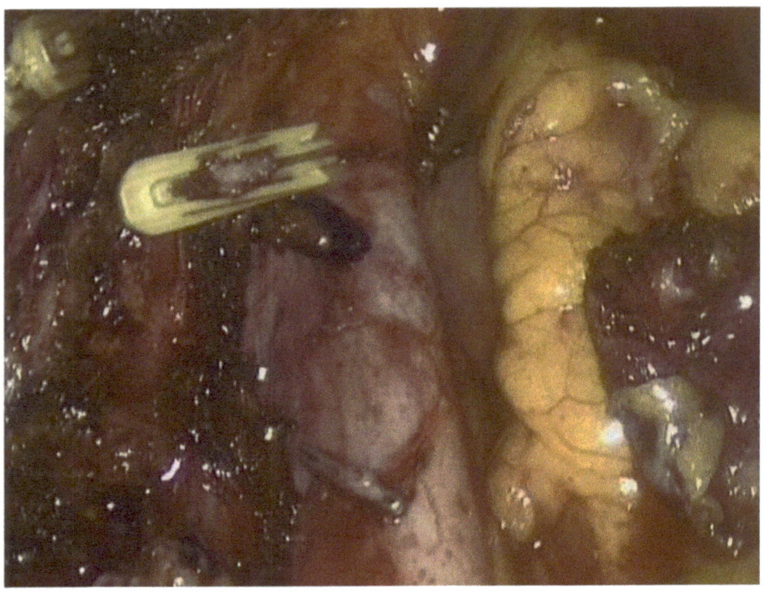

Fig. 6.93 The view of the inferior vena cava after the caudate lobe was removed

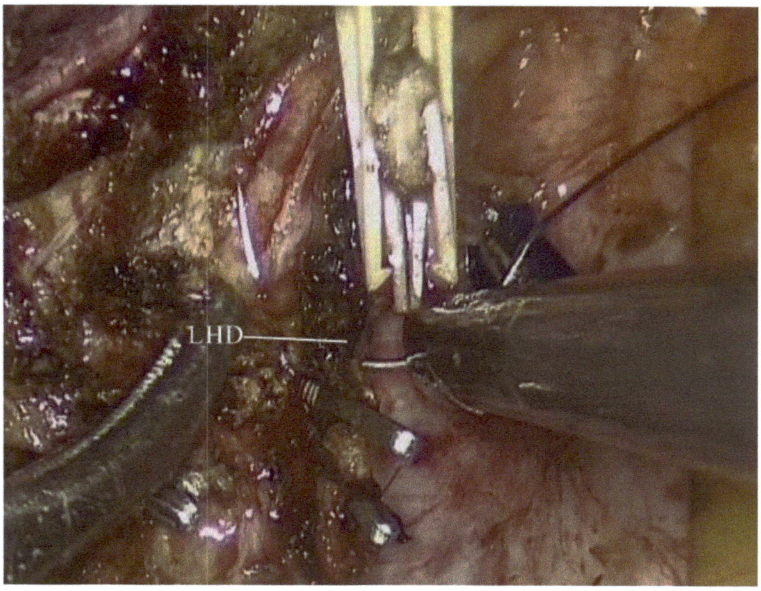

Fig. 6.94 The stump of LHD is closed by the suture

Reference

Takayama T, Makuuchi M, Watanabe K, et al. A new method for mapping hepatic subsegment: counterstaining identification technique. Surgery. 1991;109:226–9.

7 Laparoscopic Non-anatomical Liver Resection

We began to explore the technique of laparoscopic hepatectomy by curettage and aspiration (LHCA) in August 1998. For the purpose of safe dissection of the liver parenchyma, the laparoscopic Peng's multifunctional operative dissector (LPMOD) (Cai et al. 2006) was designed. Blunt dissection is the major point of this technique. Liver parenchyma can be crashed and be aspirated immediately with LPMOD, and intrahepatic ducts and small vessels can be preserved and be safely dissected for ligation. Massive bleeding could be avoided by the meticulous dissection with this instrument.

In non-anatomical liver resection, laparoscopic ultrasound is used as a conventional procedure to locate tumors or intrahepatic stones replacing the use of the surgeons' hands. Furthermore, the laparoscopic ultrasound is more accurate than the surgeons' hands and can calculate the size and depth of tumors. It can be repeated in the course of parenchyma transection to secure an enough free margin for malignancies or to make a proper transection line to completely remove intrahepatic stones.

7.1 Indications and Contraindications

Indications include superficial benign tumors less than 5 cm in diameter, superficial malignant tumors less than 3 cm in diameter or multiple malignant tumors in an area less than 3 cm in depth requiring local resection of tumors or segmentectomy, peripheral lesions (segments VI, VII) of intrahepatic stones with irreversible diseases (biliary strictures or severe parenchymal fibrosis or atrophy) requiring segmentectomy, and liver function of Child A to B. Contraindications include malignant tumors involving porta hepatis (PH) or close to major vessels or hepatic ducts (HDs), history of biliary surgeries such as exploration of the common bile duct (CBD) or cholangiojejunostomy (cholecystectomy is not regarded as a contraindication), extrahepatic bile duct stricture, or acute suppurative cholangitis.

X. Cai, *Laparoscopic Hepatectomy: Atlas and Techniques*,
DOI 10.1007/978-94-017-9840-2_7,

7.2 Patient Position and Trocars' Position

Patients are placed in the supine position under general anesthesia. Three surgeons are needed in the operation. The senior surgeon stands on the left side of the patient, one assistant surgeon stands on the right side of the senior surgeon controlling the aspiration device, and the other assistant surgeon stands on the right side of the patient. Four entries are made. A supraumbilical 10-mm trocar is inserted as the observation port. A 12-mm trocar is inserted below the xiphoid as the main manipulation port for right liver lesions or is inserted below the left costal margin for left liver lesions. And two 5-mm trocars are inserted at the right flank area as assistant manipulation ports (Fig. 7.1).

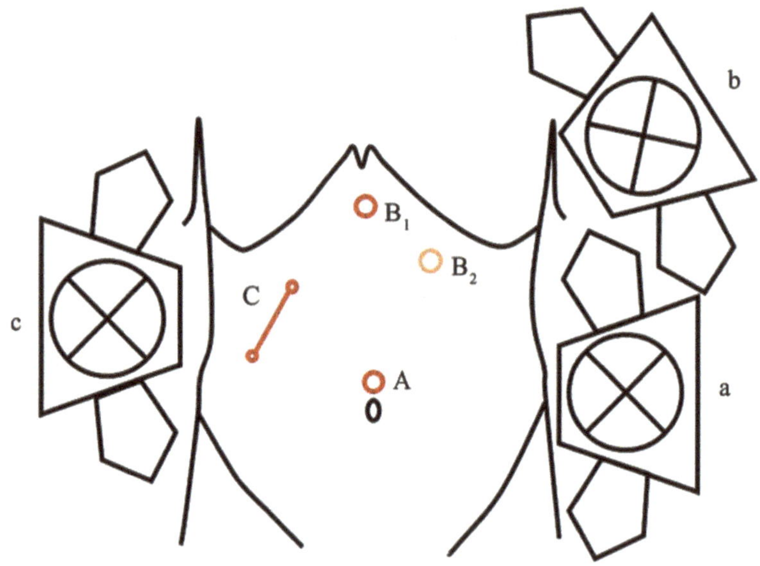

Fig. 7.1 Trocars' position and surgeons' position. (*A*) Observation port; (*B*$_1$) Main manipulation port for right liver lesions; (*B*$_2$) Main manipulation port for left liver lesions; (*C*) Two assistant ports and the incision for removing specimen; (**a**) The senior surgeon stands on the left side of the patient; (**b**) One assistant surgeon stands on the right side of the senior surgeon controlling the aspiration device; (**c**) The other assistant surgeon stands on the right side of the patient

7.3 Laparoscopic Local Resection for Tumors in the Right Anterior Section

See Figs. 7.2, 7.3, 7.4, 7.5, 7.6, 7.7, 7.8, 7.9, 7.10, 7.11, 7.12, 7.13, 7.14, 7.15, 7.16, 7.17, 7.18, 7.19, 7.20, 7.21, 7.22, 7.23, 7.24, 7.25, 7.26, 7.27, 7.28, 7.29, and 7.30.

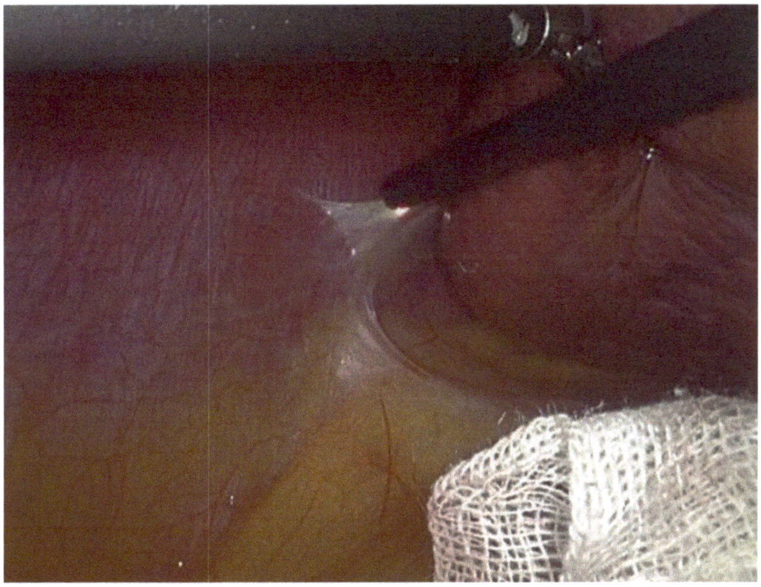

Fig. 7.2 The liver is mobilized to the left and the right triangle ligament (RTL) is divided with LPMOD

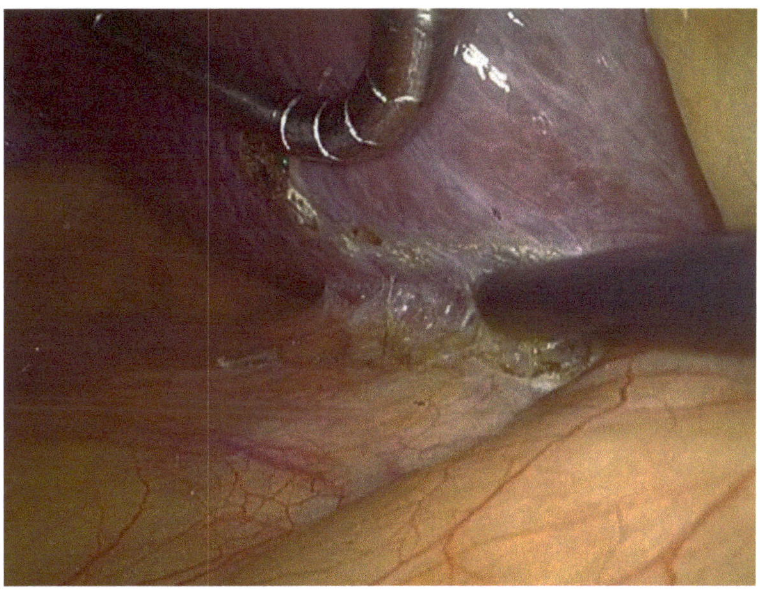

Fig. 7.3 The right lobe of the liver (RLL) is elevated with a laparoscopic liver retractor, and the hepatorenal ligament (HRL) is divided with LPMOD

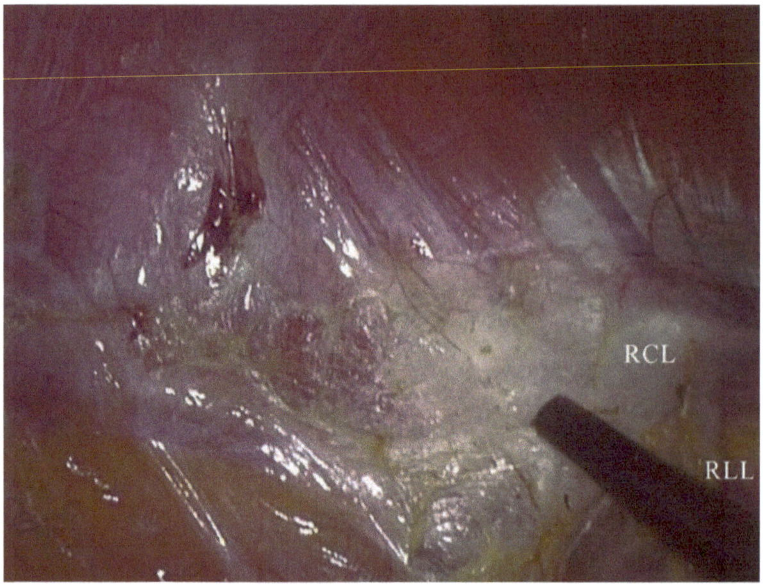

Fig. 7.4 The RLL is mobilized downward, and the right coronary ligament (*RCL*) is divided with LPMOD

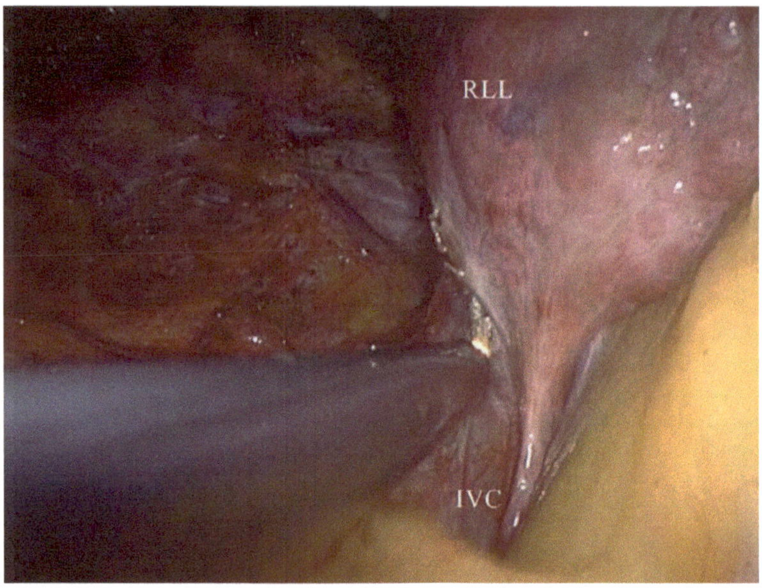

Fig. 7.5 The RLL is freed and is mobilized to the left, then the RLL is dissected from the inferior vena cava (*IVC*)

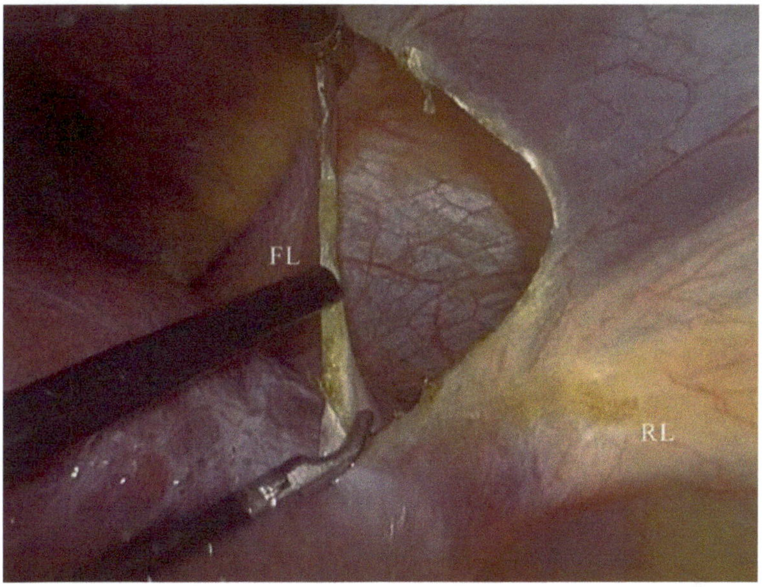

Fig. 7.6 The falciform ligament (*FL*) is divided with LPMOD

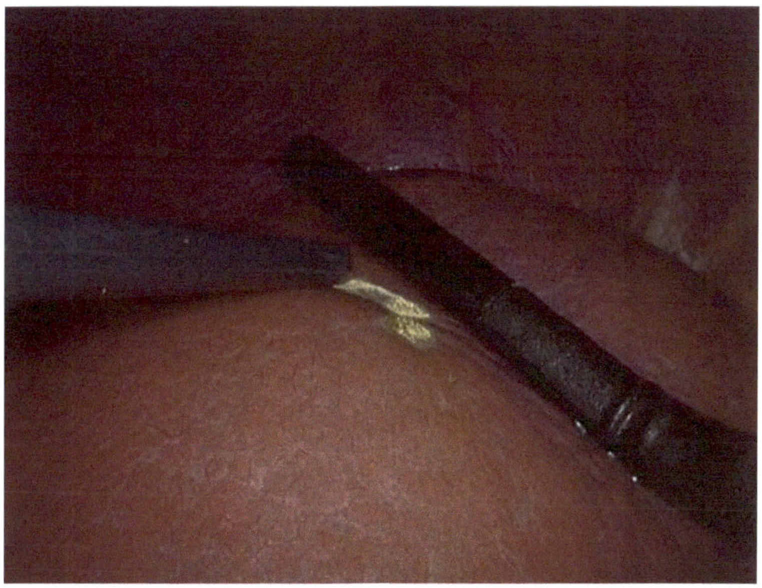

Fig. 7.7 The tumor (hemangioma) is located with the laparoscopic ultrasound

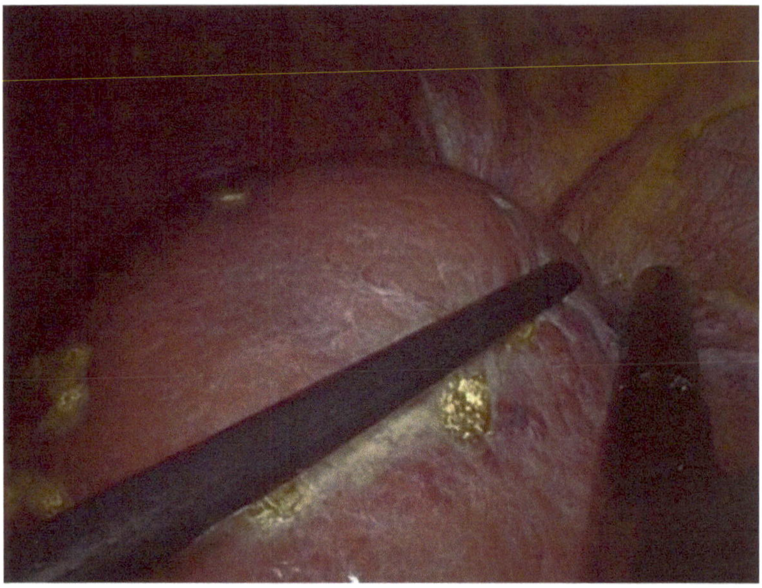

Fig. 7.8 The transection line is marked on the liver surface with LPMOD according to the guidance of laparoscopic ultrasound

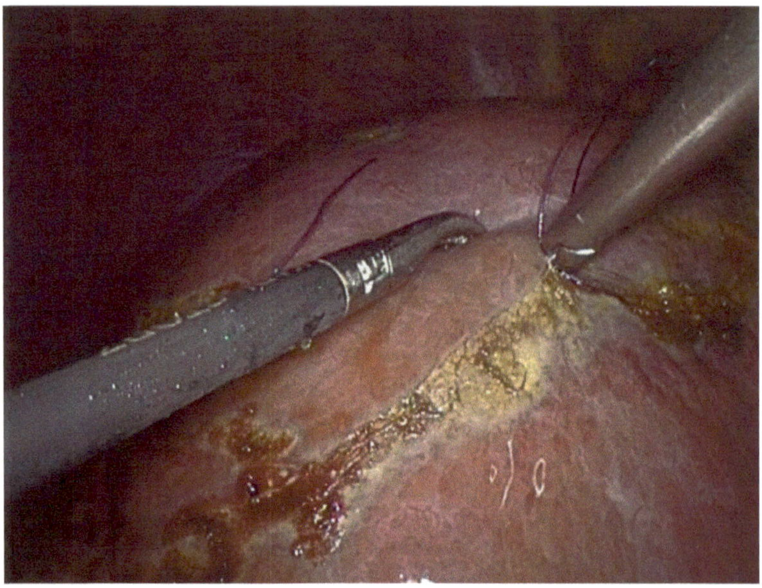

Fig. 7.9 A suture is executed on liver capsule for the mobilization of the lesion

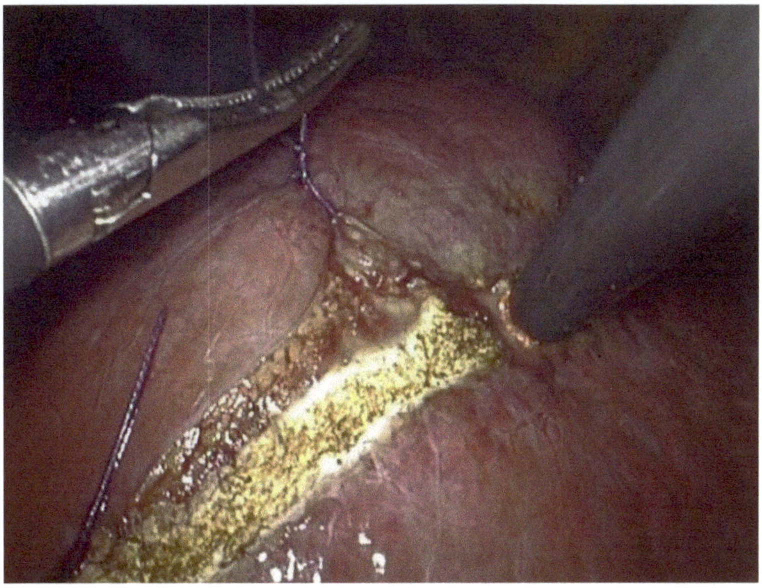

Fig. 7.10 The lesion is lifted by drawing sutures, and the liver capsule is cut with LPMOD

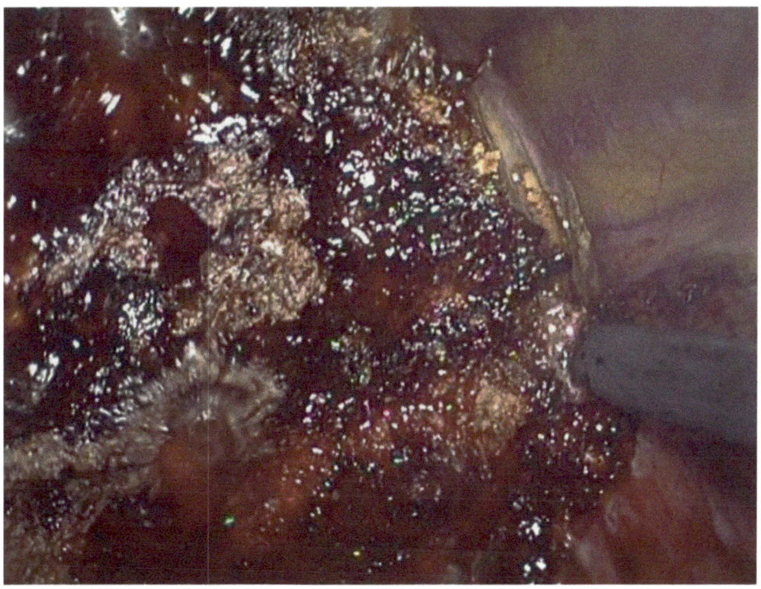

Fig. 7.11 Liver parenchyma is transected with LPMOD along the left side of the lesion

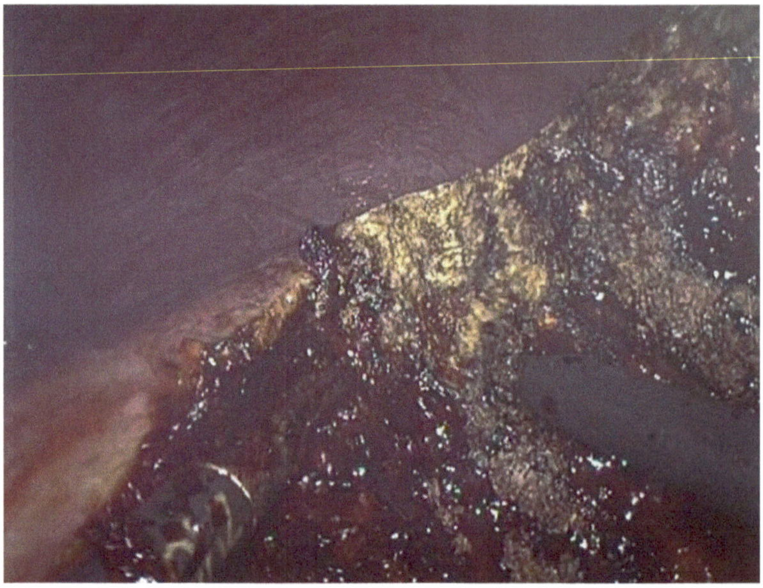

Fig. 7.12 Liver parenchyma is transected with LPMOD along the right side of the lesion

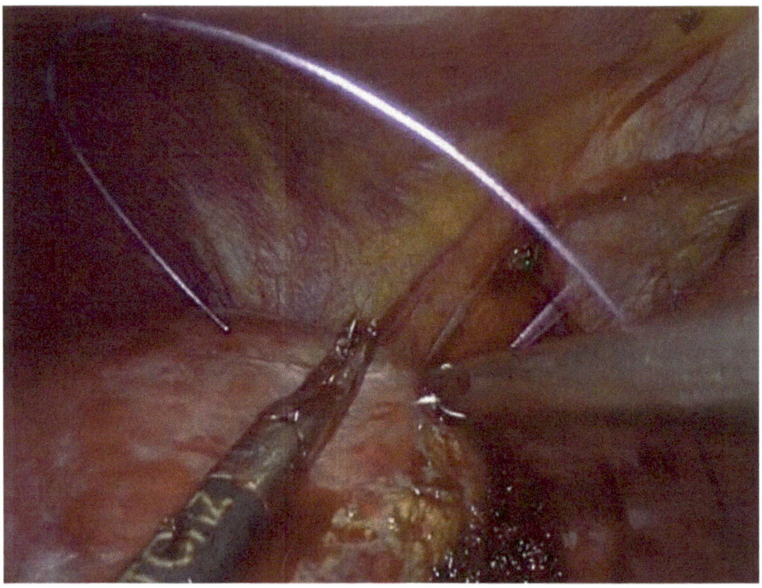

Fig. 7.13 Another suture is executed on the capsule at the back of the lesion

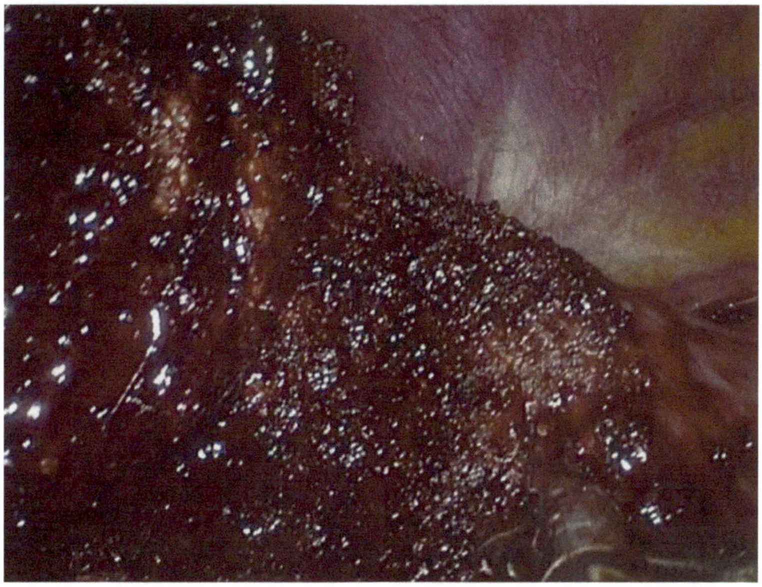

Fig. 7.14 The lesion is lifted by drawing the suture

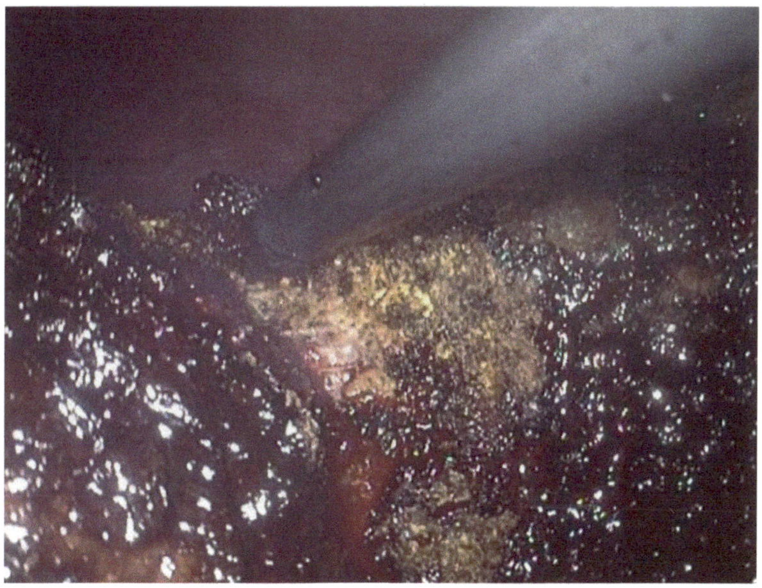

Fig. 7.15 A branch of the hepatic vein is visualized in the transection of the liver

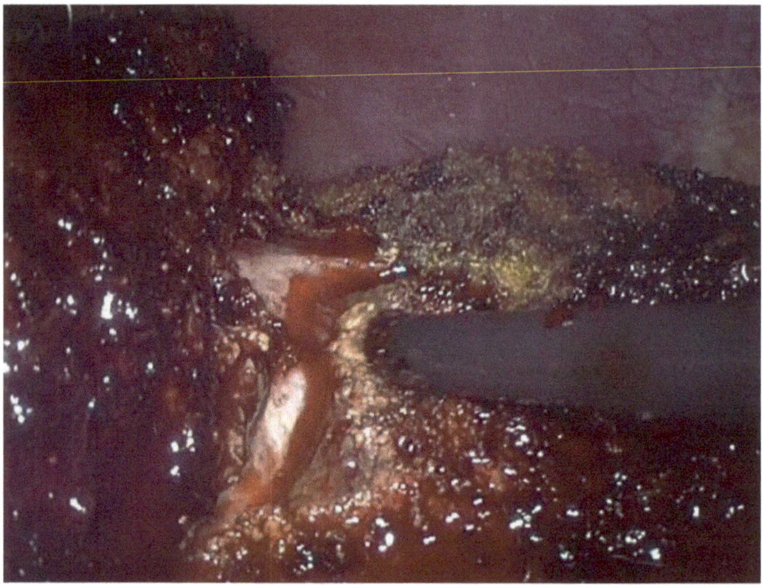

Fig. 7.16 The branch of the hepatic vein and the left wall of the hemangioma are dissected with LPMOD

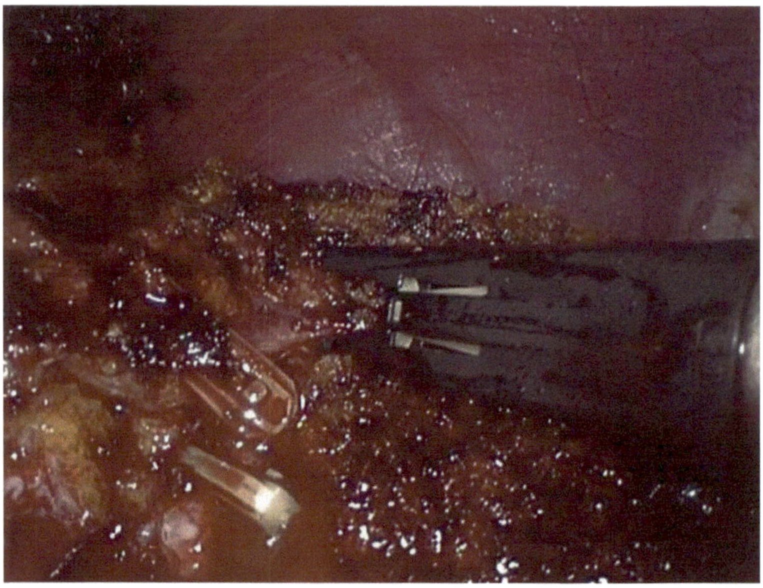

Fig. 7.17 The branch of the hepatic vein is clamped with an absorbable clip

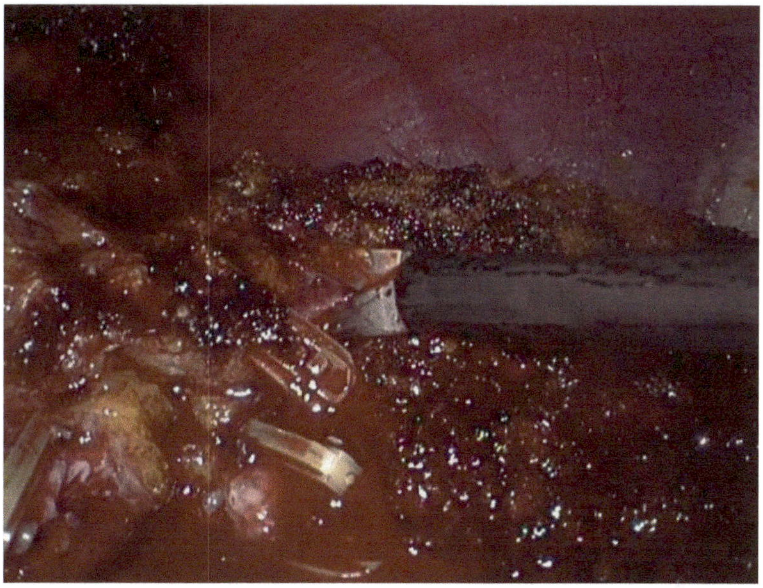

Fig. 7.18 The branch of the hepatic vein is divided

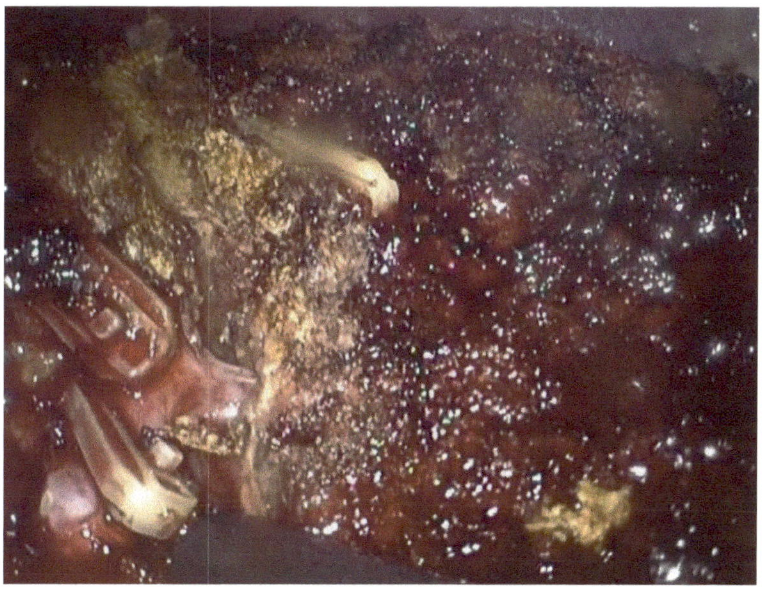

Fig. 7.19 Another branch of the hepatic vein is visualized in the transection of the liver parenchyma

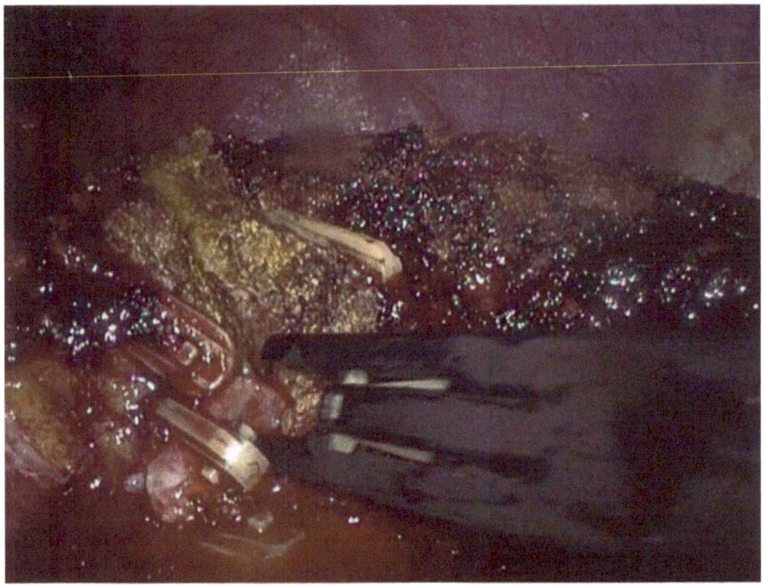

Fig. 7.20 The branch of the hepatic vein is clamped with an absorbable clip

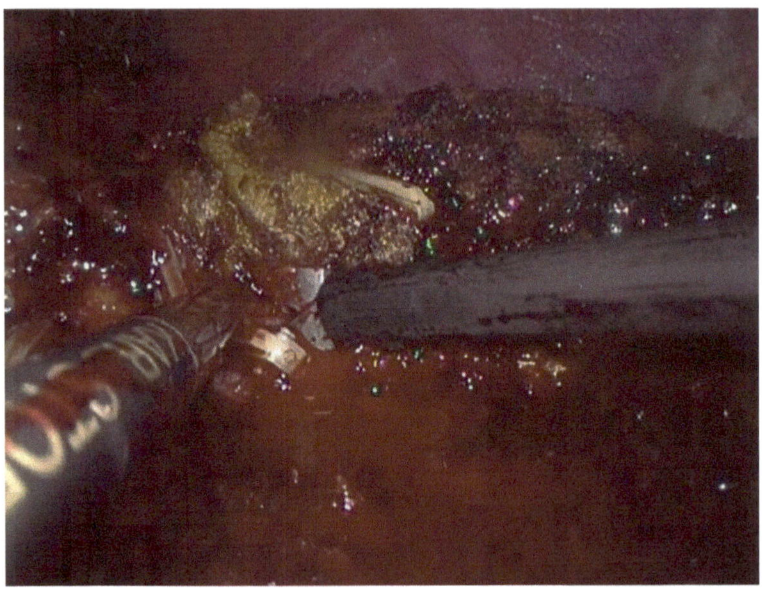

Fig. 7.21 The branch of the hepatic vein is divided

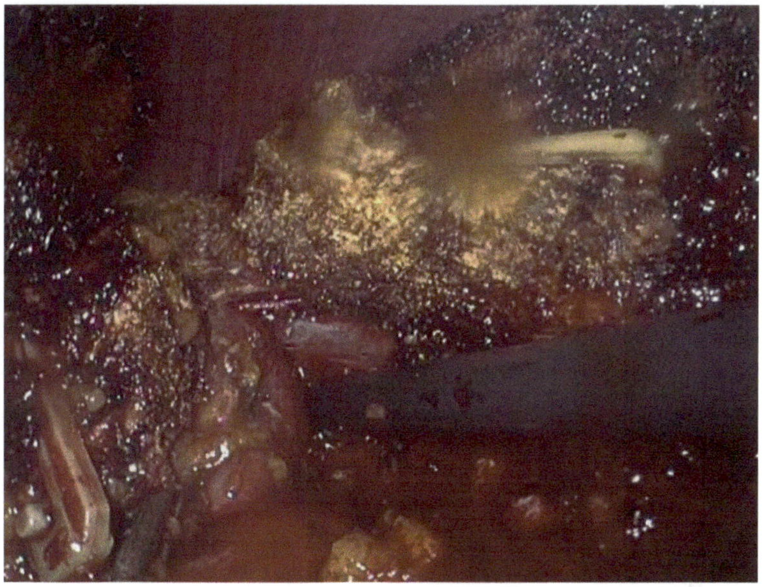

Fig. 7.22 Liver parenchyma is transected along the left wall of the hemangioma and the branches of the hepatic veins to the hemangioma are dissected with LPMOD

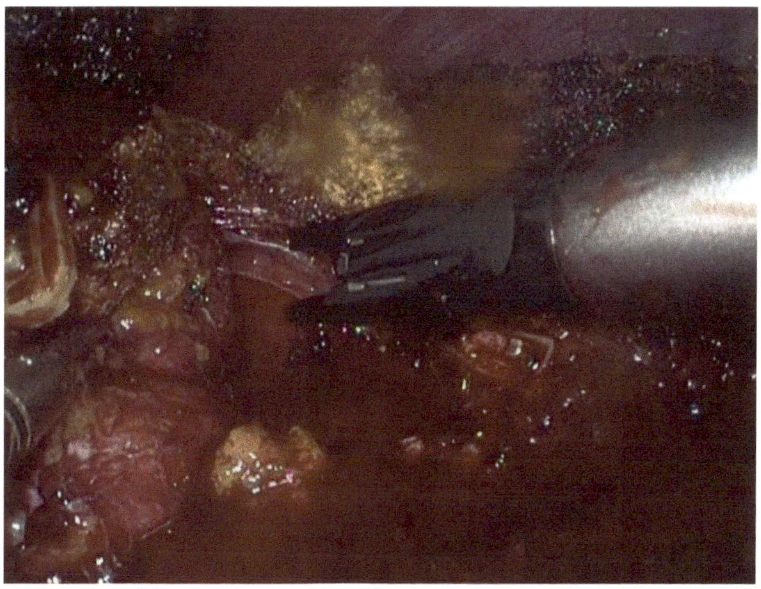

Fig. 7.23 One branch of the hepatic vein is clamped with an absorbable clip

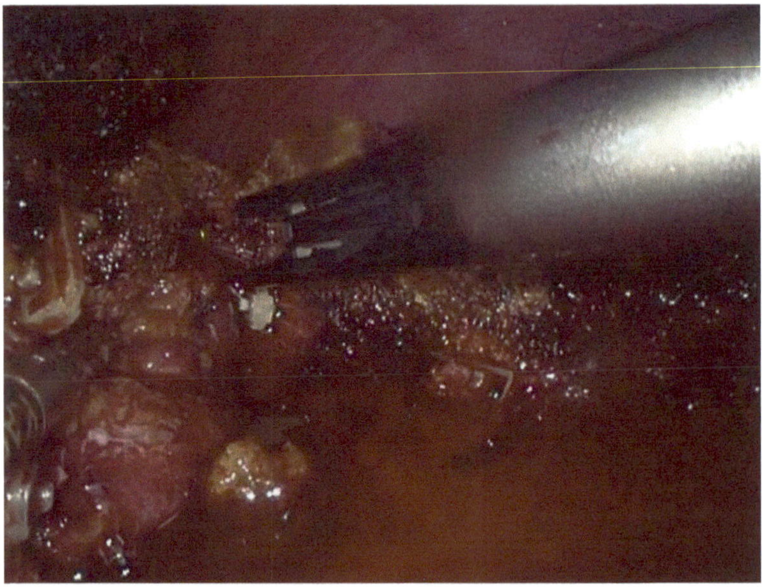

Fig. 7.24 Another branch of the hepatic vein is clamped with an absorbable clip

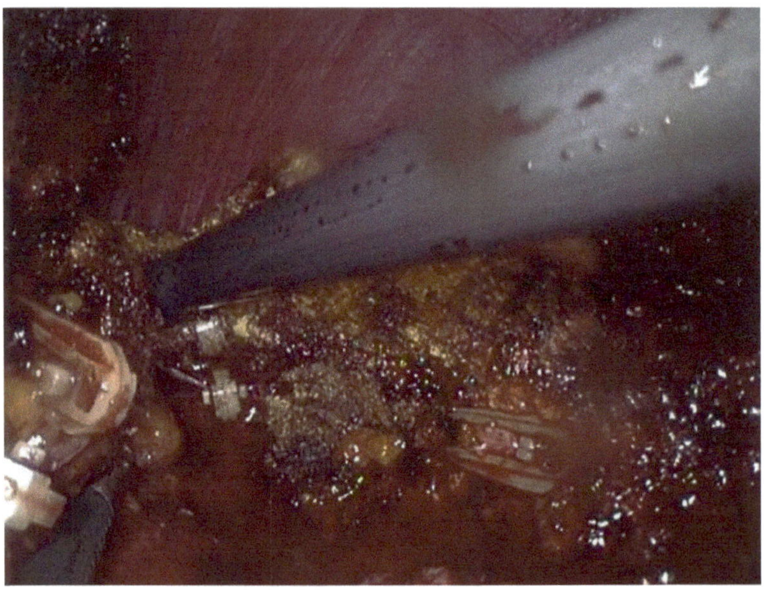

Fig. 7.25 These clamped branches of the hepatic vein are divided with LPMOD

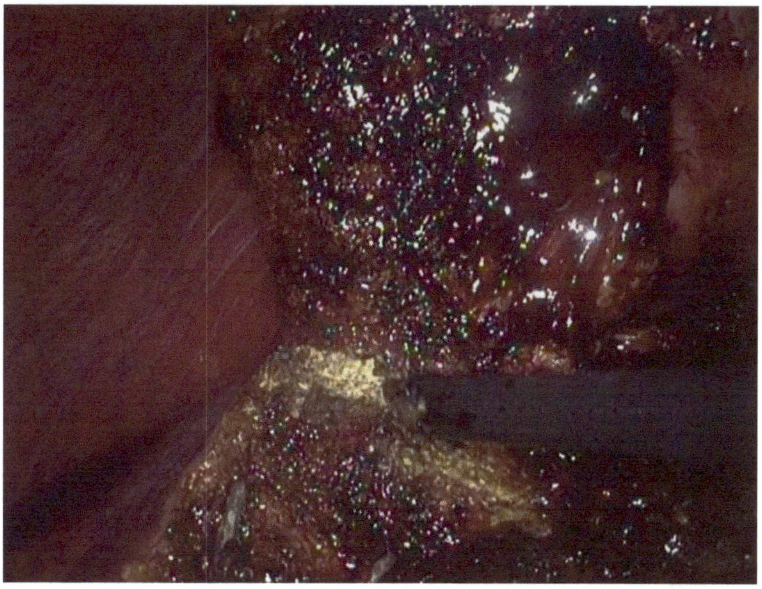

Fig. 7.26 The lesion is lifted and the liver parenchyma is transected with LPMOD along the right wall of the hemangioma

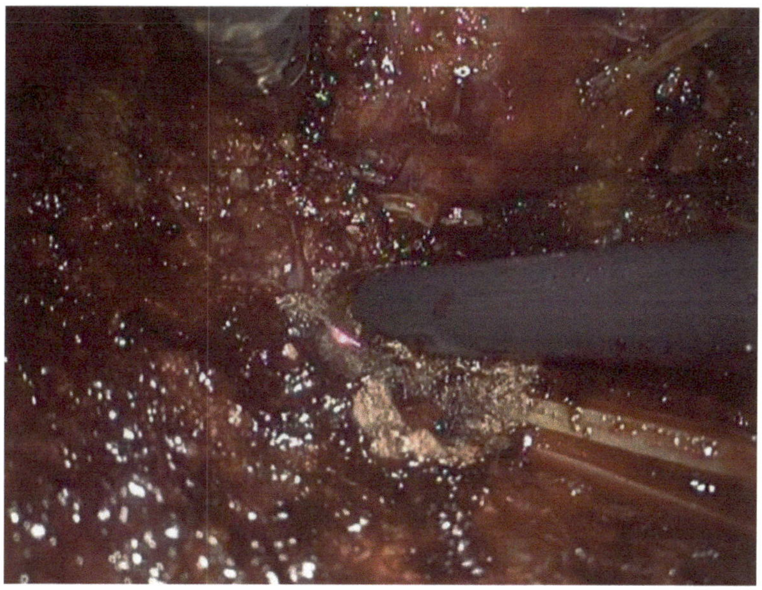

Fig. 7.27 A small vessel is dissected with LPMOD

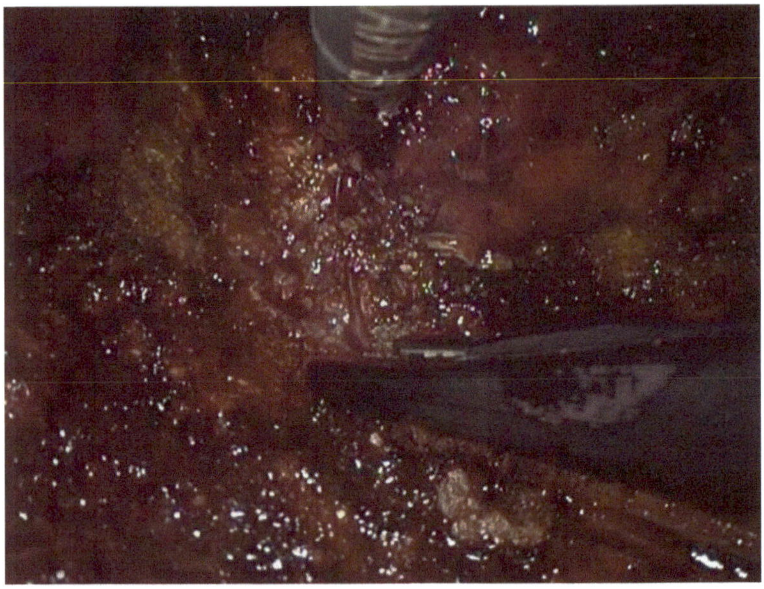

Fig. 7.28 The small vessel is clamped with LPMOD

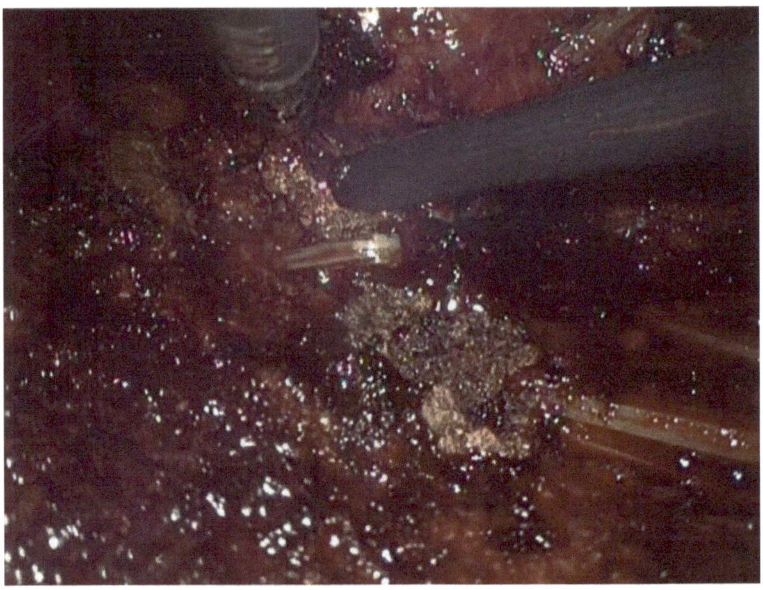

Fig. 7.29 The small vessel is divided and is followed by complete resection of the hemangioma

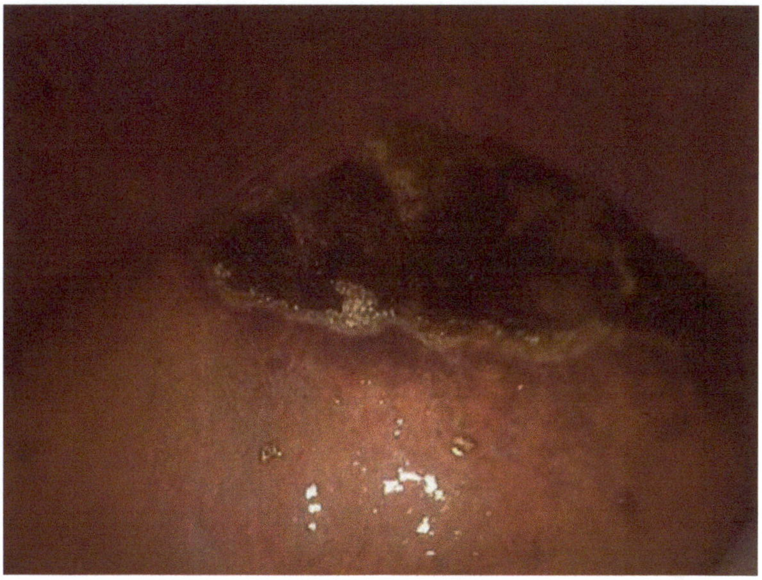

Fig. 7.30 The view of the row surface

7.4 Laparoscopic Local Resection for Multiple Tumors in Segment IV

See Figs. 7.31, 7.32, 7.33, 7.34, 7.35, 7.36, 7.37, 7.38, 7.39, 7.40, 7.41, 7.42, 7.43, 7.44, 7.45, 7.46, 7.47, 7.48, 7.49, 7.50, 7.51, 7.52, 7.53, 7.54, 7.55, 7.56, and 7.57.

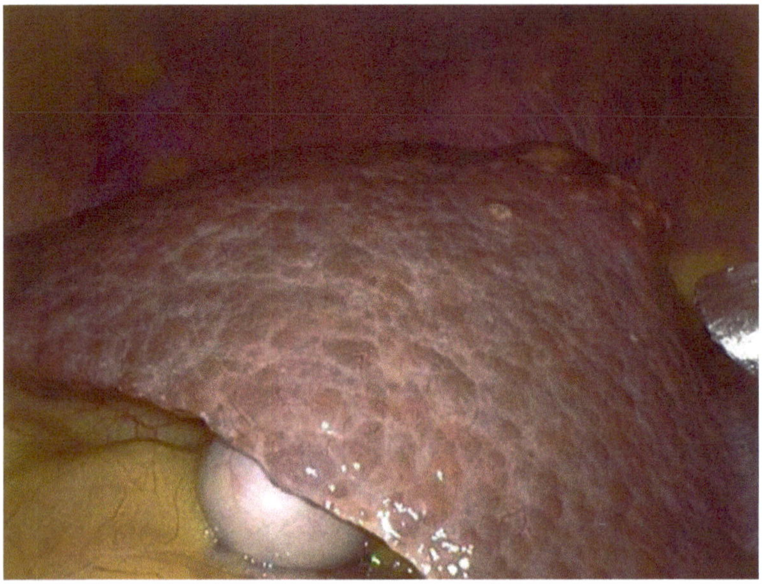

Fig. 7.31 Multiple tumors, as well as liver cirrhosis, are observed on the surface of segment IV

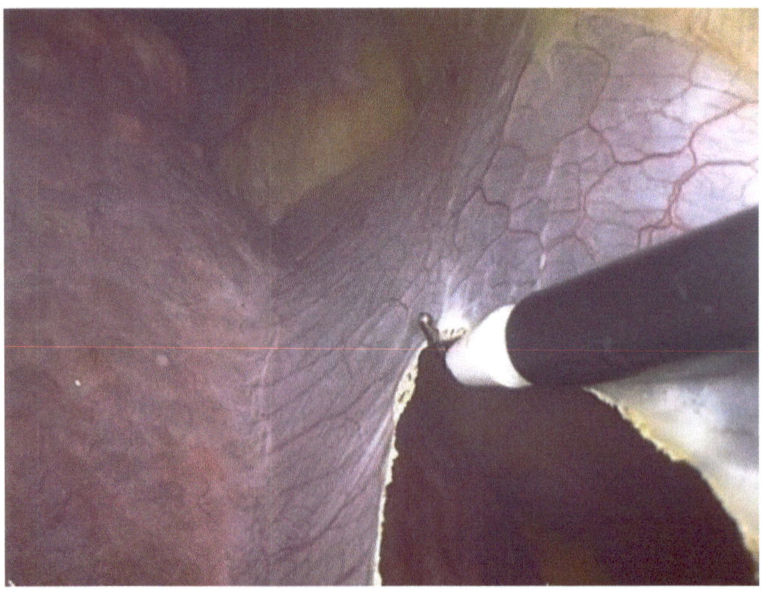

Fig. 7.32 The round ligament (RL) and the falciform ligament are divided

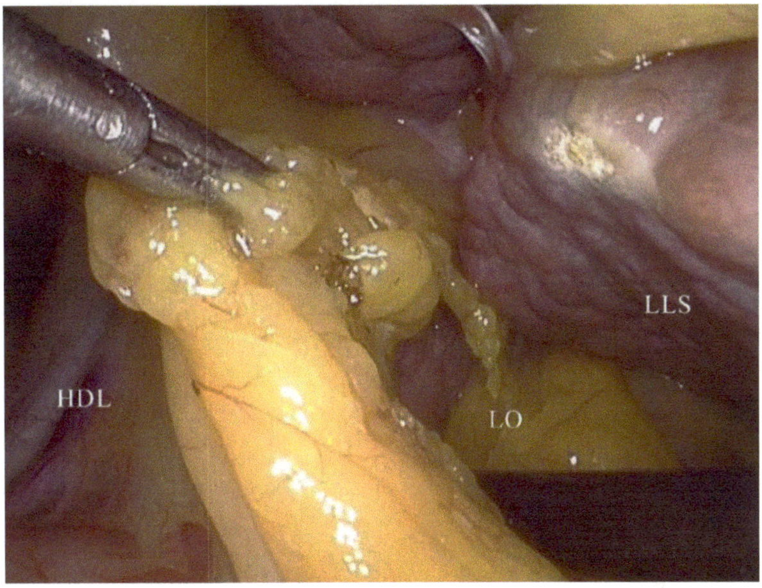

Fig. 7.33 The part of lesser omentum (*LO*) close to the hepatoduodenal ligament (*HDL*) is divided with LPMOD

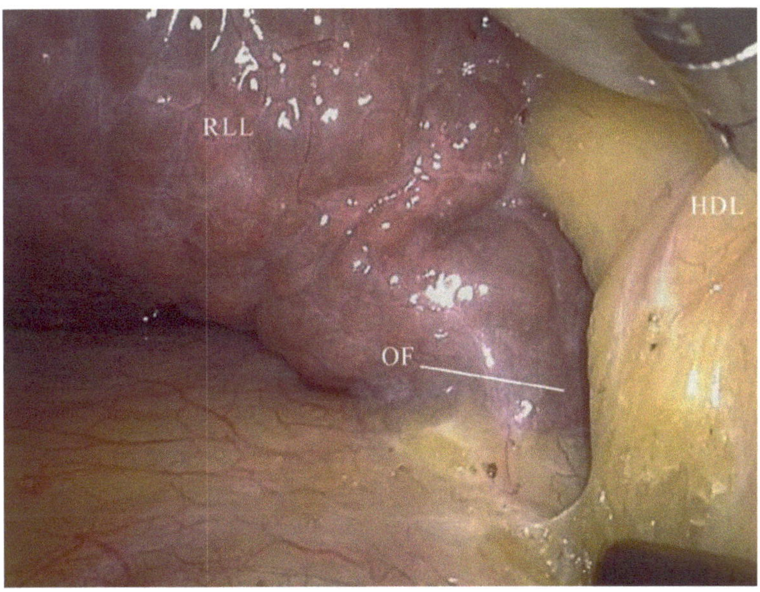

Fig. 7.34 The HDL is mobilized to expose the omental foramen (*OF*)

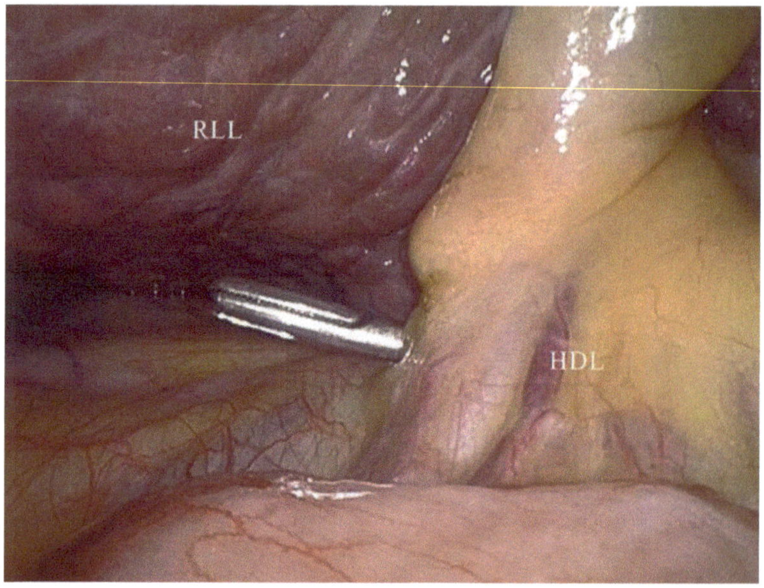

Fig. 7.35 A lithotomy forceps which is used in the open exploration of the common bile duct (CBD) is inserted through the manipulation port and is passed omental foramen

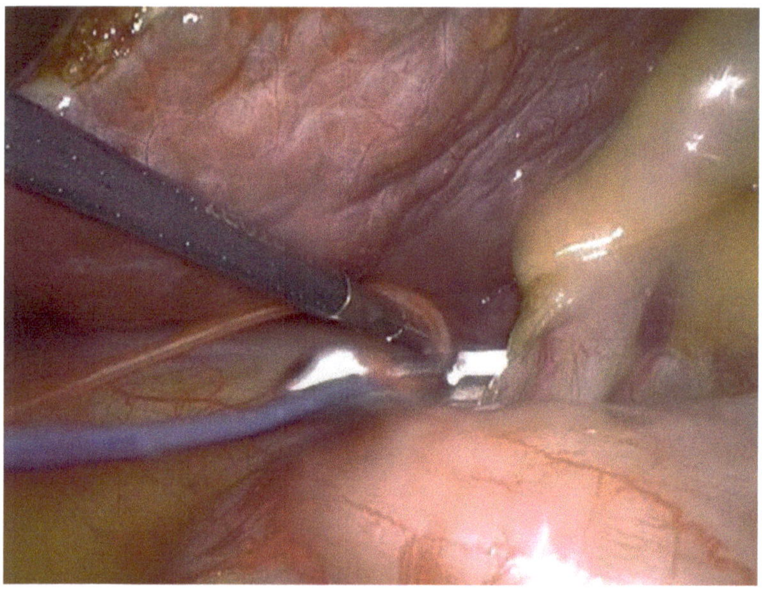

Fig. 7.36 An elastic tape and a no. 8 urinary catheter are passed through the space behind the HDL by the guidance of the lithotomy forceps

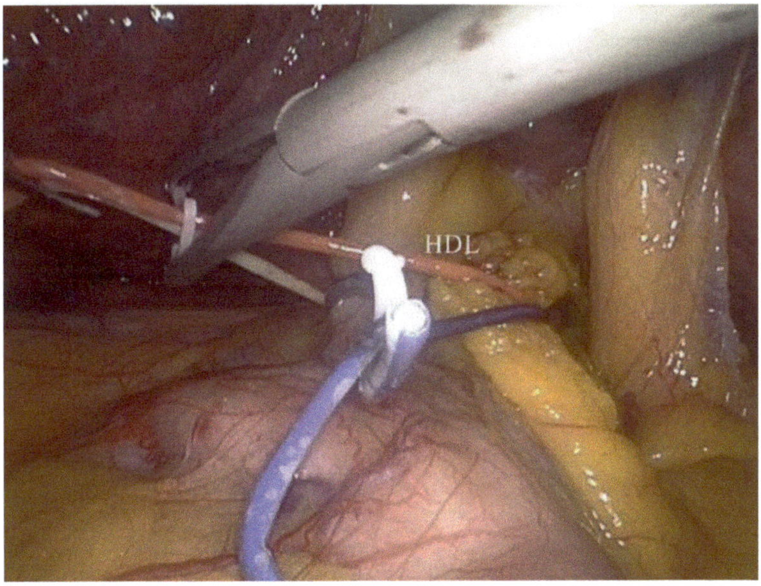

Fig. 7.37 The elastic tape and the urinary catheter are rounded the HDL and are closed with nonabsorbable polymer clips for the potential execution of total vascular occlusion

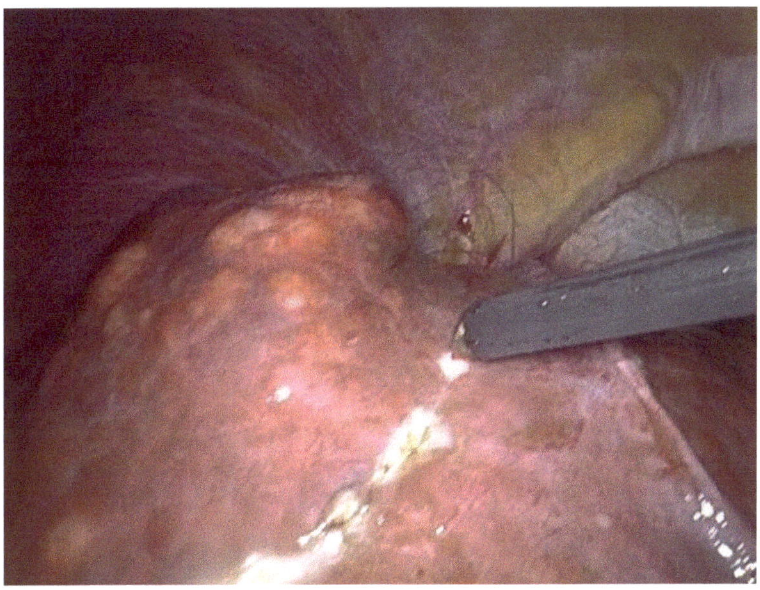

Fig. 7.38 The transection line is marked on the liver surface 10 mm to the tumors

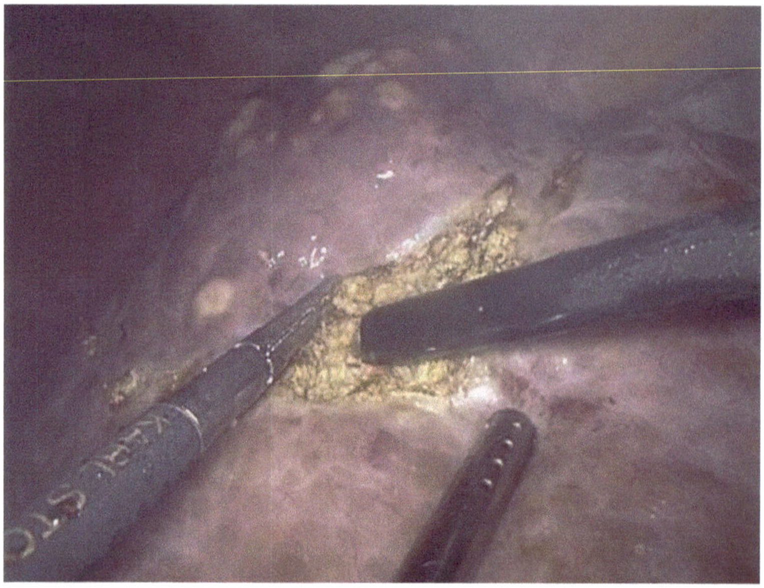

Fig. 7.39 The liver capsule is cut with LPMOD

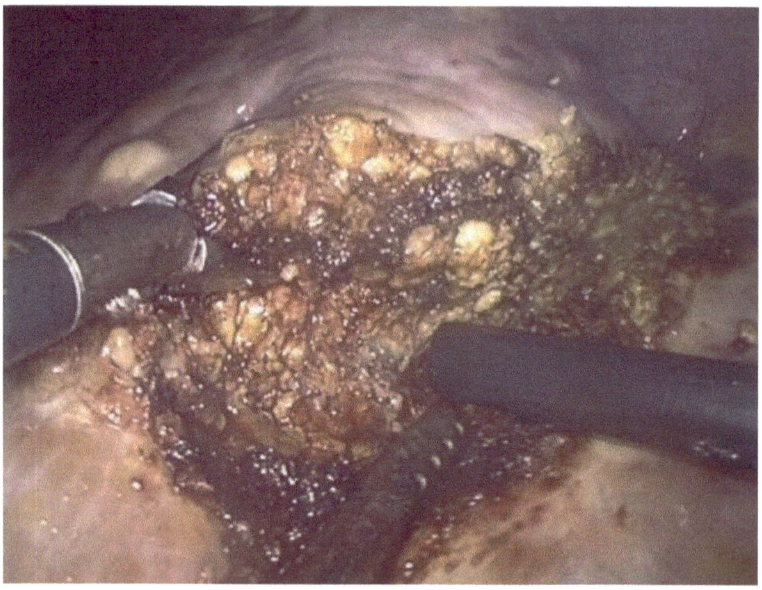

Fig. 7.40 One side of the liver parenchyma is elevated with a curved dissecting forceps, and the other side is pressed downward with the tip of aspiration tube, and the parenchyma is transected along the transection line

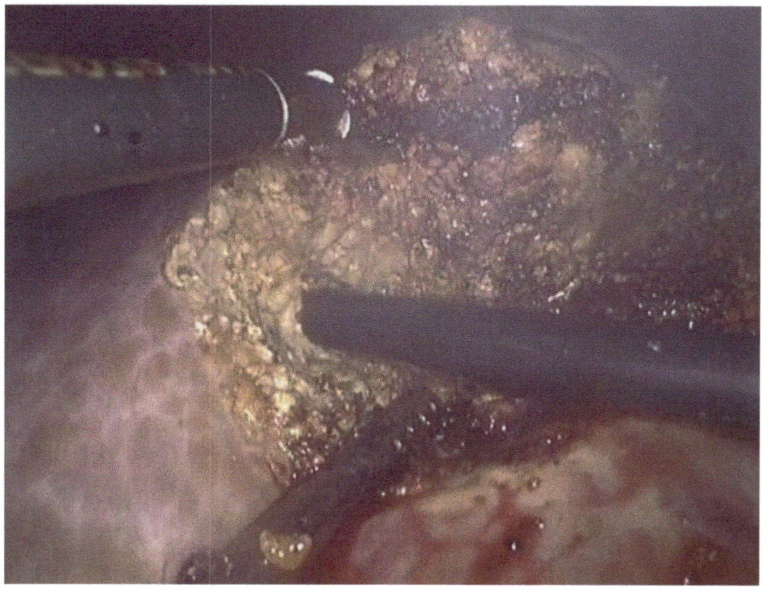

Fig. 7.41 The lesion is pushed to the left with the curved dissecting forceps, and the liver parenchyma is transected along the right side of the lesion

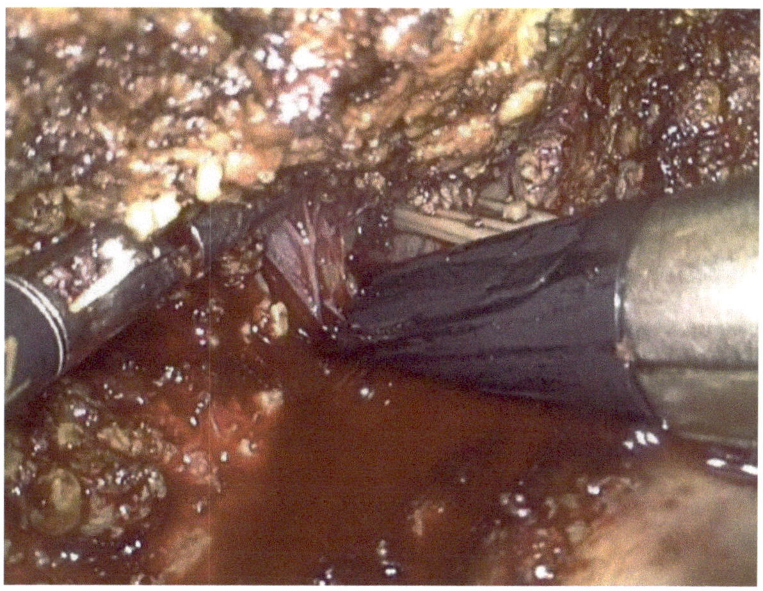

Fig. 7.42 A small vessel is dissected and is clamped with absorbable clips

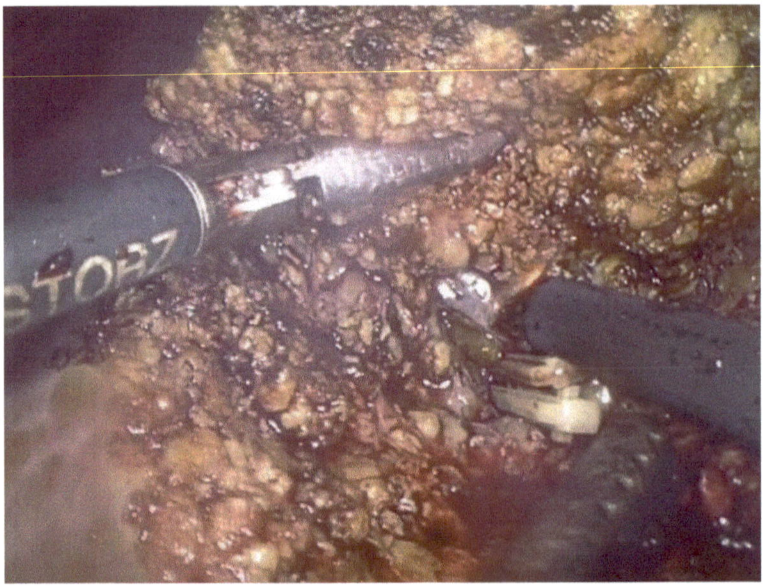

Fig. 7.43 The small vessel is transected with LPMOD after being clamped with absorbable clips

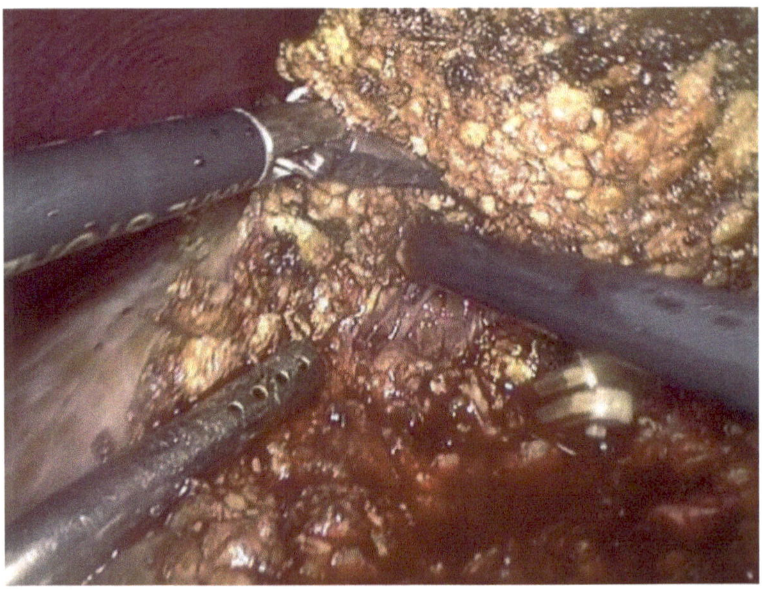

Fig. 7.44 Another small vessel is dissected with LPMOD in the transection of the liver parenchyma

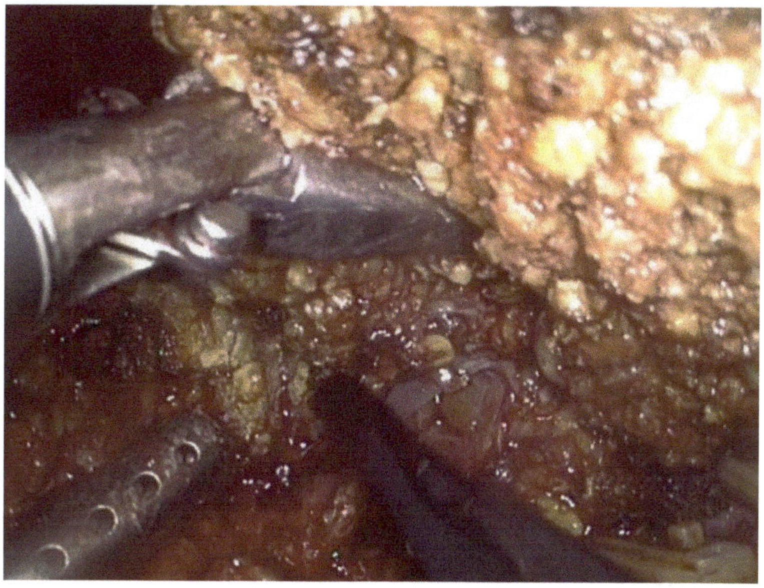

Fig. 7.45 The small vessel is clamped with an absorbable clip

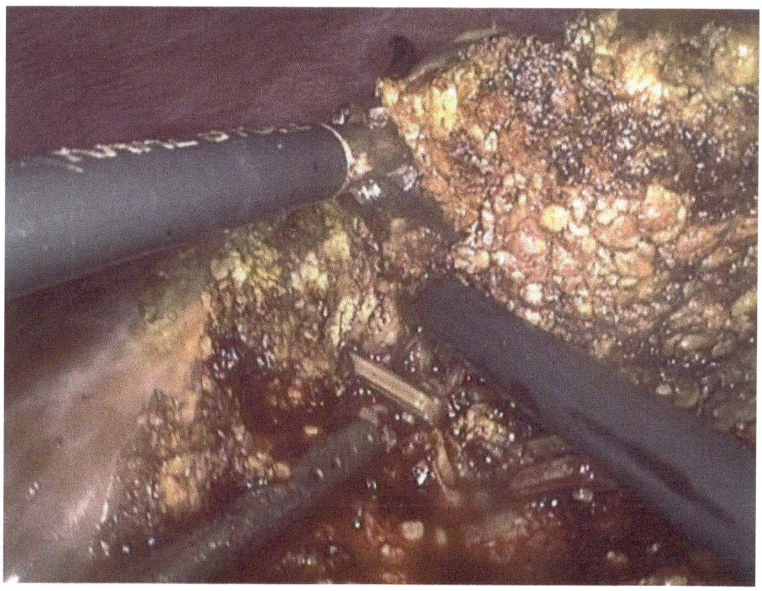

Fig. 7.46 The small vessel is divided with LPMOD

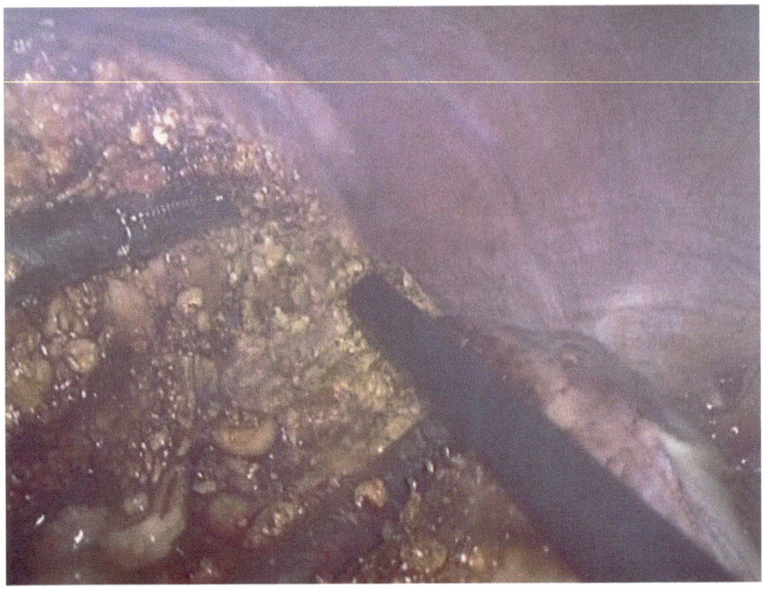

Fig. 7.47 The lesion is mobilized to the right, and the liver parenchyma is transected along the left side of the lesion

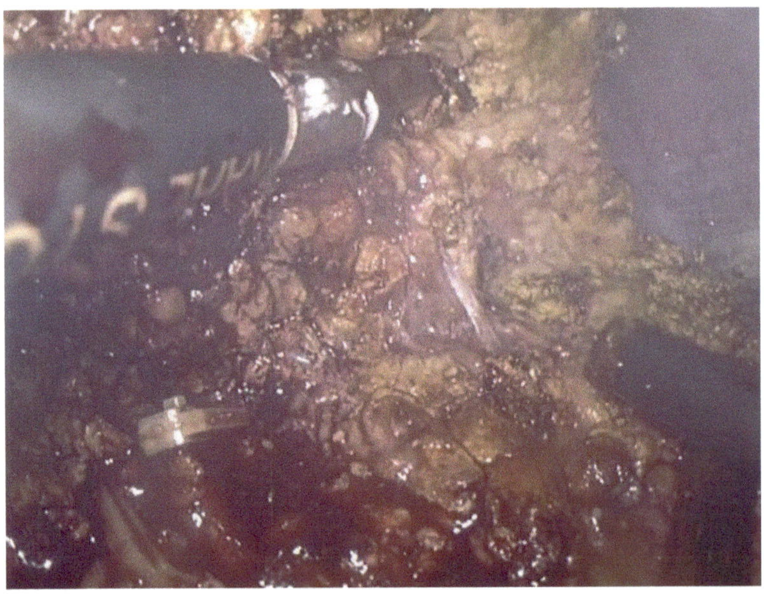

Fig. 7.48 A small vessel is dissected with LPMOD

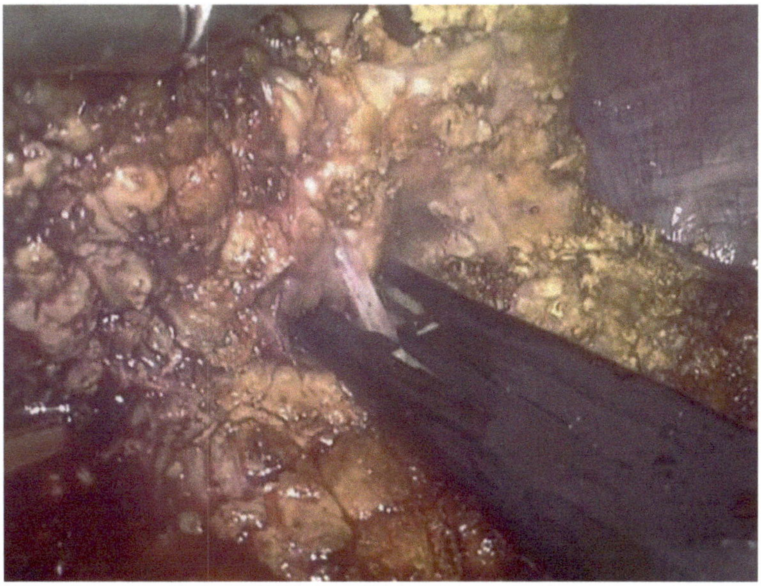

Fig. 7.49 The small vessel is clamped with an absorbable clip

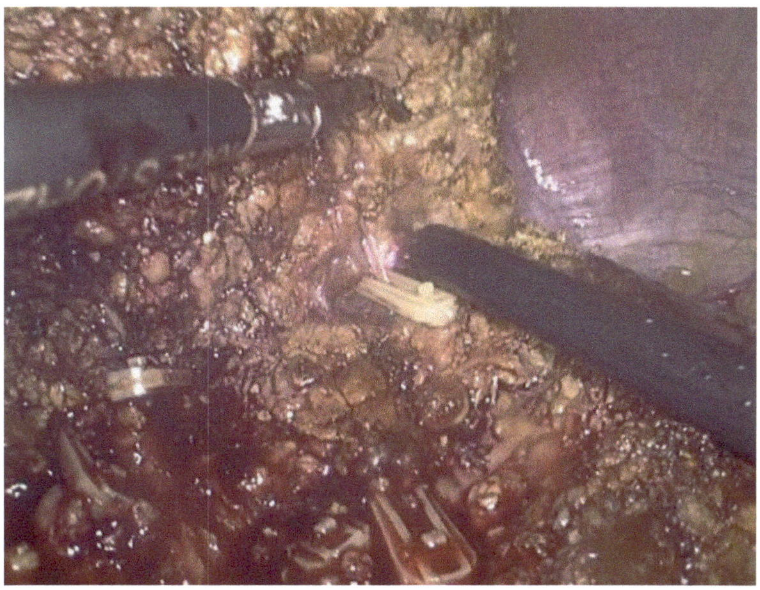

Fig. 7.50 The small vessel is transected with LPMOD

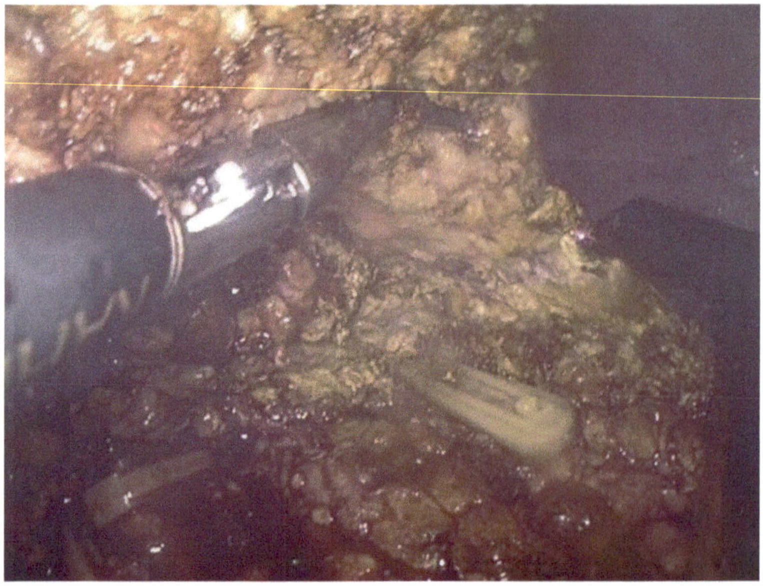

Fig. 7.51 After lateral sides of the lesion were divided, the lesion is elevated with a curved dissecting forceps and is transected with LPMOD

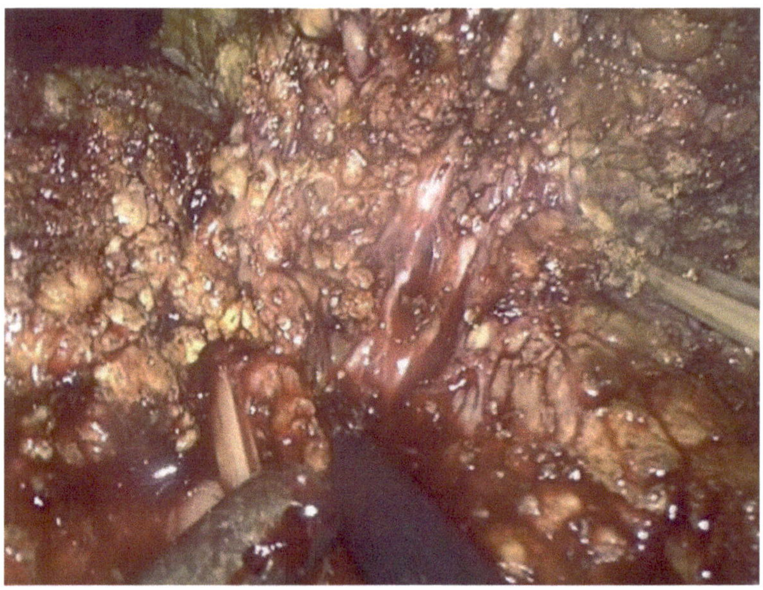

Fig. 7.52 The artery to tumors is dissected

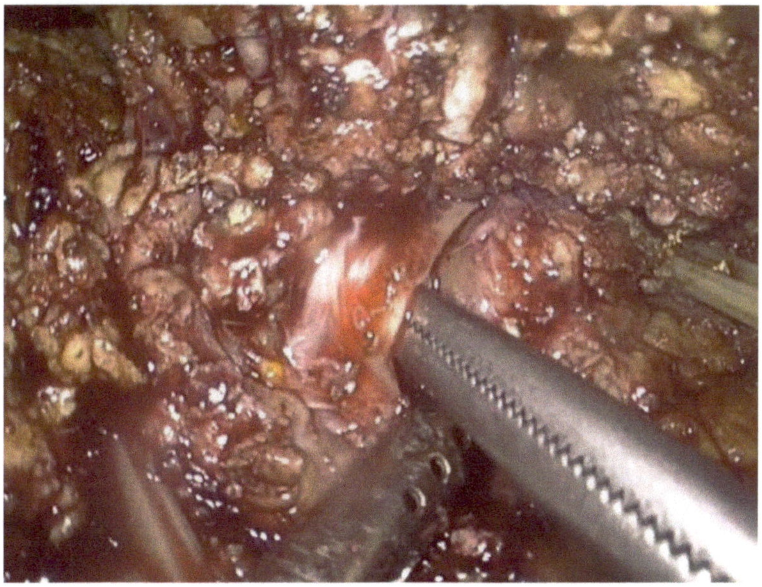

Fig. 7.53 The artery is freed with a curved dissecting forceps

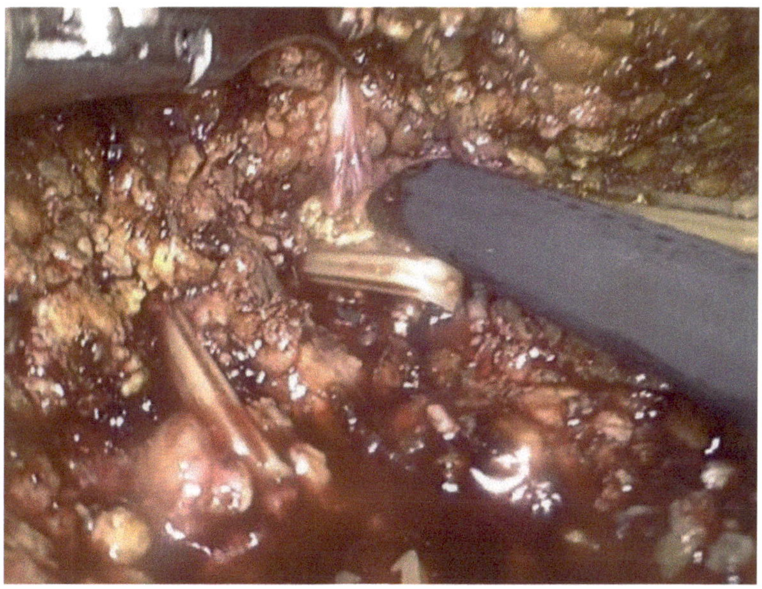

Fig. 7.54 The artery is divided with LPMOD after being clamped with an absorbable clip

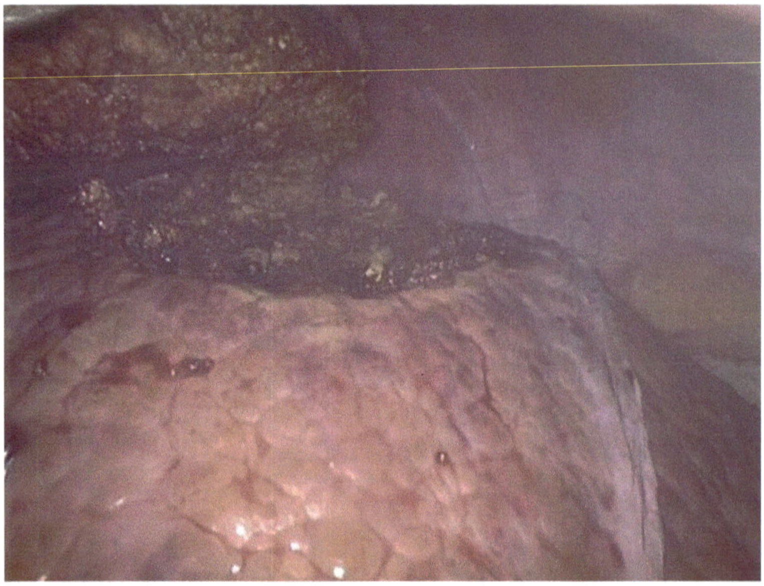

Fig. 7.55 The lesion is elevated, and it is followed by the resection of the lesion

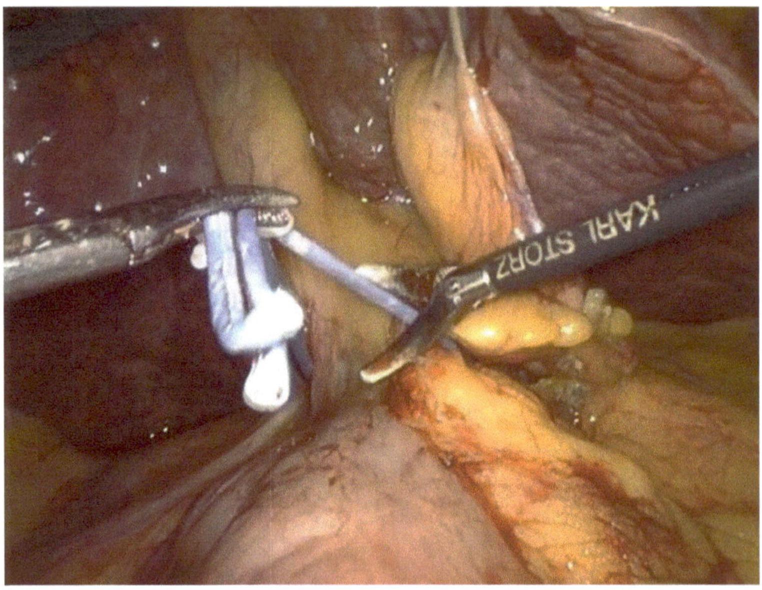

Fig. 7.56 After the tumor was removed, the round-the-hepatoduodenal tapes which were placed for the potential execution of total vascular occlusion are removed

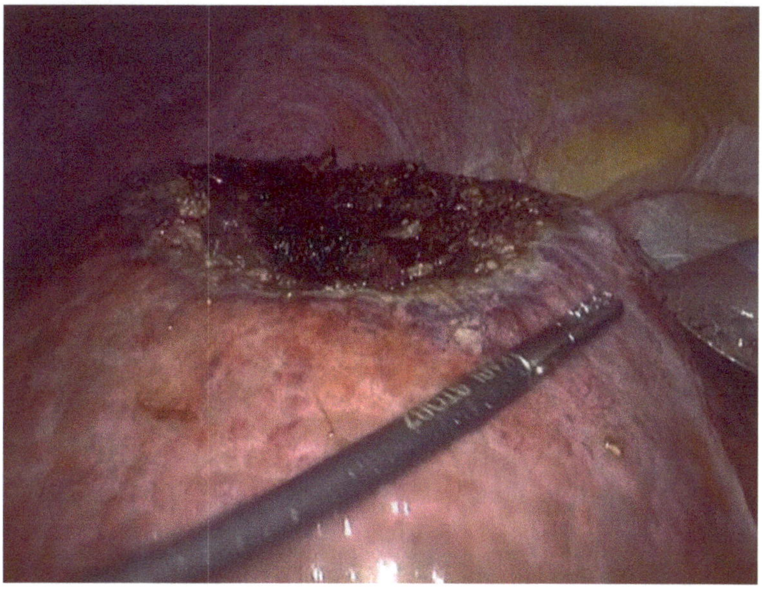

Fig. 7.57 The view of the raw surface after the lesion was removed

7.5 Laparoscopic Bisegmentectomy (Segment VI, VII)

See Figs. 7.58, 7.59, 7.60, 7.61, 7.62, 7.63, 7.64, 7.65, 7.66, 7.67, 7.68, 7.69, 7.70, 7.71, 7.72, 7.73, 7.74, 7.75, 7.76, 7.77, 7.78, 7.79, 7.80, and 7.81.

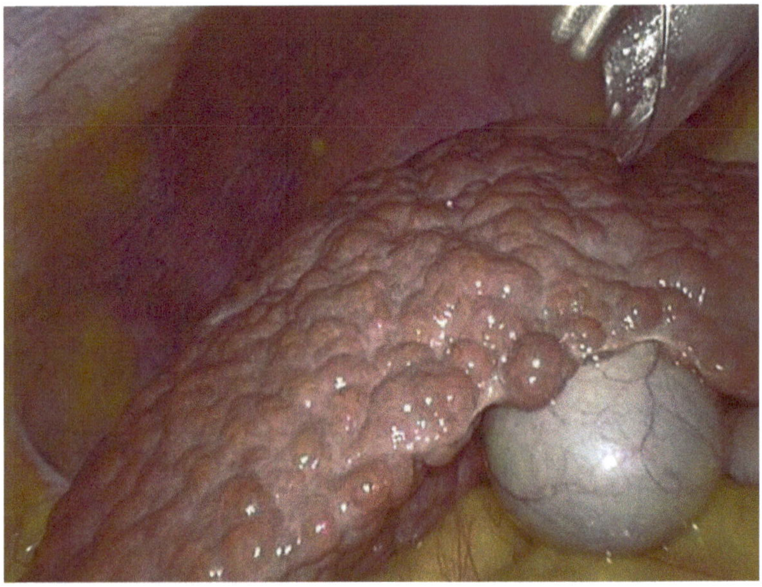

Fig. 7.58 Nodular liver cirrhosis is observed on the liver surface

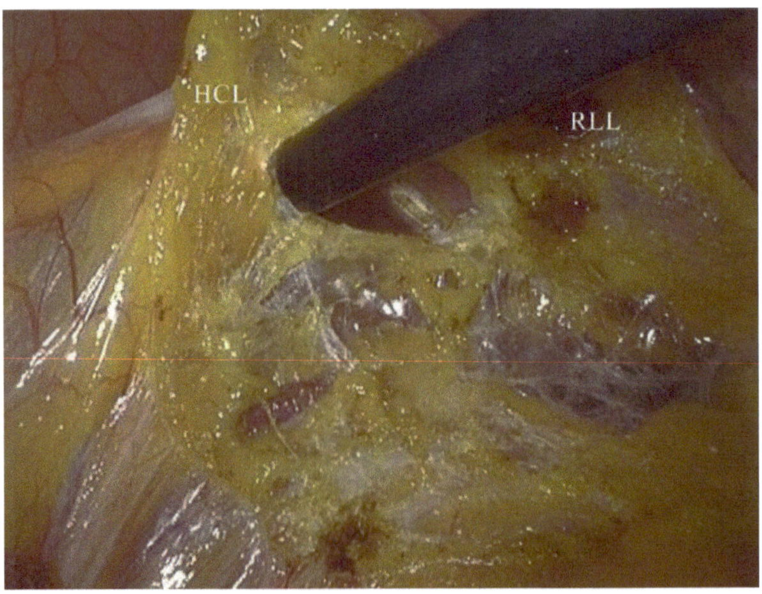

Fig. 7.59 The liver is mobilized upward, and the hepatocolic ligament (*HCL*) is divided with LPMOD

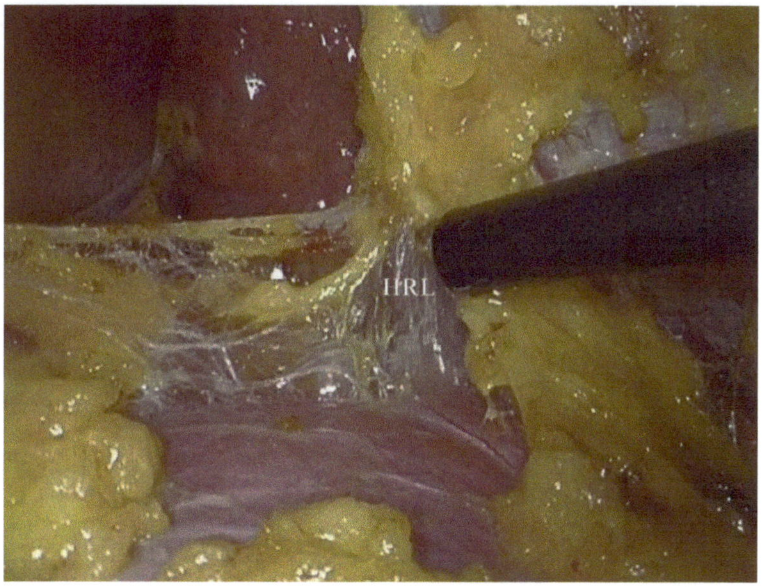

Fig. 7.60 The HRL is divided with LPMOD

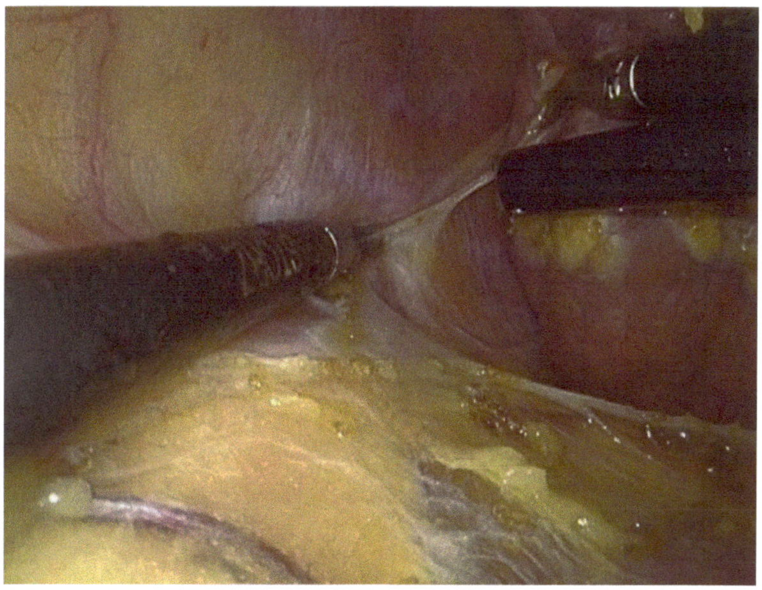

Fig. 7.61 The RLL is mobilized to the right, and the RTL is divided with LPMOD

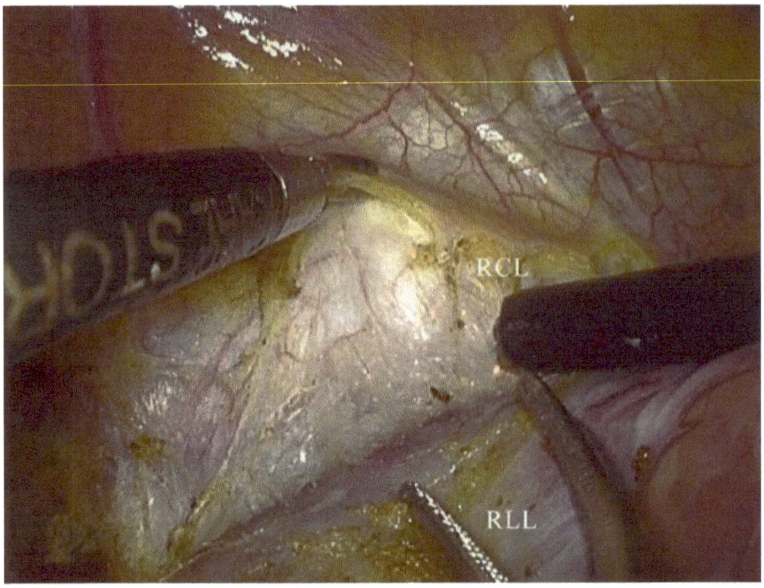

Fig. 7.62 The RLL is pressed downward, and the RCL is divided with LPMOD

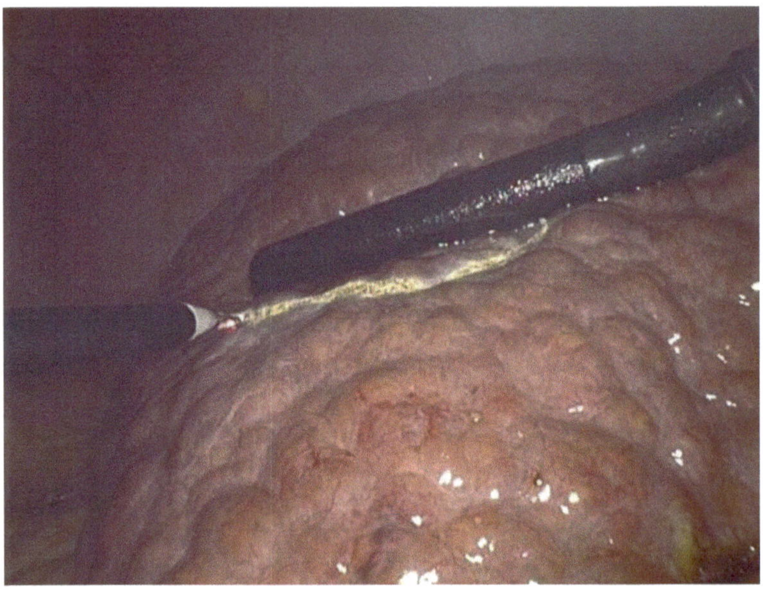

Fig. 7.63 Laparoscopic ultrasound is performed to locate the liver tumor, and the tumor location is marked on the liver surface according to the guidance of the laparoscopic ultrasound

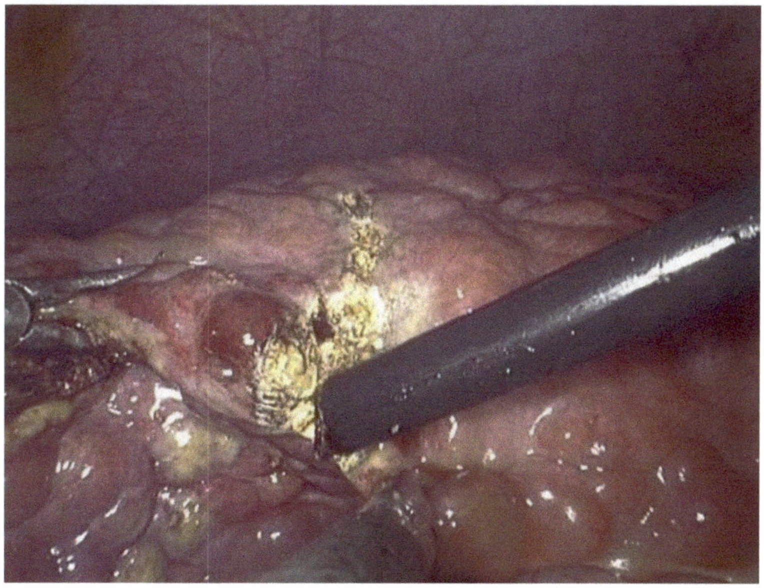

Fig. 7.64 Liver parenchyma is transected with LPMOD

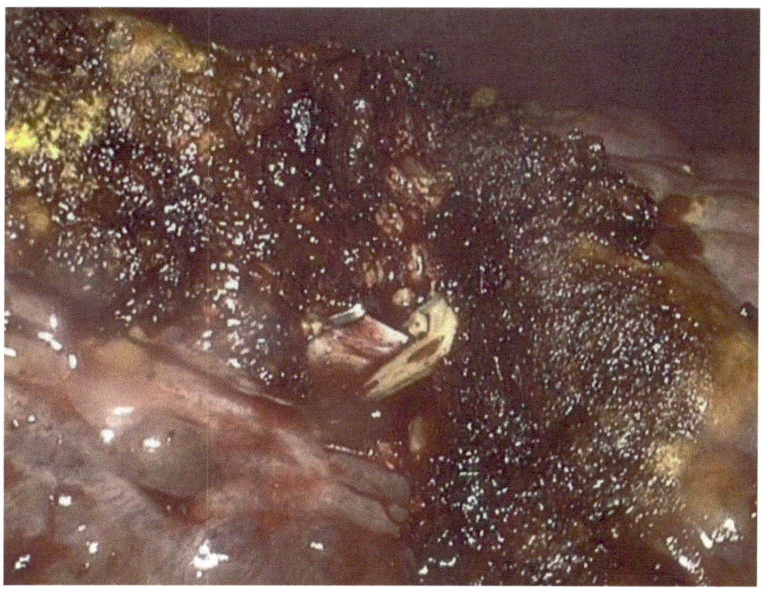

Fig. 7.65 A branch of the right hepatic artery (RHA) is dissected and is clamped with an absorbable clip, and a titanic clip is applied on the distal portion of the branch of the RHA

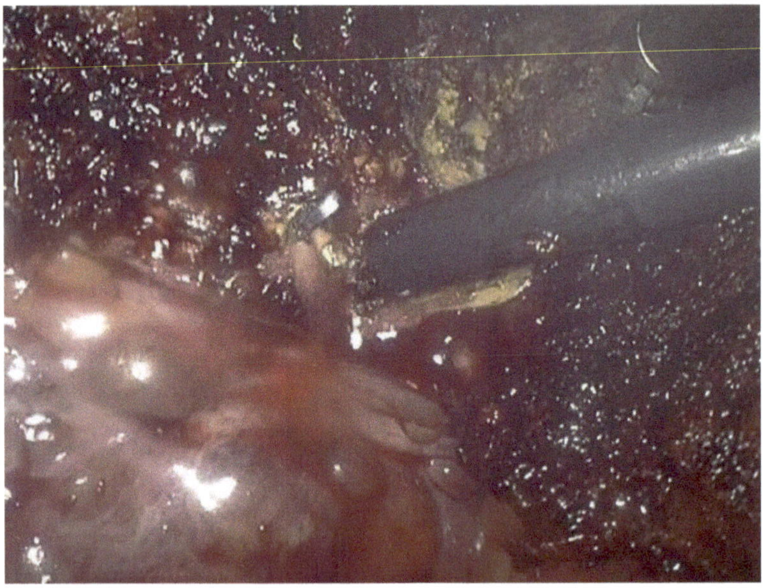

Fig. 7.66 The branch of RHA is divided between the clips with LPMOD

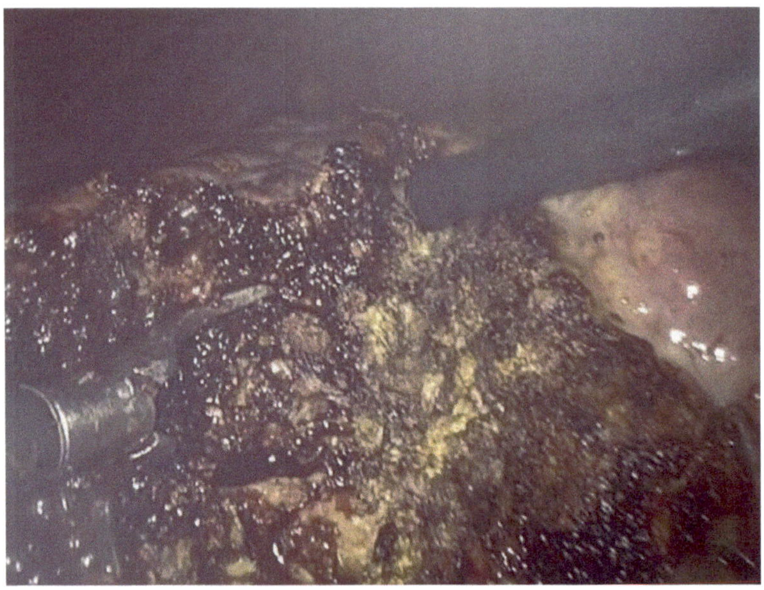

Fig. 7.67 Liver parenchyma is transected with LPMOD

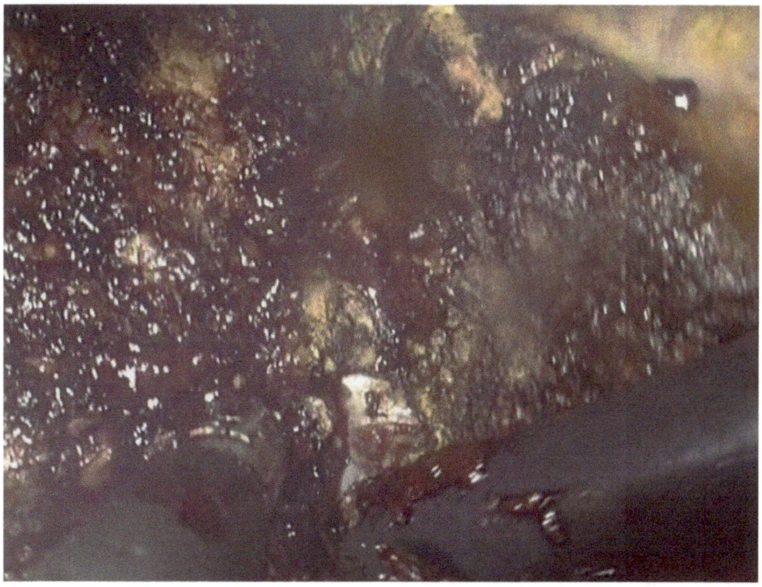

Fig. 7.68 A branch of the hepatic vein is dissected with LPMOD

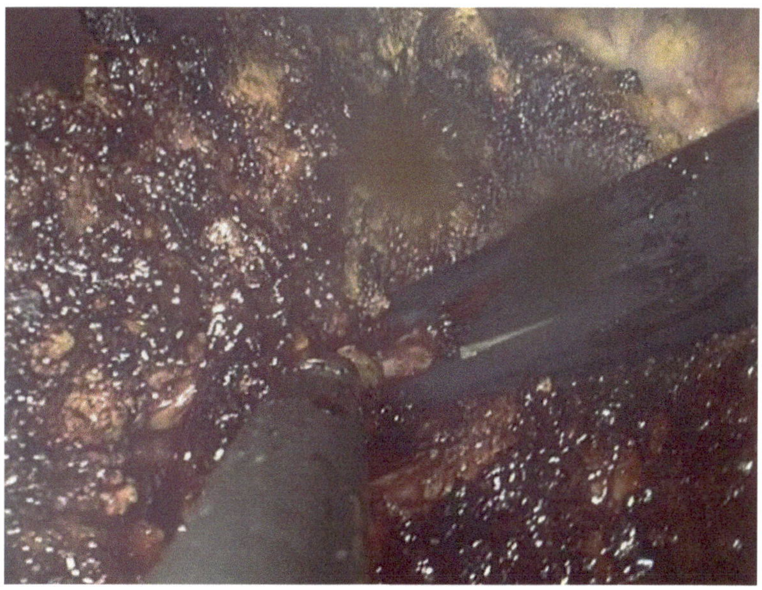

Fig. 7.69 The branch of the hepatic vein is clamped with an absorbable clip

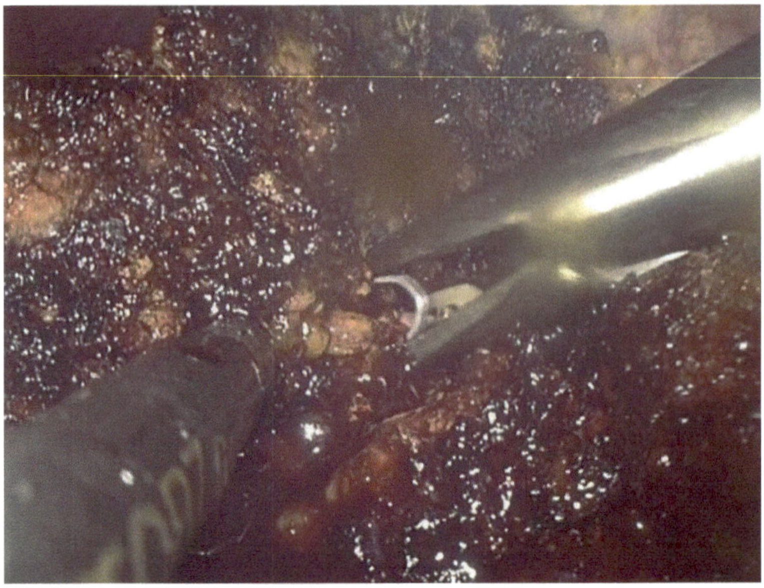

Fig. 7.70 A titanic clip is applied on the distal portion of the branch of the hepatic vein

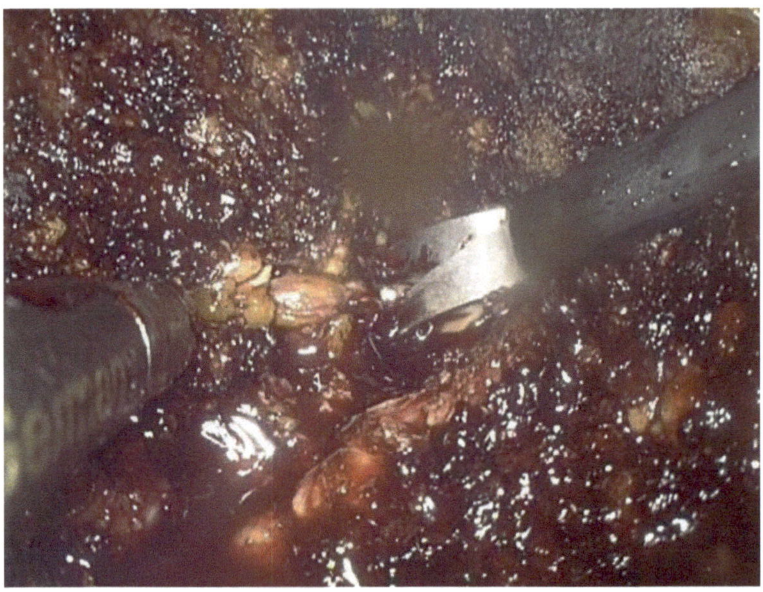

Fig. 7.71 The branch of the hepatic vein is divided

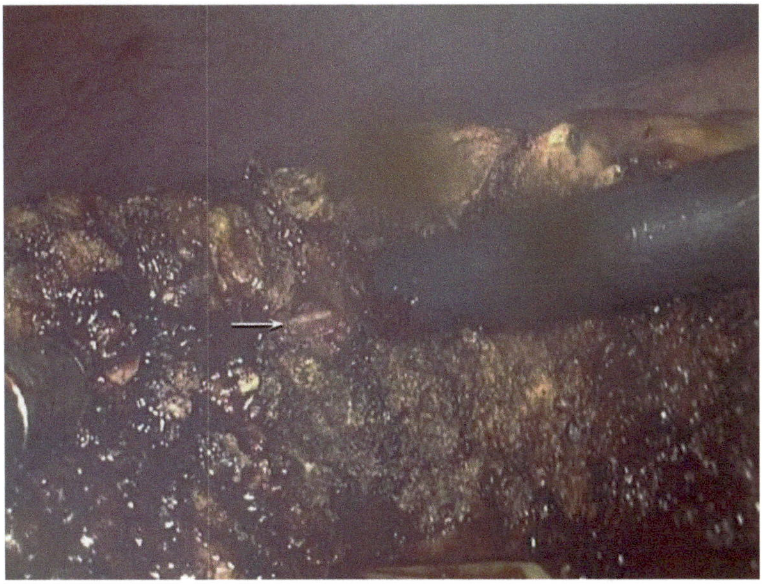

Fig. 7.72 A small vessel (*arrow*) is dissected in liver transection

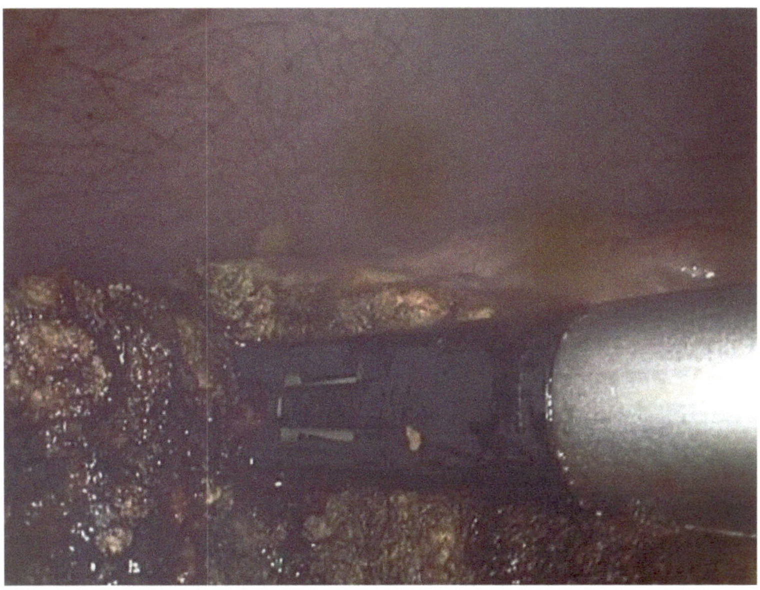

Fig. 7.73 The small vessel is clamped with an absorbable clip

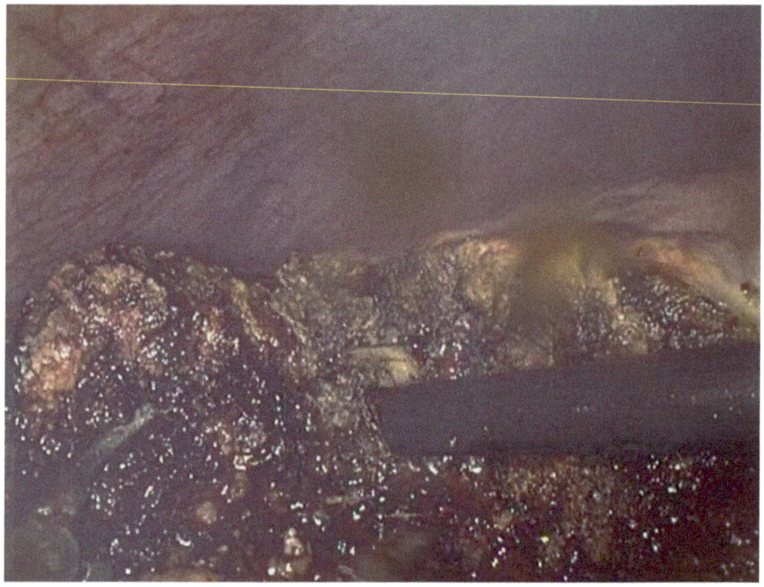

Fig. 7.74 The small vessel is divided with LPMOD

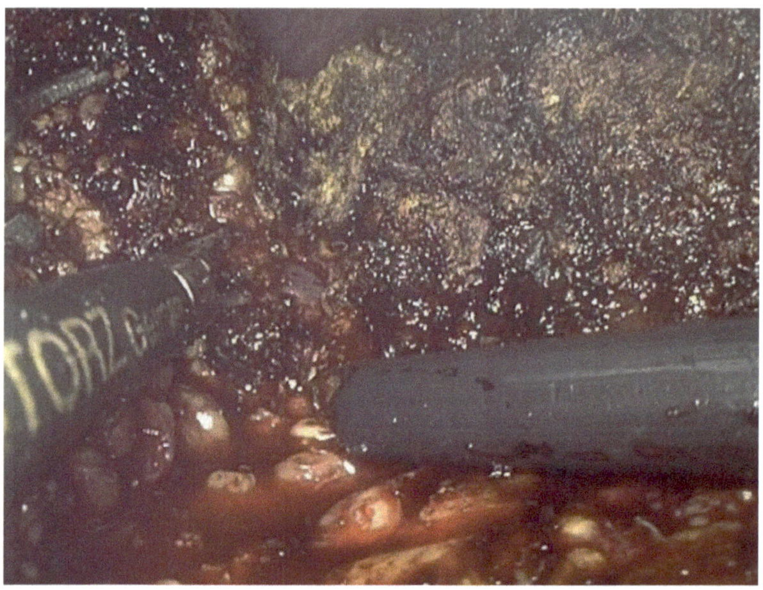

Fig. 7.75 Another small vessel is dissected with LPMOD

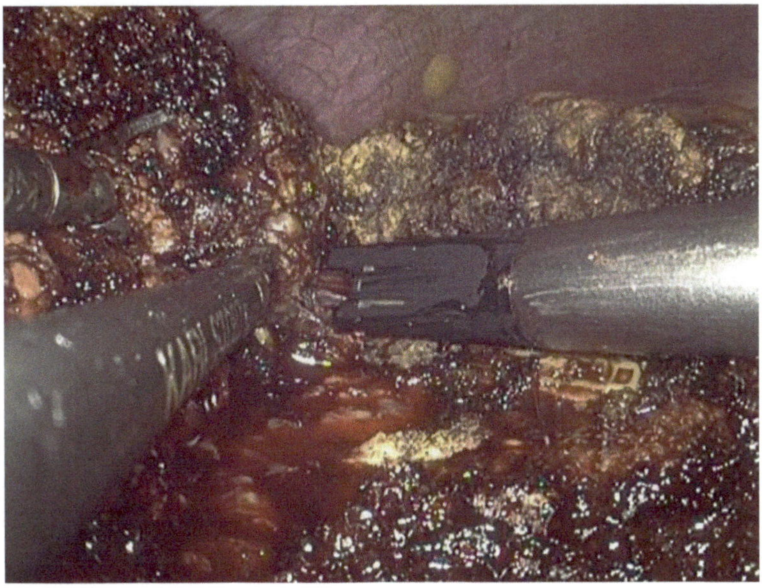

Fig. 7.76 The small vessel is clamped with an absorbable clip

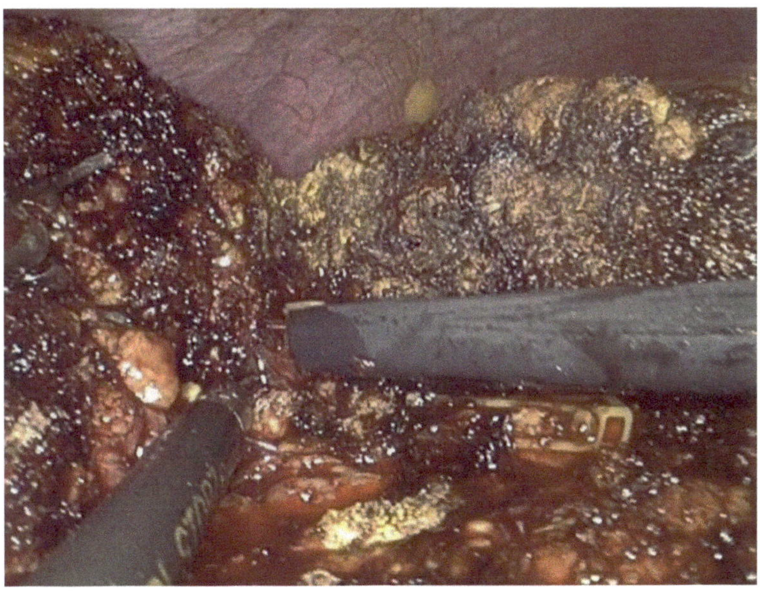

Fig. 7.77 The small vessel is divided with LPMOD

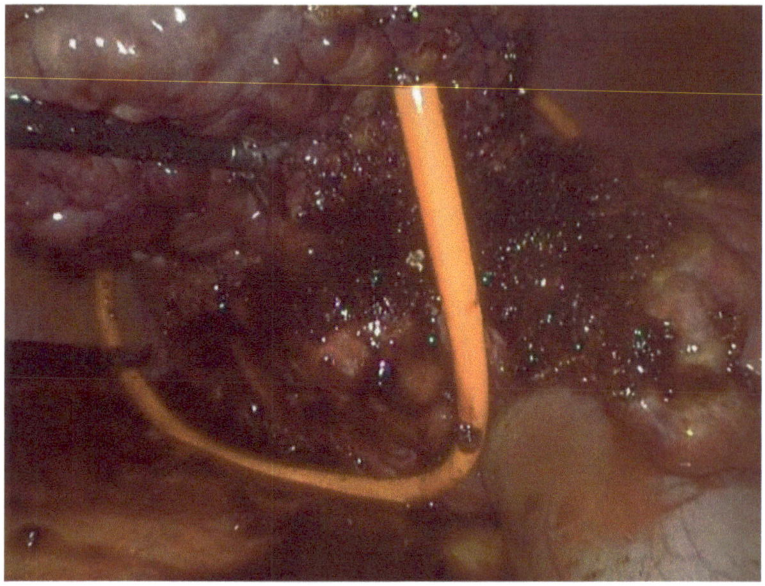

Fig. 7.78 The right posterior section is elevated with a laparoscopic grasping forceps, and a urinary catheter is rounded the transection plane

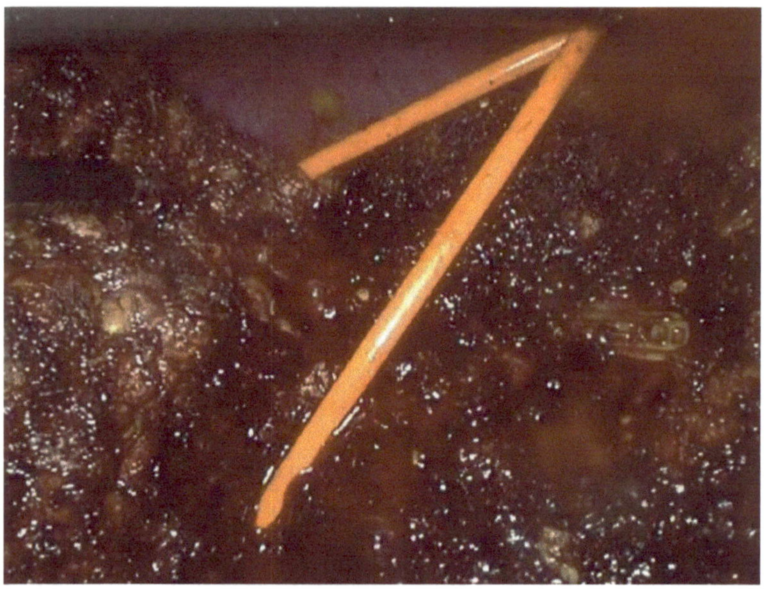

Fig. 7.79 The transection plane is lifted with the "round-the-liver" tape

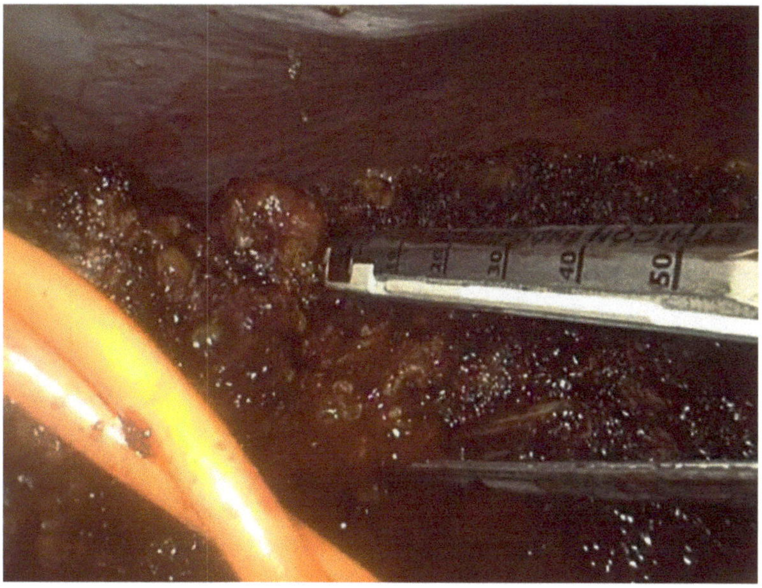

Fig. 7.80 The remaining liver parenchyma and branches of the hepatic vein are transected with a laparoscopic linear staple

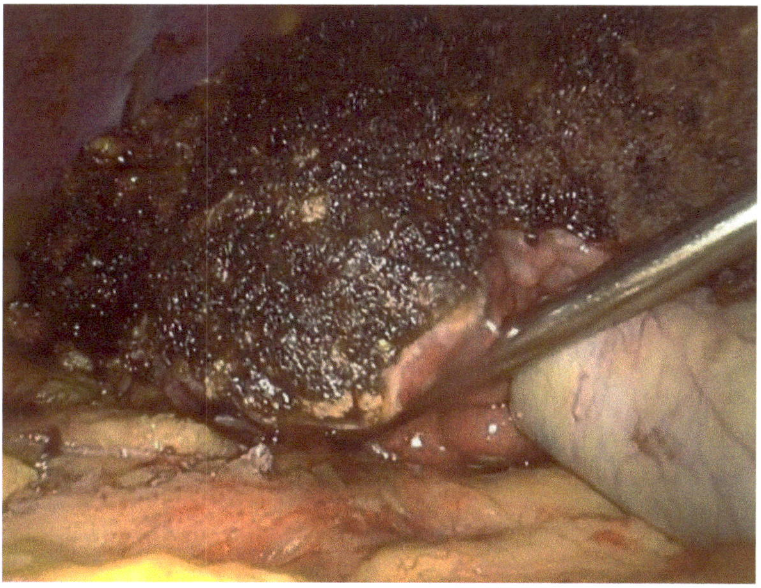

Fig. 7.81 The view of the transection plane after the right posterior section was removed

Reference

Cai XJ, Yu H, Liang X, et al. Laparoscopic hepatectomy by curettage and aspiration: experiences of 62 cases. Surg Endosc. 2006;20:1531–5.

Two-Stage Completely Laparoscopic Hemihepatectomy: Completely Laparoscopic ALPPS Using Round-the-Liver Ligation

8

The safety of liver resection mainly depends on the function of the future liver remnant (FLR). Inadequate volume of FLR is associated with a significant increase in postoperative liver failure, especially in patients with liver cirrhosis. Even though laparoscopic hepatectomy could decrease the surgical trauma, it still could not solve the problem of inadequate volume of FLR. In clinical practice, surgical indications for patients with small volumes of FLR are always difficult to make because of the conflict between safety and oncological radicality. Two effective methods for increasing volume of FLR are adopted. One is portal vein ligation or percutaneous portal vein embolization, and the other is a two-stage surgery. However, these methods require several weeks for liver regeneration before the resection of liver malignancy. The risk of tumor progression during the waiting time is of concern by surgeons (Hayashi et al. 2007; Kokudo et al. 2001). Recently, a new "two-stage" operation which was named as "associating liver partition with portal vein ligation for staged hepatectomy (ALPPS)" by de Santibañes and Clavien (2012) has drawn the attention of surgeons. This method enables the rapid growth of FLR. However, the complication of bile leakage increased. In Schnitzbauer's report (Schnitzbauer et al. 2012), bile leakage was observed in 24 % of the patients and the mortality was 12 %. The safety of the ALPPS was questioned by some surgeons (Kokudo and Shindoh 2013). The procedure of the in situ splitting of the liver was supposed to the major cause of the high occurrence rate of biliary leakage. This procedure was modified by Robles Campos et al. (2013). A round-the-liver ligation was executed to replace liver splitting to avoid the complication of biliary leakage and simplify the procedure as well (Fig. 8.1).

Totally laparoscopic ALPPS was described by Machado et al. in a letter to the editor in 2012. Differing from his cases, we adopted the execution of the round-the-liver ligation to replace the in situ splitting of the liver that could avoid postoperative bile leakage and might simplify the operation. Laparoscopic meticulous dissection is the point of the first-stage operation. The aspiration tube and 90°-angle forceps are good instruments for blunt dissection which could safely free the branches of portal vein (PV) and hepatic veins. The ligation would become loose after the first-stage operation for the gradual atrophy of the liver parenchyma under the ligature, so it is necessary to tighten the ligation a few days after the first-stage operation.

In 2014, completely laparoscopic ALPPS using round-the-liver ligation was performed on patients with an estimated volume of FLR lower than 40 % to achieve a radical resection of multiple liver malignancies, and a rapid increase of FLR volume was observed. Theoretically, the

Electronic supplementary material The online version of this chapter at (doi: 10.1007/978-94-017-9840-2_8) contains supplementary material, which is available to authorized users.

X. Cai, *Laparoscopic Hepatectomy: Atlas and Techniques*,
DOI 10.1007/978-94-017-9840-2_8,

advantage of minimal invasion of laparoscopic surgery would decrease surgical trauma and lead to a lower occurrence rate of postoperative liver failure. The adoption of round-the-liver which replaced liver splitting could avoid biliary leakage and simplify the first-stage operation and finally could lead to decreases in perioperative morbidity and mortality. However, this procedure is still in the exploration stage. The value of this procedure should be further evaluated.

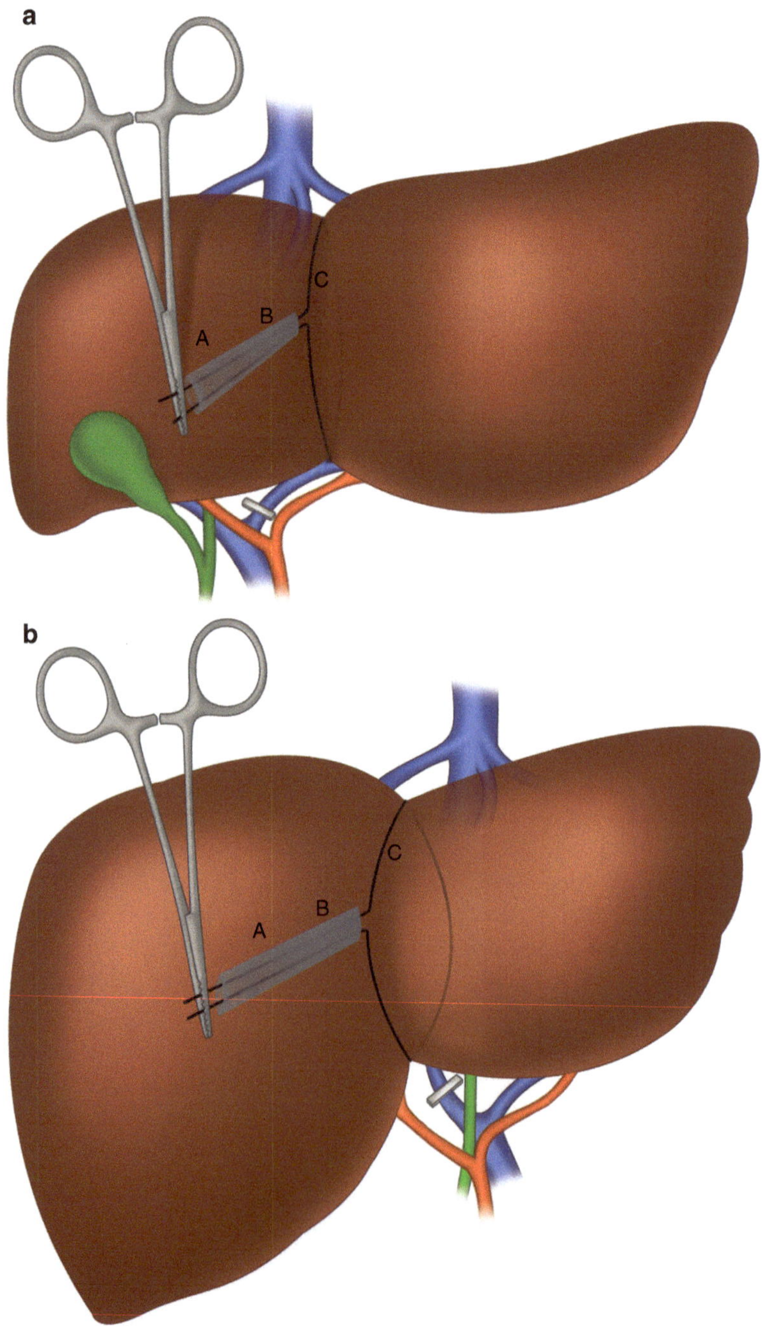

Fig. 8.1 Placement of the round-the-liver ligature in the two-stage completely laparoscopic left hemihepatectomy (**a**) and the two-stage completely laparoscopic right hemihepatectomy (**b**). (*a*) Abdominal wall; (*b*) Thoracic tube; (*c*) Round-the-liver ligature

8.1 Indications and Contraindications

Indications include liver tumors requiring left hemihepatectomy, estimated volume of FLR lower than 40 %, and with liver cirrhosis and liver function of Child A to B classification. The contraindication is malignant tumor involving porta hepatic (PH).

8.2 Patient Position and Trocars' Position

Patients are placed in the supine position under general anesthesia. Three surgeons are needed in the operation. The senior surgeon stands on the left side of the patient, one assistant surgeon stands on the right side of the senior surgeon controlling the aspiration device, and the other assistant surgeon stands on the right side of the patient. Four entries are made. A supraumbilical 10-mm trocar is inserted as the observation port. A 12-mm trocar is inserted below the xiphoid as the main manipulation port for right liver lesions or is inserted below the left costal margin for left liver lesions. And two 5-mm trocars are inserted at the right flank area as assistant manipulation ports (Fig. 8.2).

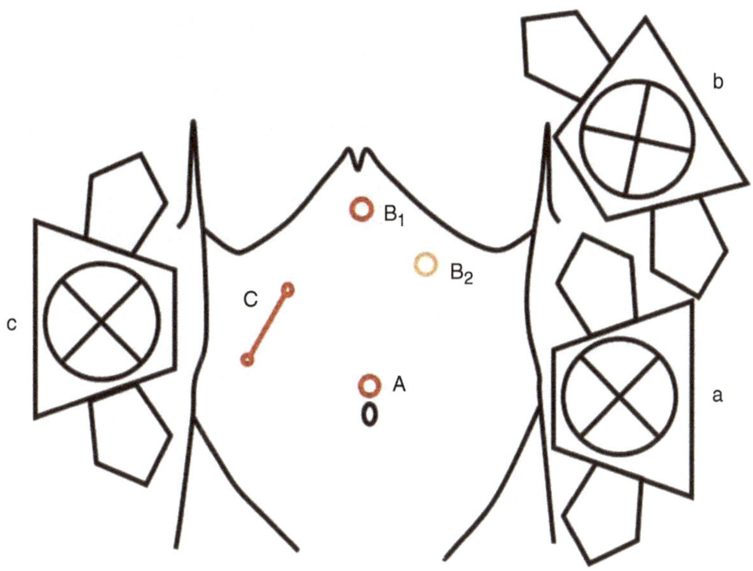

Fig. 8.2 Trocars' position and surgeons' position. (*A*) Observation port; (B_1) Main manipulation port for right liver lesions; (B_2) Main manipulation port for left liver lesions; (*C*) Two assistant ports and the incision for removing specimen; (**a**) The senior surgeon stands on the left side of the patient; (**b**) One assistant stands on the right side of the senior surgeon controlling the aspiration device; (**c**) The other assistant surgeon stands on the right side of the patient

8.3 Two-Stage Laparoscopic Left Hemihepatectomy

The first-stage operation: laparoscopic ALPPS using round-the-liver ligation (Figs. 8.3, 8.4, 8.5, 8.6, 8.7, 8.8, 8.9, 8.10, 8.11, 8.12, 8.13, 8.14, 8.15, 8.16, 8.17, 8.18, 8.19, 8.20, 8.21, 8.22, 8.23, 8.24, 8.25, 8.26, 8.27, 8.28, 8.29, 8.30, 8.31, and Video 8.1).

The second-stage operation: laparoscopic left hemihepatectomy (Figs. 8.32, 8.33, 8.34, 8.35, 8.36, 8.37, 8.38, 8.39, 8.40, 8.41, 8.42, 8.43, and Video 8.2).

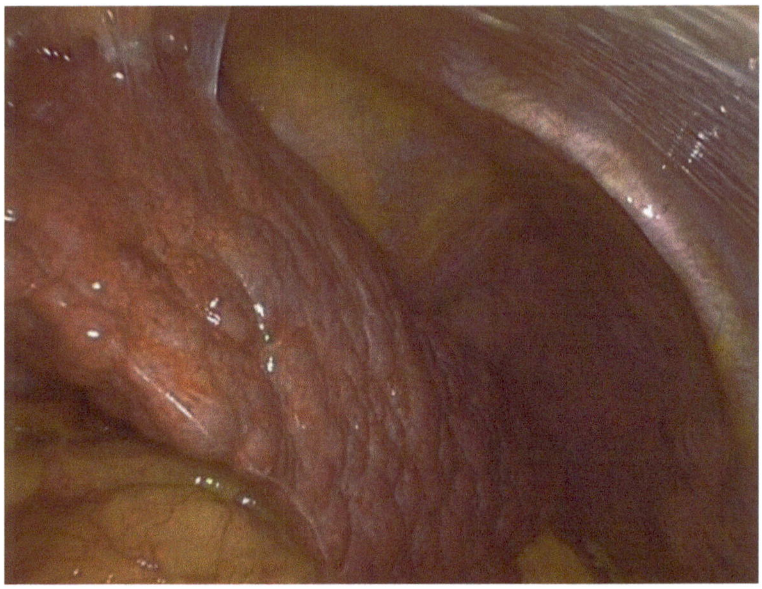

Fig. 8.3 The patient has severe liver cirrhosis due to a hepatitis B infection and the hepatocellular carcinoma in the segment IV which was confirmed by liver biopsy. The estimated volume of FLR is 38.8 %, and his liver function classification is Child A

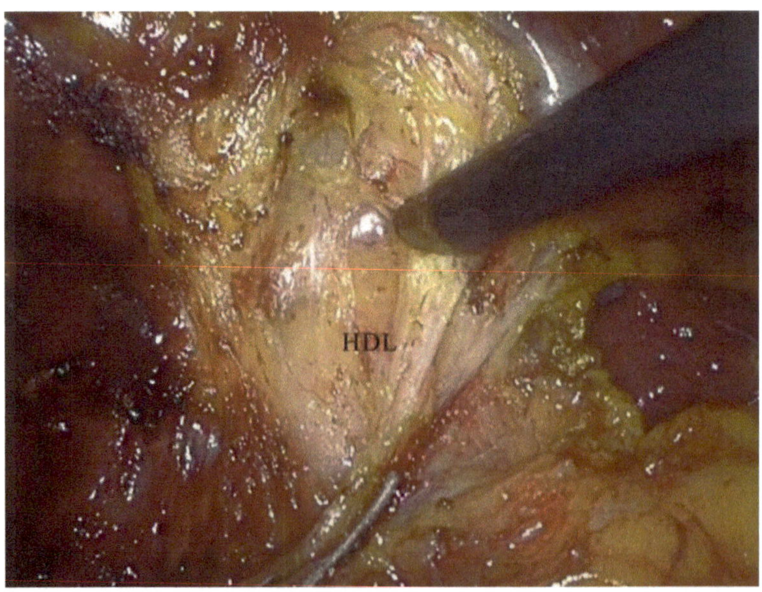

Fig. 8.4 The liver is mobilized upward, and the hepatoduodenal ligament (*HDL*) is dissected with LPMOD

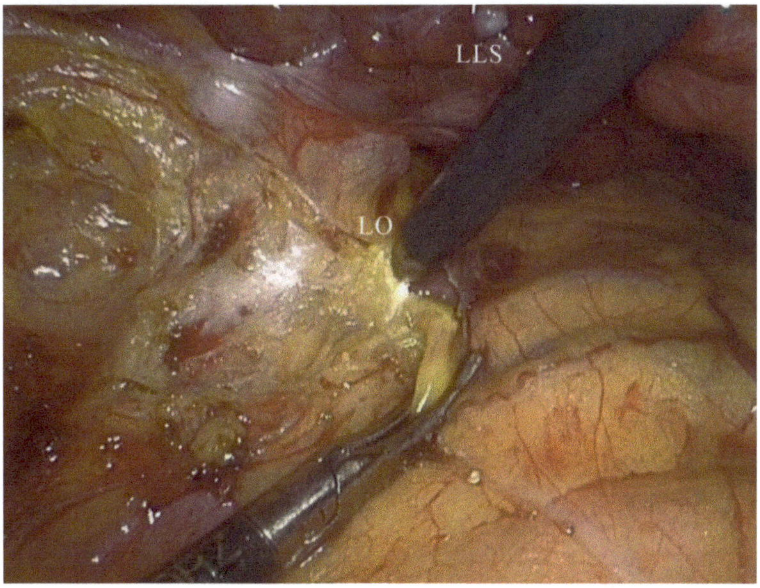

Fig. 8.5 The lesser omentum (*LO*) is partly divided with LPMOD

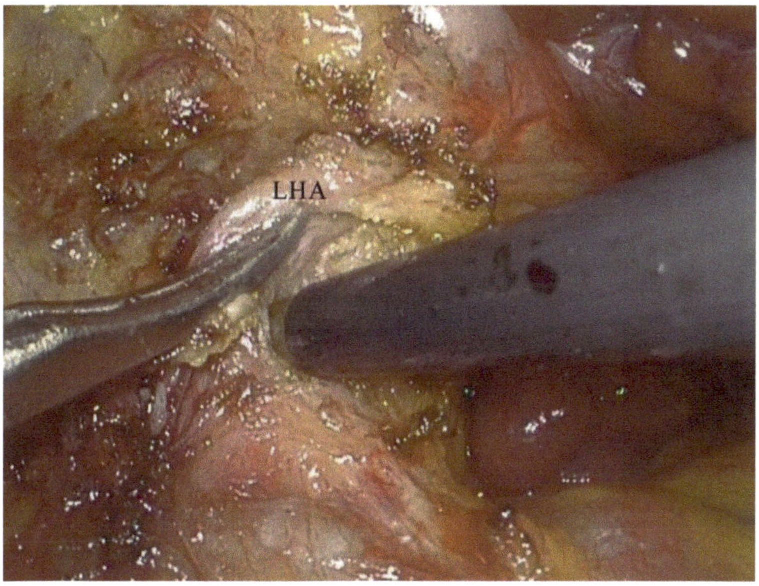

Fig. 8.6 The left hepatic artery (*LHA*) is visualized in the dissection of hepatoduodenal ligament

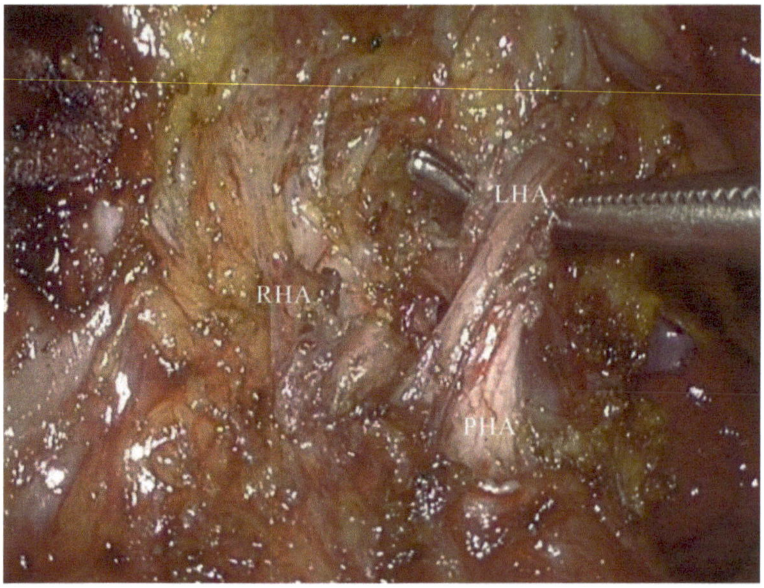

Fig. 8.7 The LHA is freed with a 90°-curved dissecting forceps

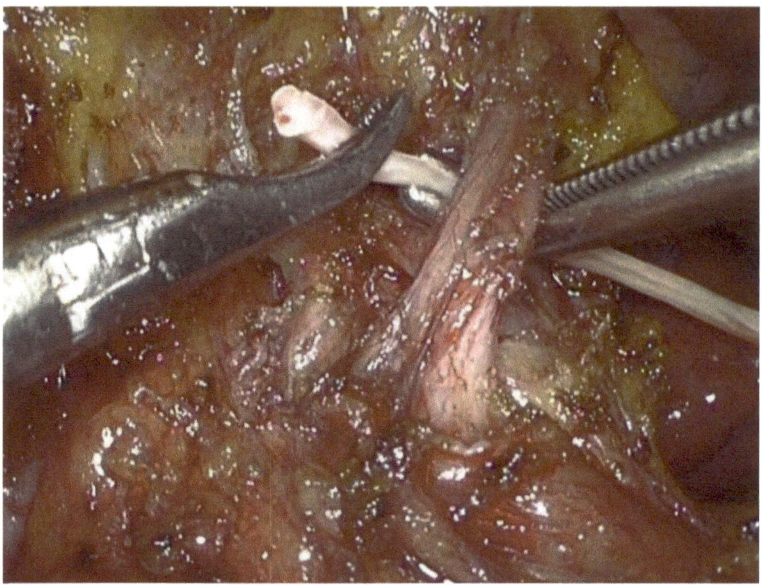

Fig. 8.8 An elastic tape is passed through the back of the LHA

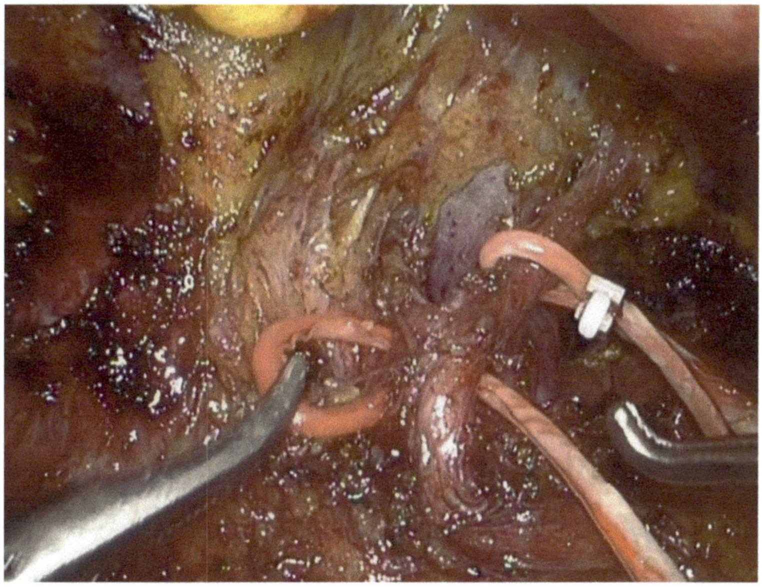

Fig. 8.9 Another elastic tape is passed through the back of the proper hepatic artery

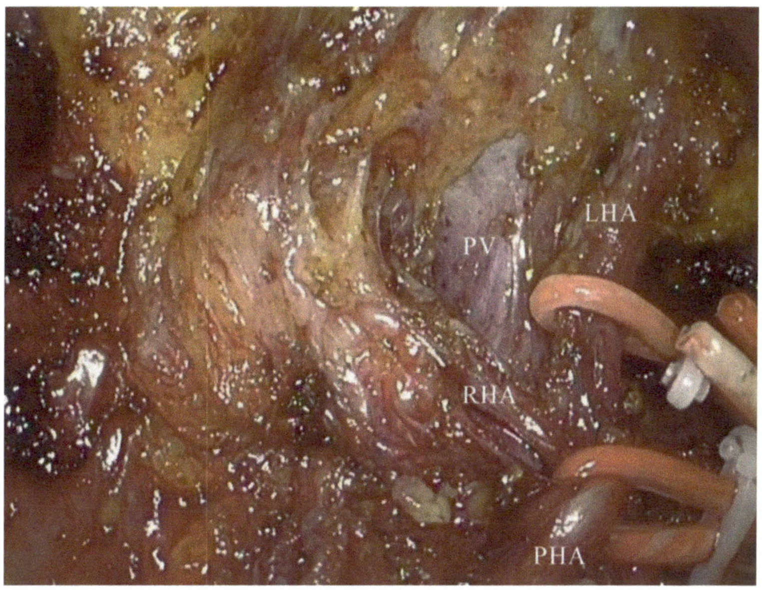

Fig. 8.10 The proper hepatic artery and the LHA are mobilized to the left, and the portal vein (*PV*) is exposed

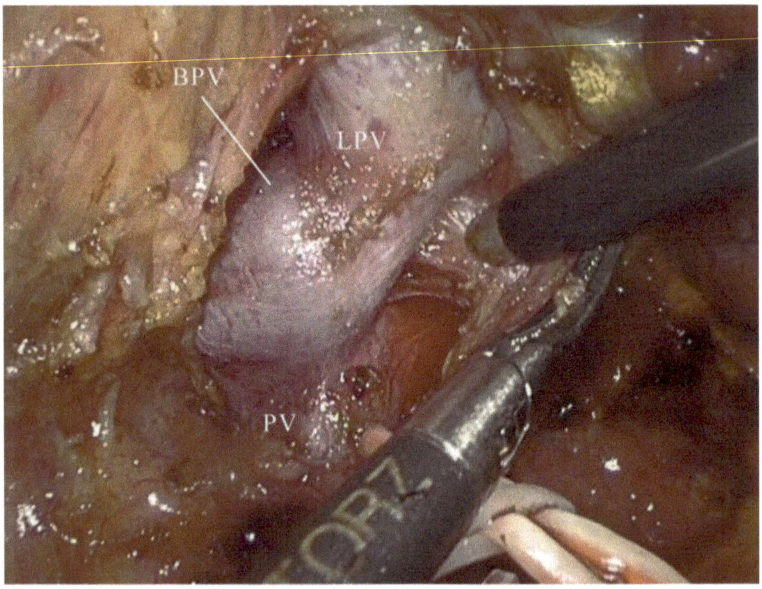

Fig. 8.11 The left branch of the portal vein (*LPV*) is dissected with LPMOD, and the bifurcation of the portal vein (*BPV*) is identified

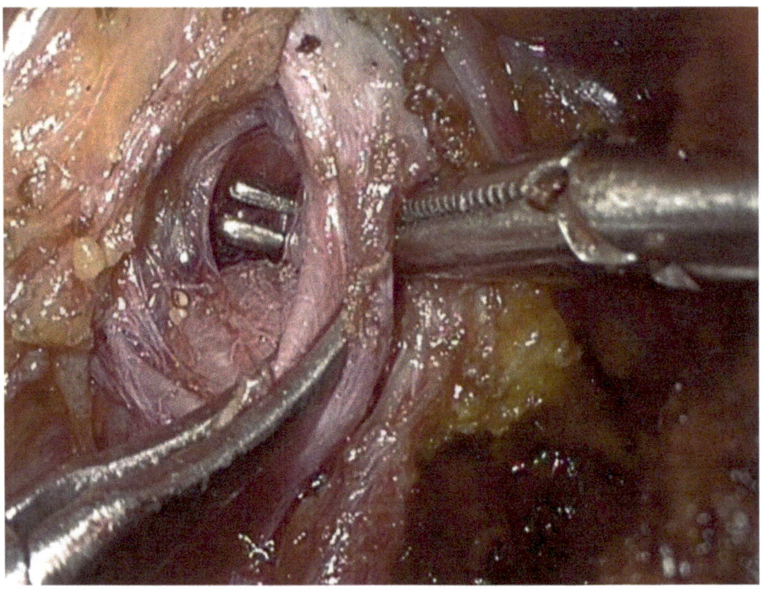

Fig. 8.12 The LPV is freed with a 90°-curved dissecting forceps

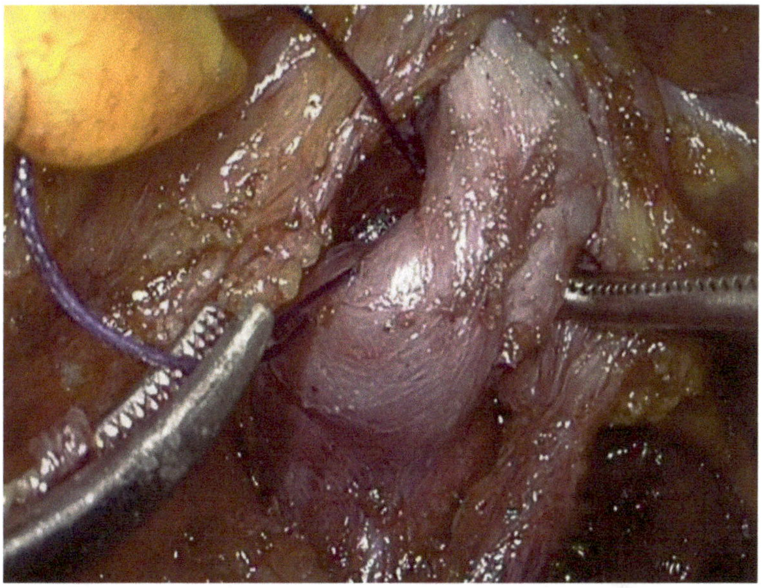

Fig. 8.13 A suture is passed through the back of the LPV with the guidance of the curved dissecting forceps

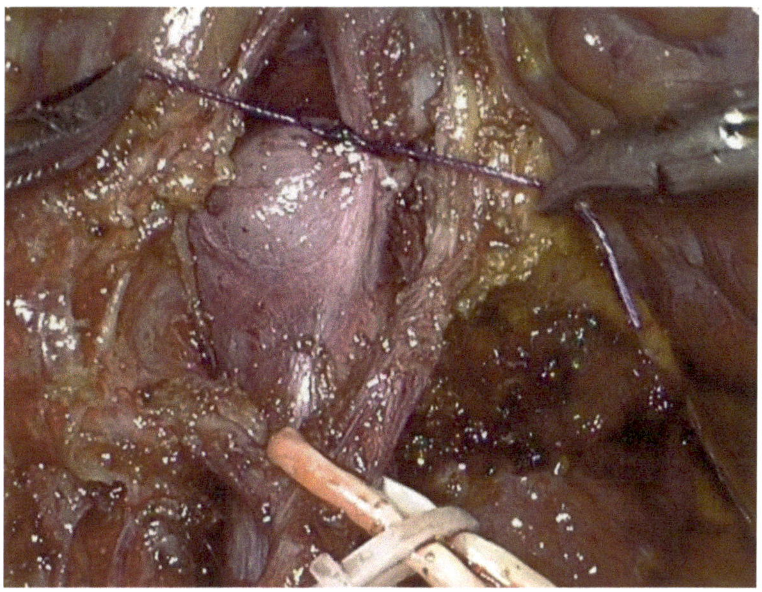

Fig. 8.14 The LPV is ligated

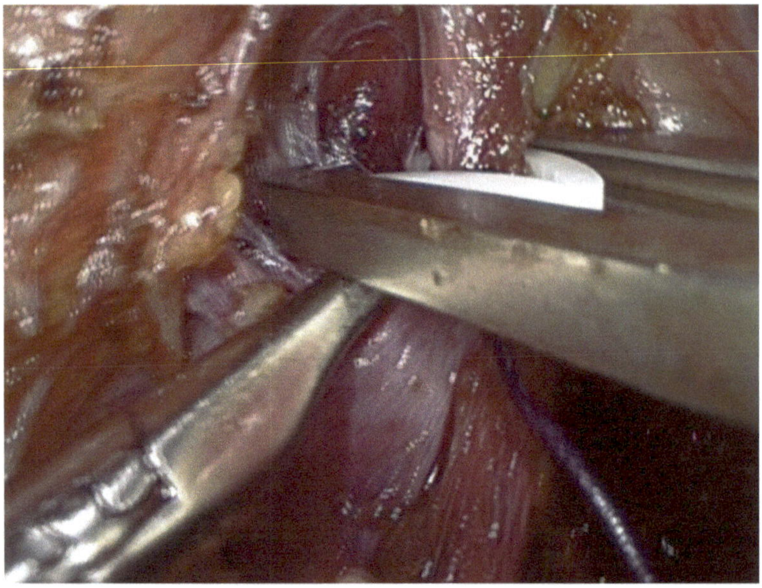

Fig. 8.15 An absorbable clip is applied on the LPV to secure the ligation

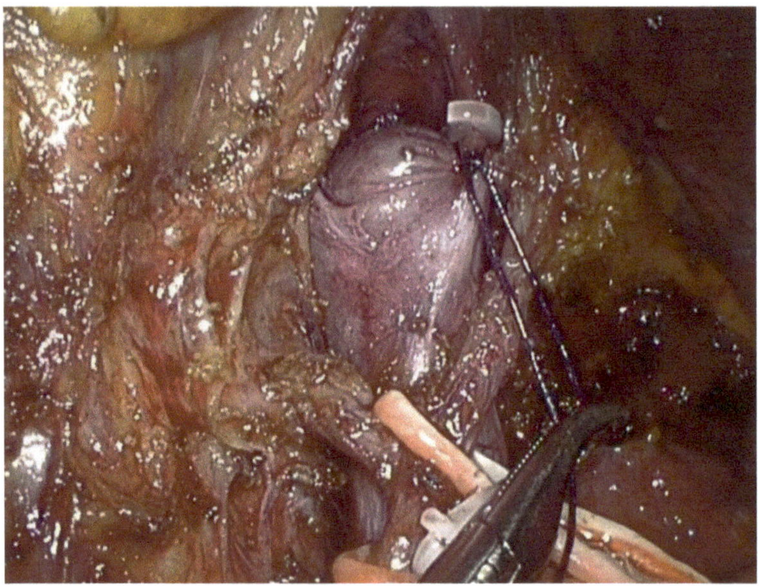

Fig. 8.16 The view of the LPV after being ligated and clamped

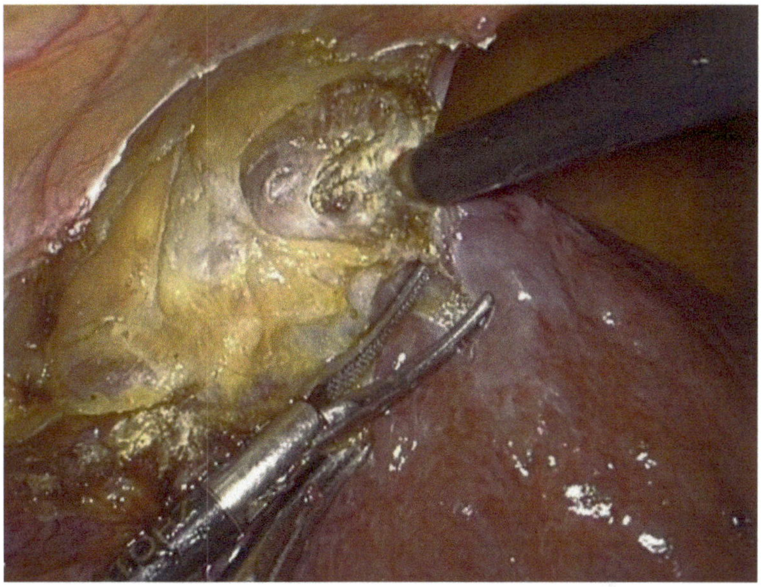

Fig. 8.17 The adhesion and the falciform ligament (FL) are divided with LPMOD

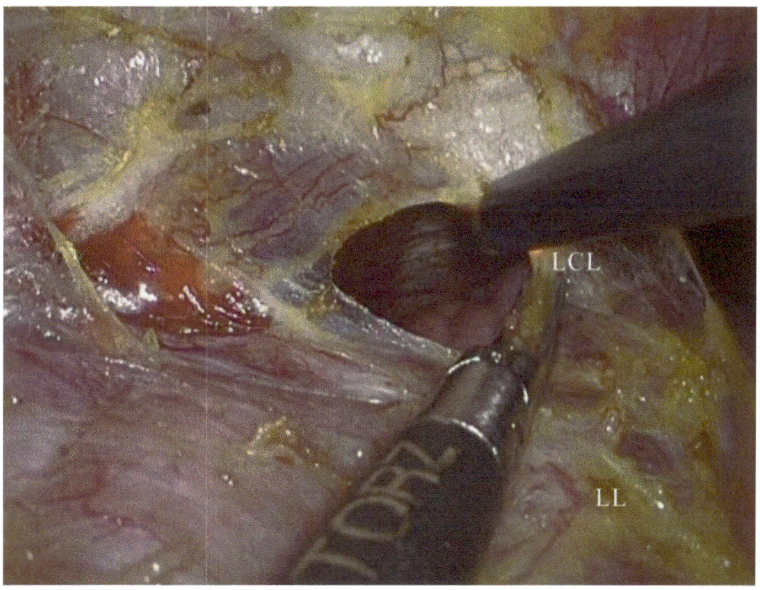

Fig. 8.18 The left coronary ligament (*LCL*) is divided with LPMOD

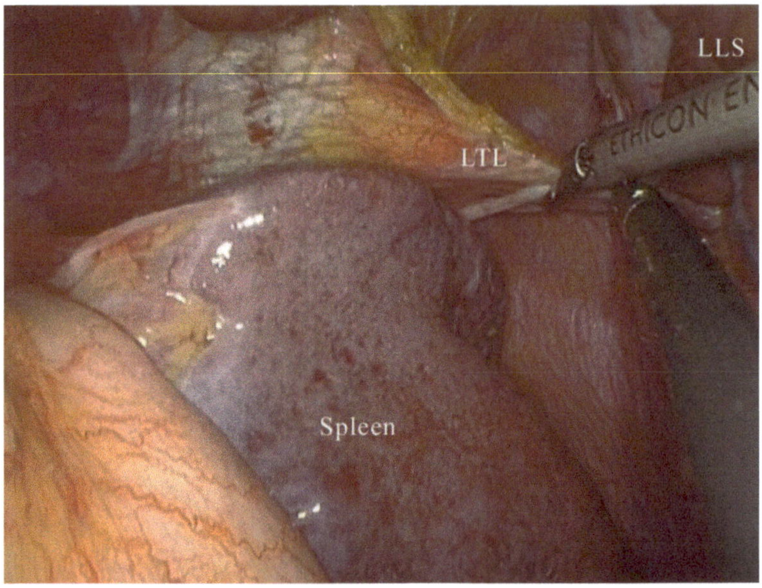

Fig. 8.19 The left triangle ligament (*LTL*) is divided with a ultrasonic scalpel

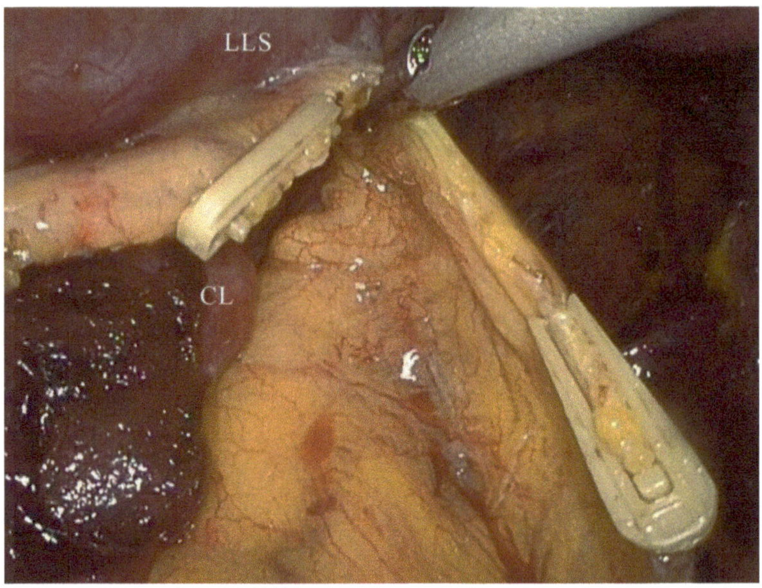

Fig. 8.20 The lesser omentum is further divided with the ultrasonic scalpel

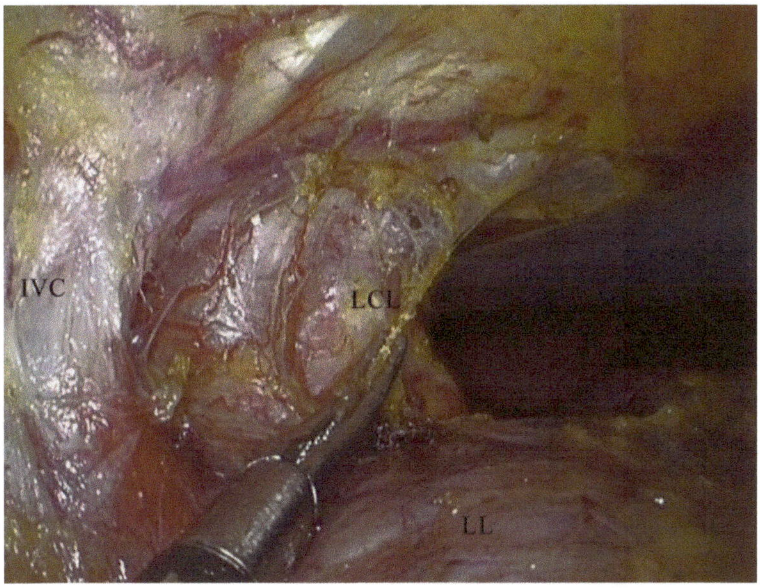

Fig. 8.21 The LCL is further divided with LPMOD

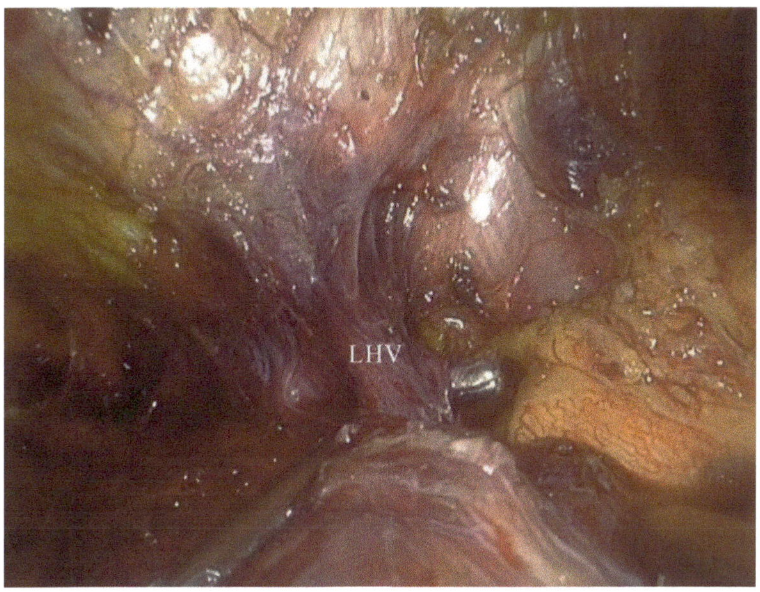

Fig. 8.22 The LHV is freed with the 10-mm 90°-curved dissecting forceps

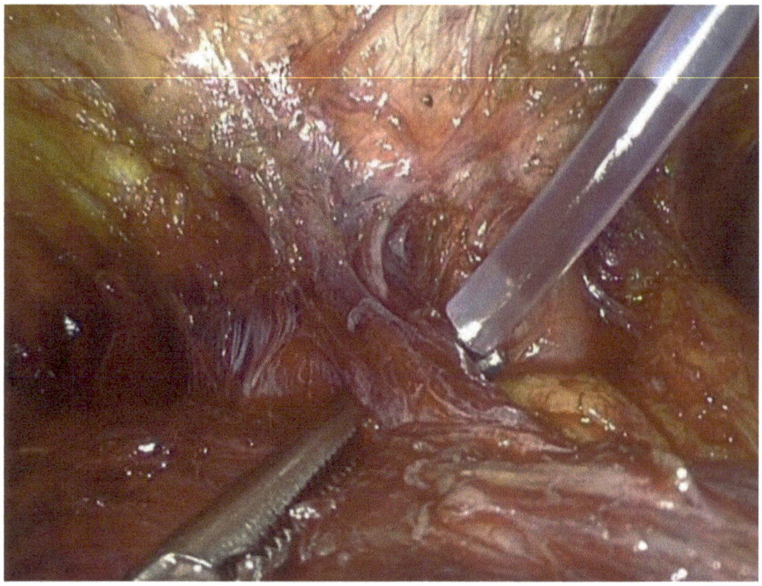

Fig. 8.23 The round-the-liver ligature, a nasogastric tube with a guide wire inside, is passed through the back of the LHV with the guidance of the curved dissecting forceps

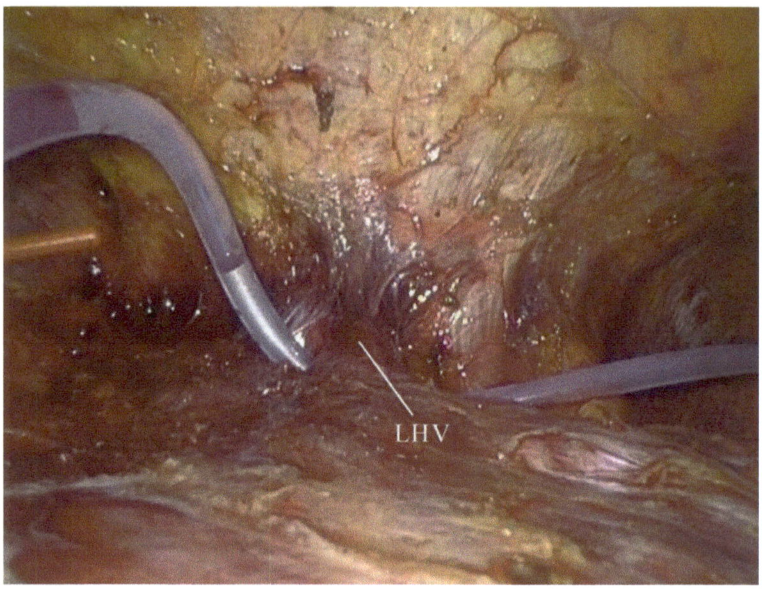

Fig. 8.24 The round-the-liver ligature has passed through the back of the LHV

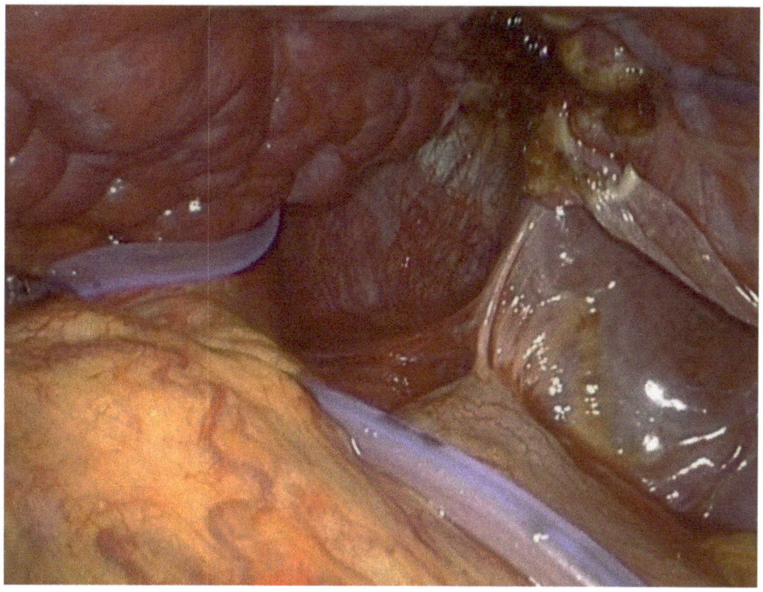

Fig. 8.25 The round-the-liver ligature is rounded the left lobe (LL) of the liver

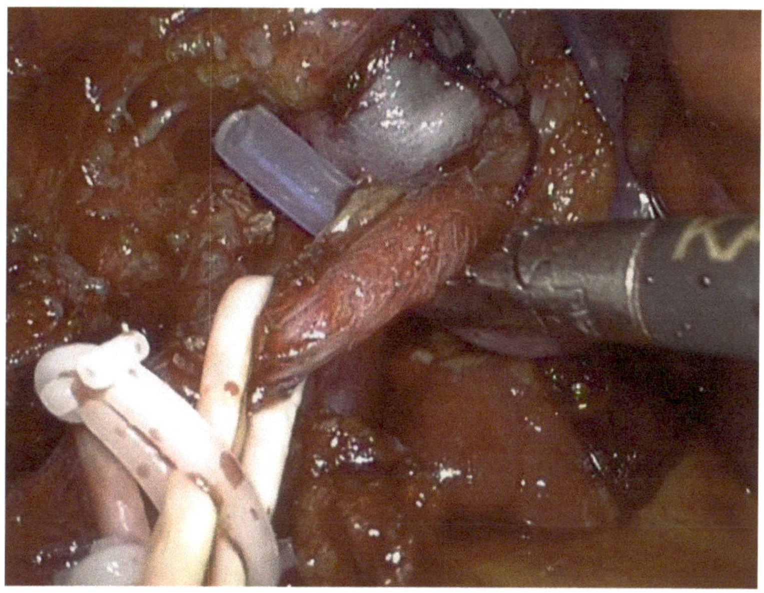

Fig. 8.26 The round-the-liver ligature is passed through the back of the left hepatic artery with the guidance of the curved dissecting forceps

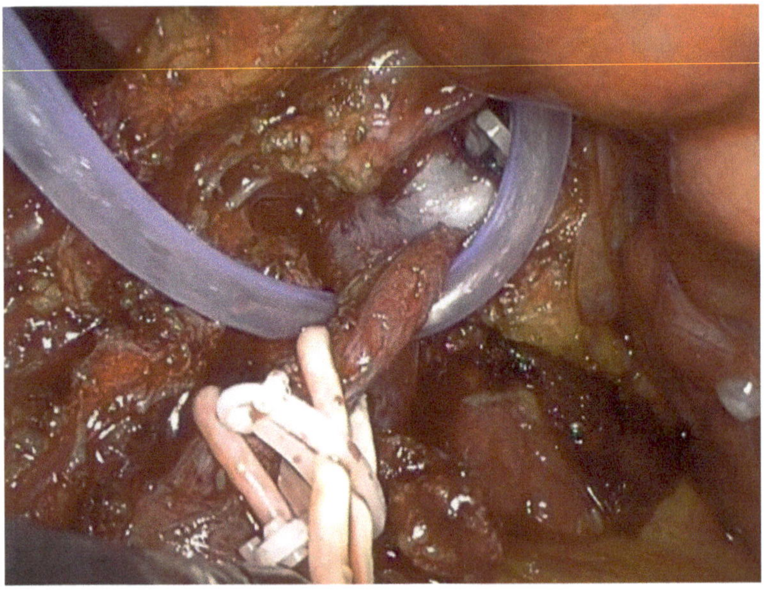

Fig. 8.27 The round-the-liver ligature has been passed through the back of the left hepatic artery

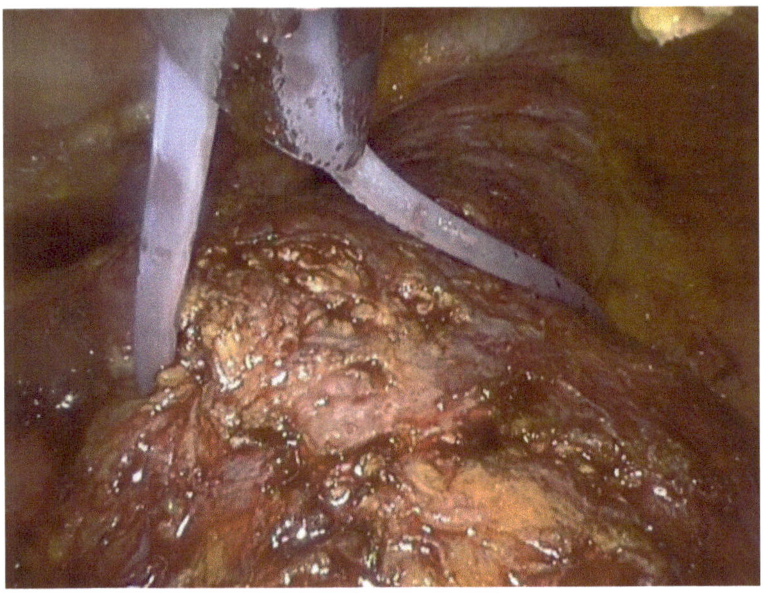

Fig. 8.28 The round-the-liver ligature is rounded the left lobe and is extracted outside the abdominal cavity through the 12-mm manipulation port

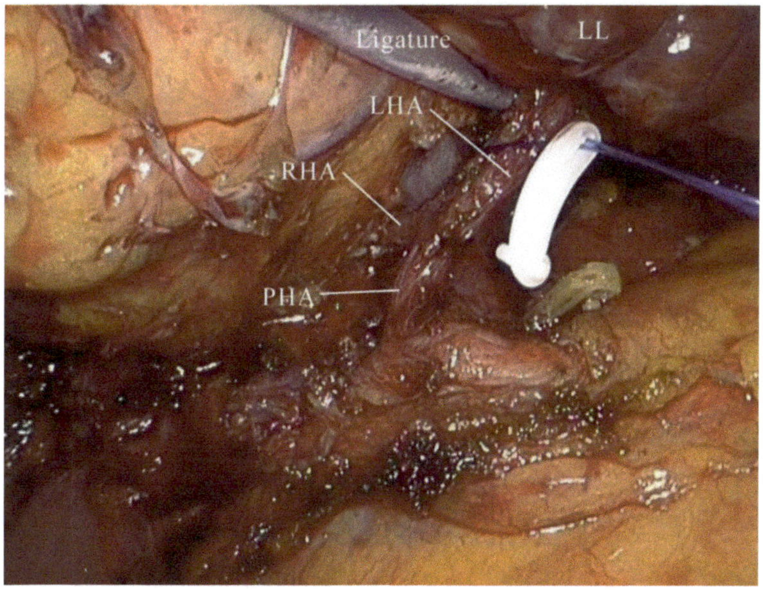

Fig. 8.29 After elastic tapes were removed, a suture is placed around the LHA for the second operation

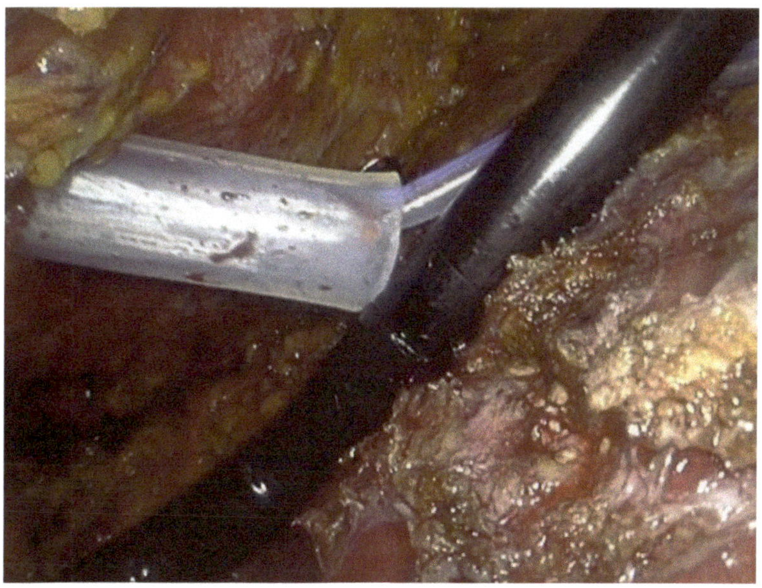

Fig. 8.30 A thoracic tube is inserted through the 12-mm trocar, and both ends of the ligature are passed through the thoracic tube. Laparoscopic ultrasound is performed to guide the placement of the round-the-liver ligature

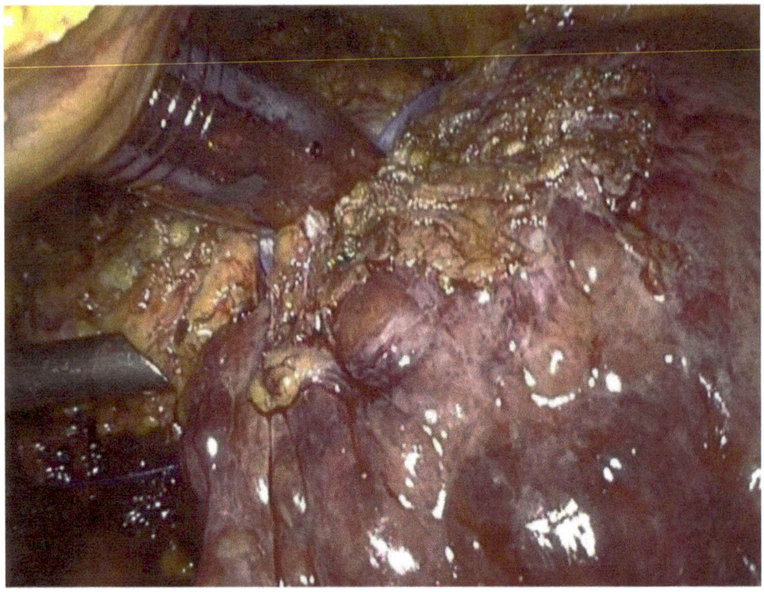

Fig. 8.31 The ligature is closed and is fixed by using the manner which is usually used in total vascular occlusion in open liver surgeries

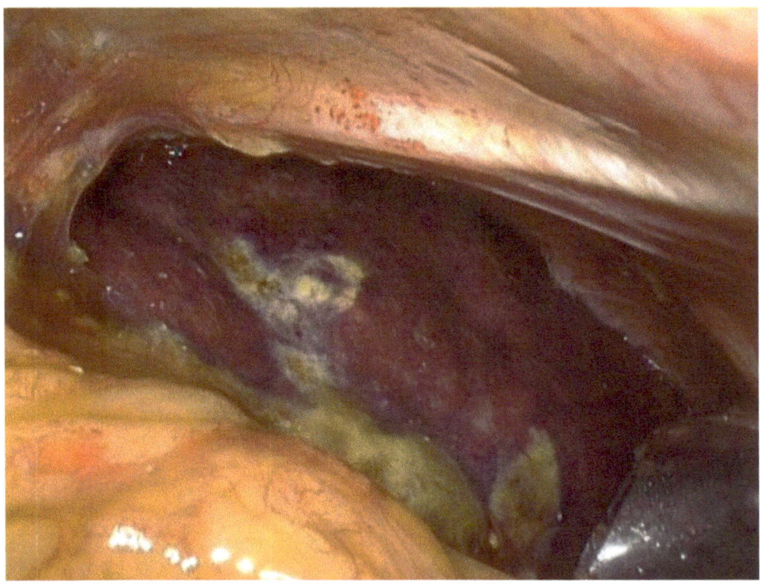

Fig. 8.32 On the 11th day after the first operation, the secondary operation is performed. Ischemic area (*white*) is visualized on the surface of the left lobe

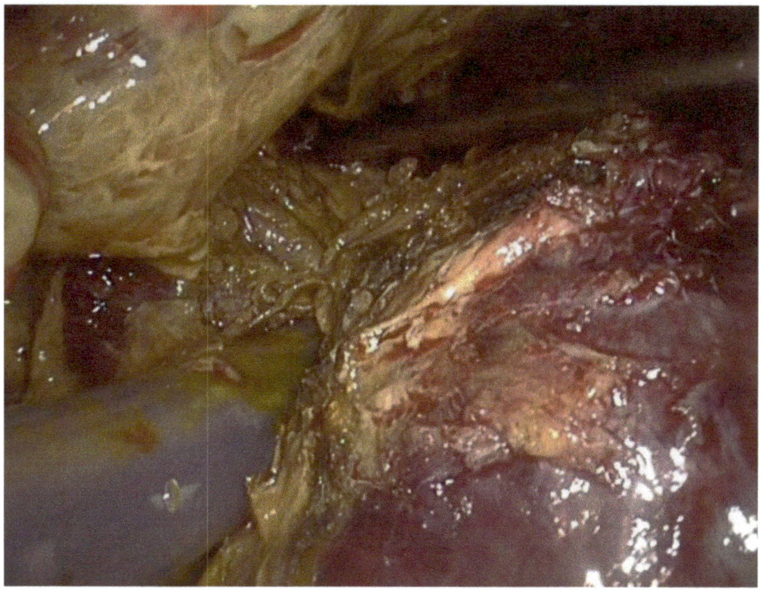

Fig. 8.33 Severe atrophy is visualized in the ligation site

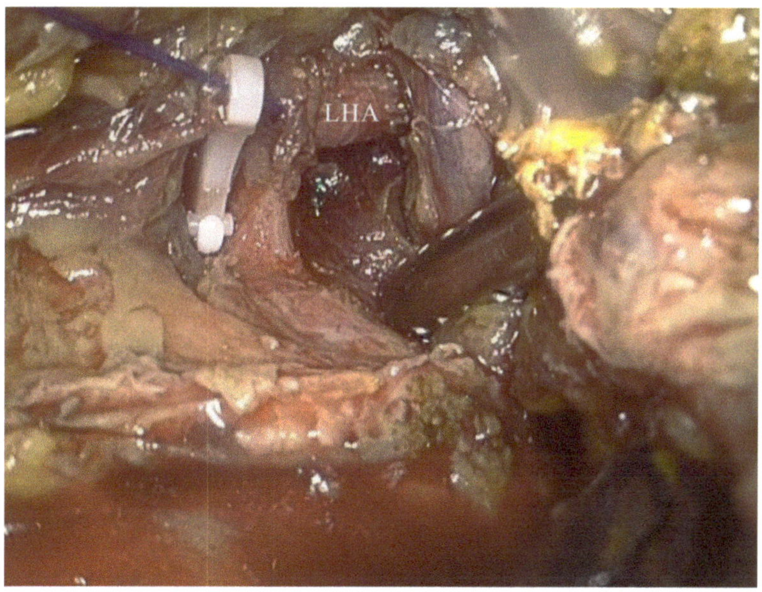

Fig. 8.34 The LHA is mobilized by pulling the suture which was placed in the first-stage operation

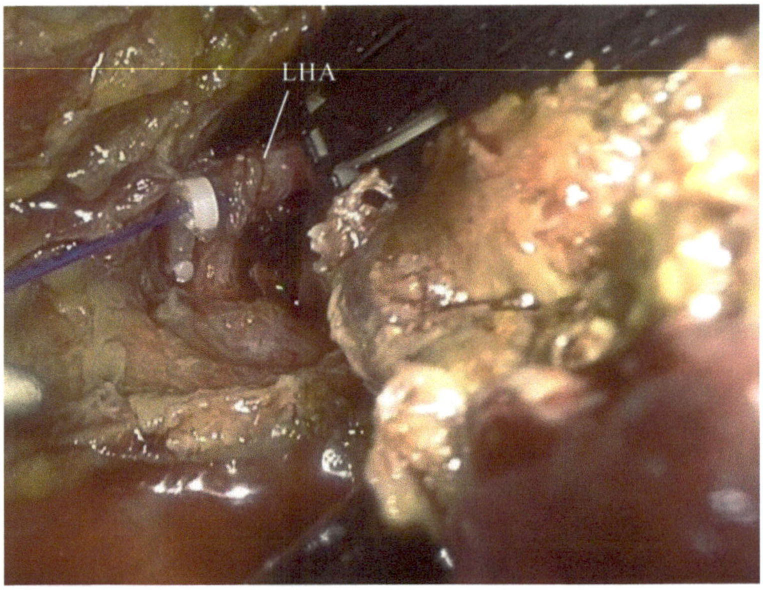

Fig. 8.35 The LHA is clamped with an absorbable clip

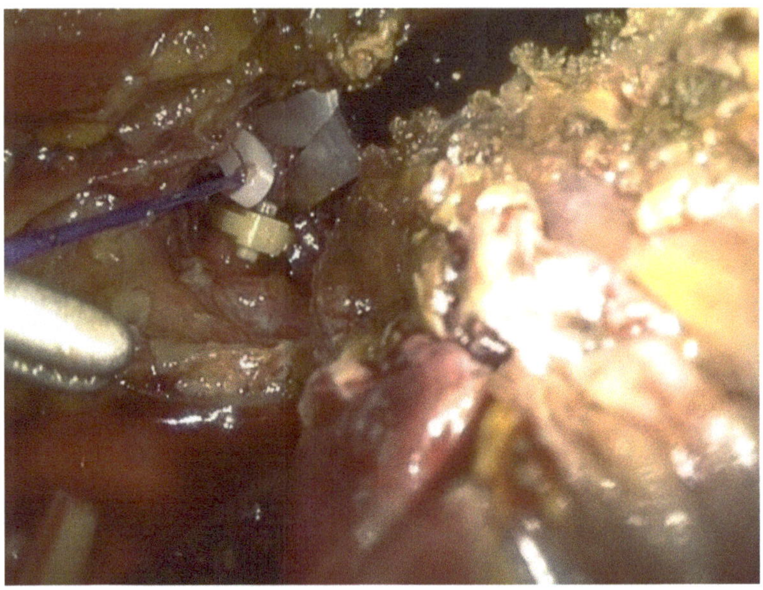

Fig. 8.36 The LHA is divided

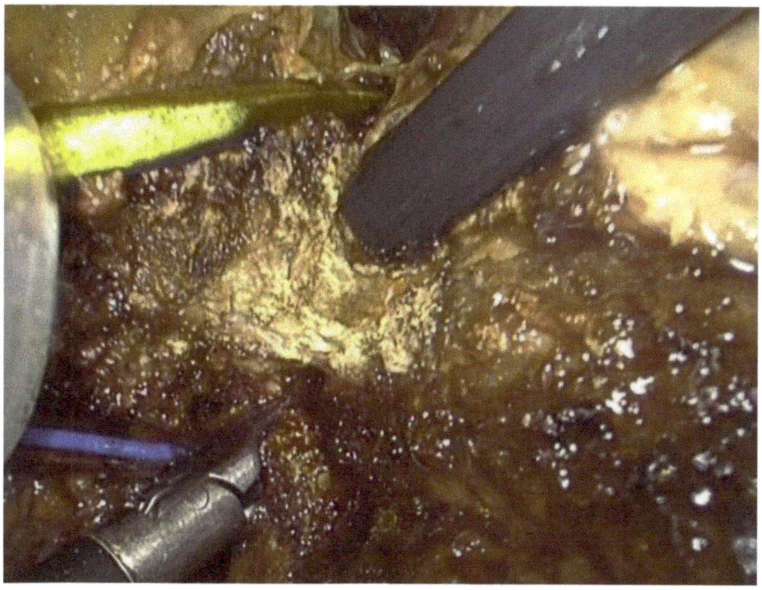

Fig. 8.37 The left lobe of the liver is mobilized by pulling the round-the-liver ligature, and the liver parenchyma is transected with LPMOD

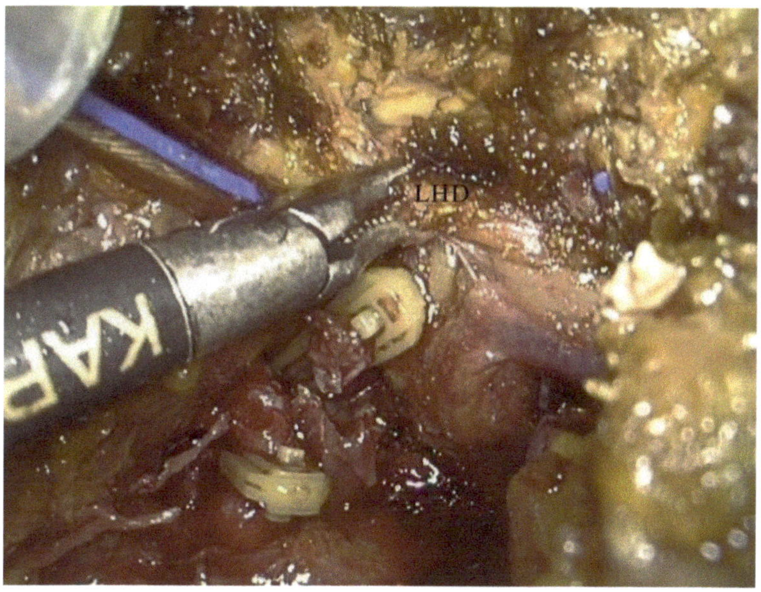

Fig. 8.38 The LHD is visualized in the transection of the liver parenchyma

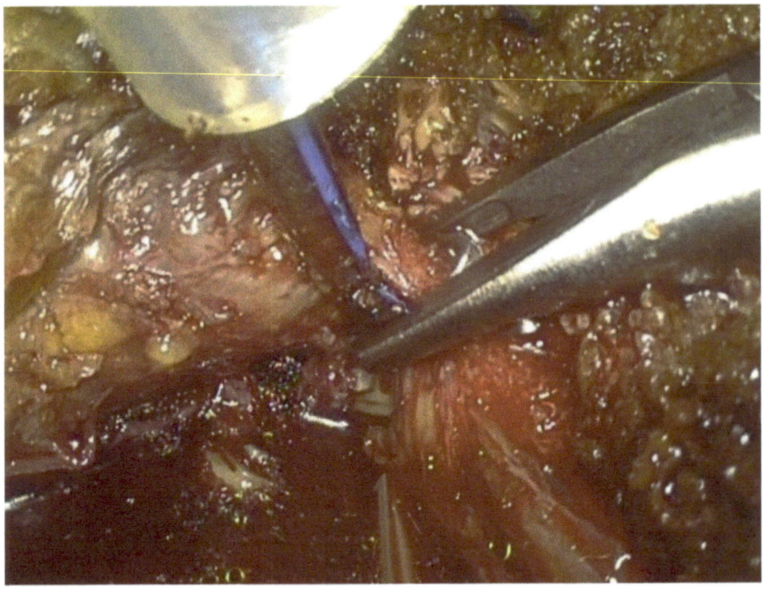

Fig. 8.39 The LHD is clamped with titanic clips

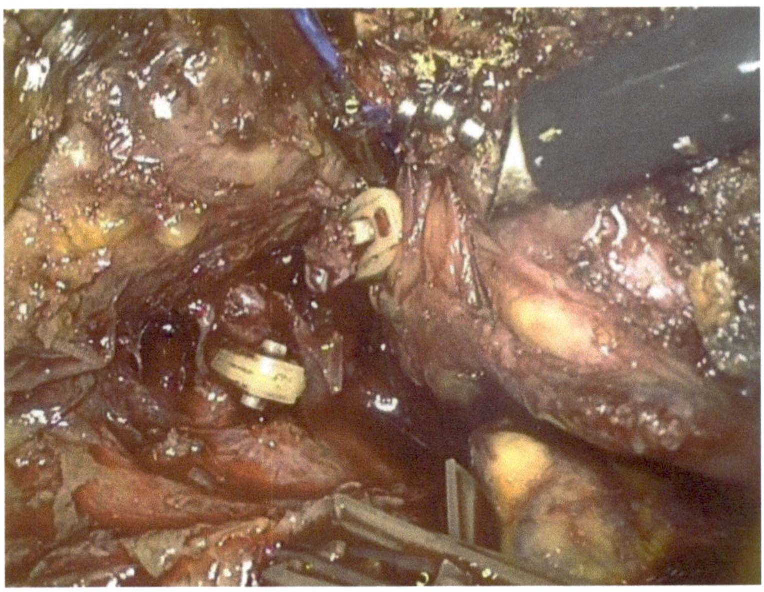

Fig. 8.40 The LHD is divided with LPMOD

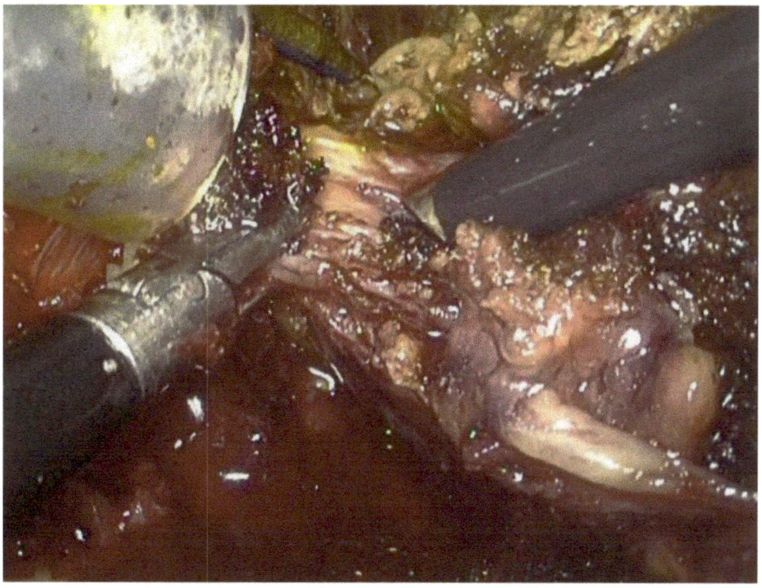

Fig. 8.41 The LPV is visualized in the transection of the liver parenchyma

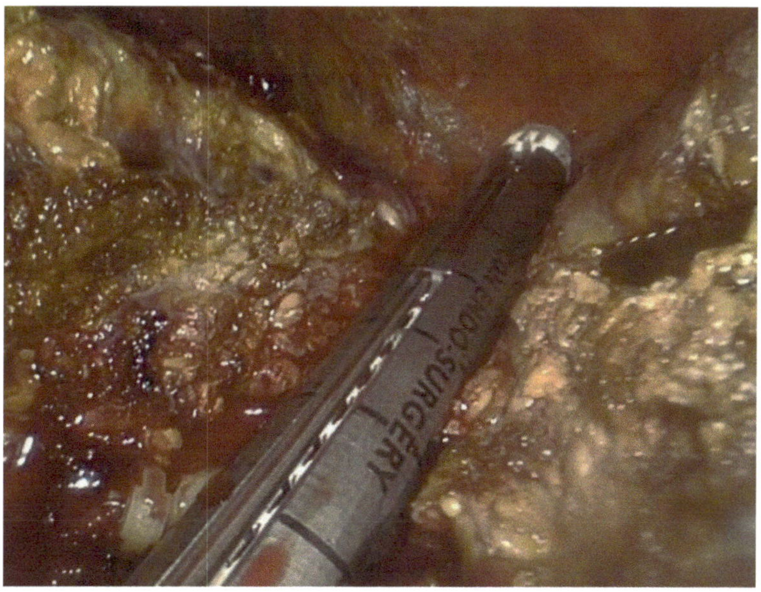

Fig. 8.42 The remaining liver parenchyma, the LPV, and the left hepatic vein (LHV) are divided with a laparoscopic linear stapler

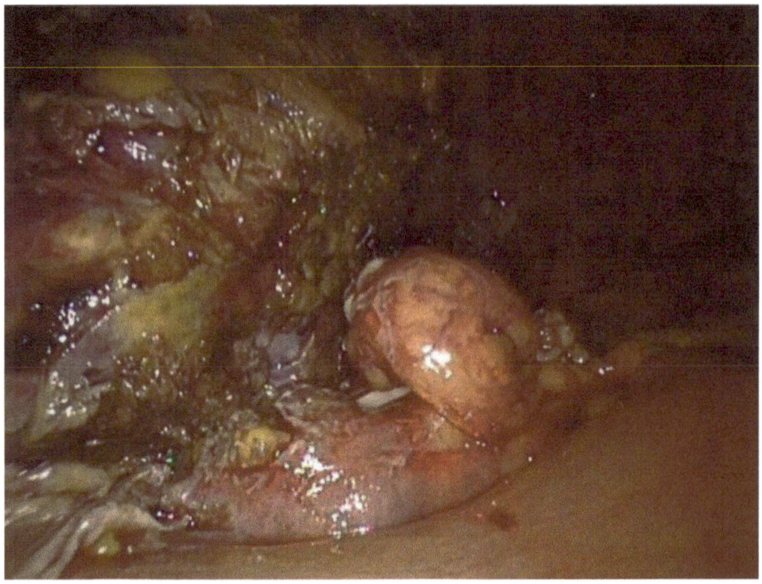

Fig. 8.43 The view of the raw surface after the left lobe of the liver was removed

8.4 Two-Stage Laparoscopic Right Hemihepatectomy

The first-stage operation: laparoscopic ALPPS using round-the-liver ligation (Figs. 8.44, 8.45, 8.46, 8.47, 8.48, 8.49, 8.50, 8.51, 8.52, 8.53, 8.54, 8.55, 8.56, 8.57, 8.58, 8.59, 8.60, 8.61, 8.62, 8.63, 8.64, 8.65, 8.66, 8.67, 8.68, 8.69, 8.70, 8.71, 8.72, 8.73, 8.74, 8.75, 8.76, 8.77, 8.78, 8.79, 8.80, 8.81, 8.82, 8.83, 8.84, 8.85, 8.86, 8.87, 8.88, 8.89, 8.90, and Video 8.3).

The second-stage operation: laparoscopic left hemihepatectomy (Figs. 8.91, 8.92, 8.93, 8.94, 8.95, 8.96, 8.97, 8.98, 8.99, 8.100, 8.101, 8.102, 8.103, 8.104, 8.105, 8.106, 8.107, 8.108, 8.109, 8.110, and Video 8.4).

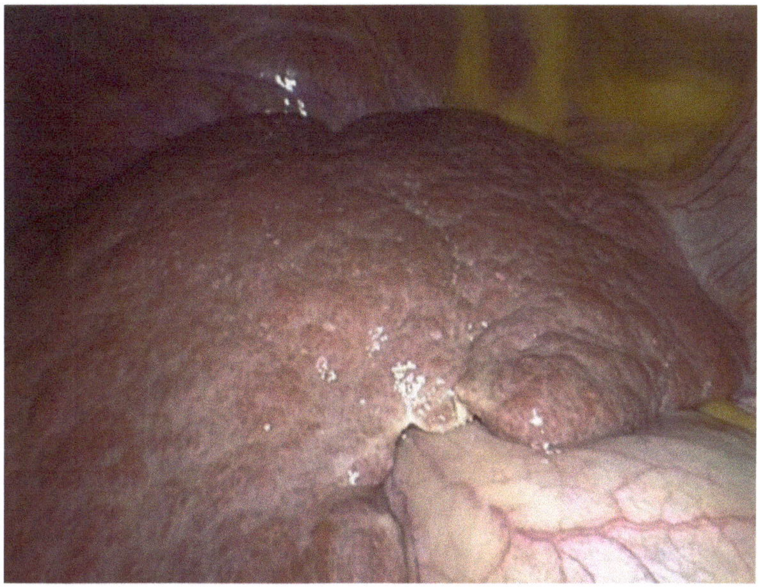

Fig. 8.44 The patient has severe liver cirrhosis due to a hepatitis B infection and multiple hepatocellular carcinomas in the right lobe which was confirmed by liver biopsy. The estimated volume of FLR is less than 35.6 %, and his liver function classification is Child A

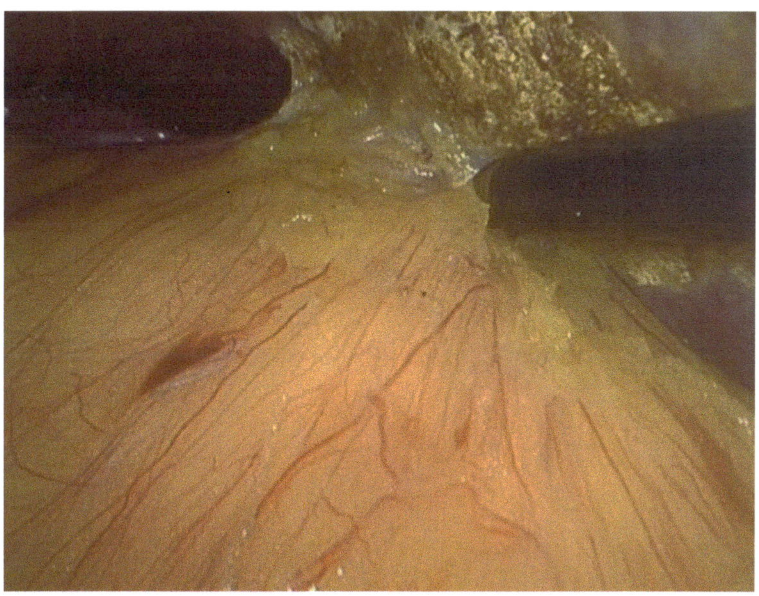

Fig. 8.45 The hepatorenal ligament (HRL) is divided with LPMOD

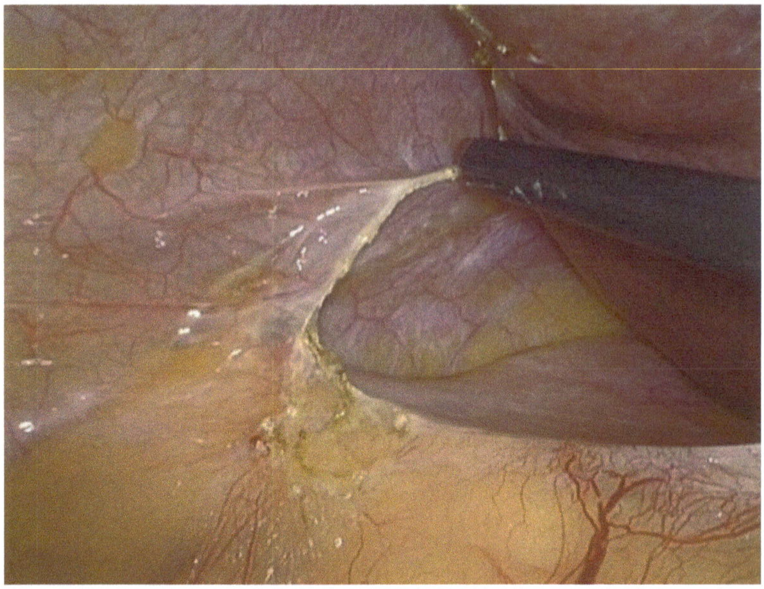

Fig. 8.46 The right lobe of the liver (RLL) is mobilized to the left, and the right triangle ligament (RTL) is divided with LPMOD

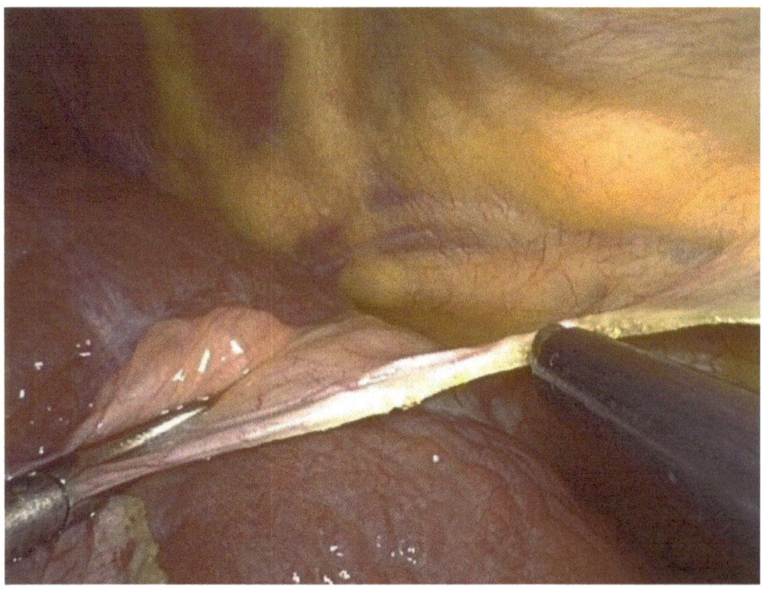

Fig. 8.47 The falciform ligament and the round ligament (RL) are divided with LPMOD

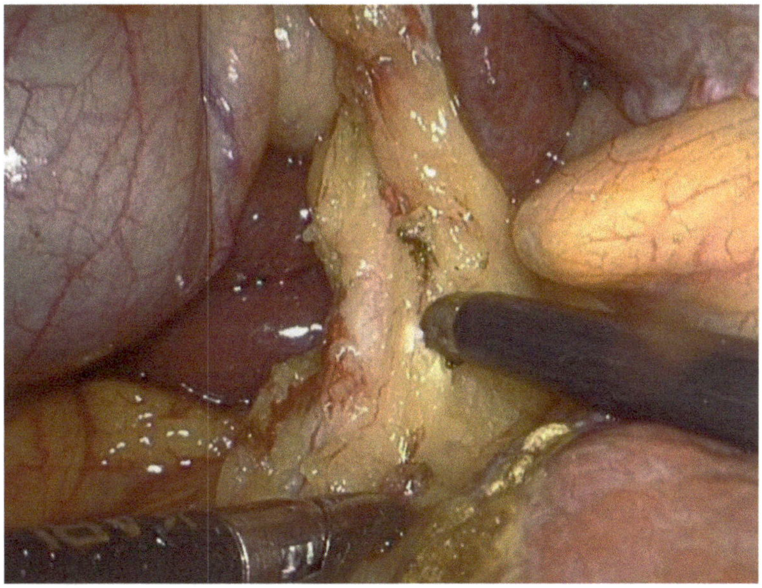

Fig. 8.48 The liver is mobilized upward, and the hepatoduodenal ligament is dissected with LPMOD

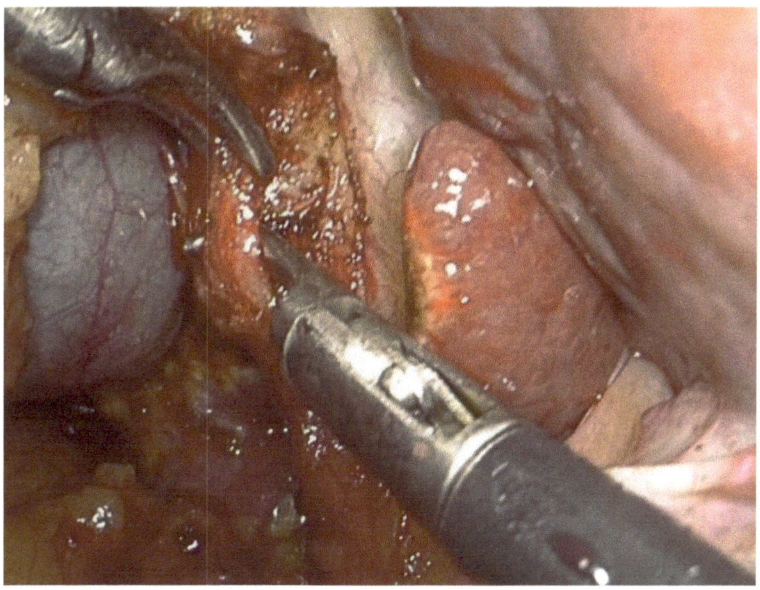

Fig. 8.49 The cystic artery (CA) is dissected with the curved dissecting forceps

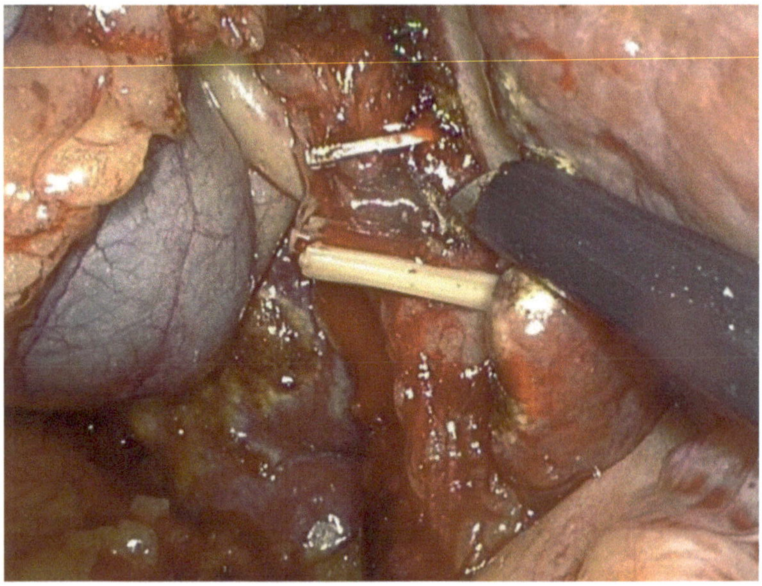

Fig. 8.50 After being clamped with clips, the cystic artery is divided with LPMOD

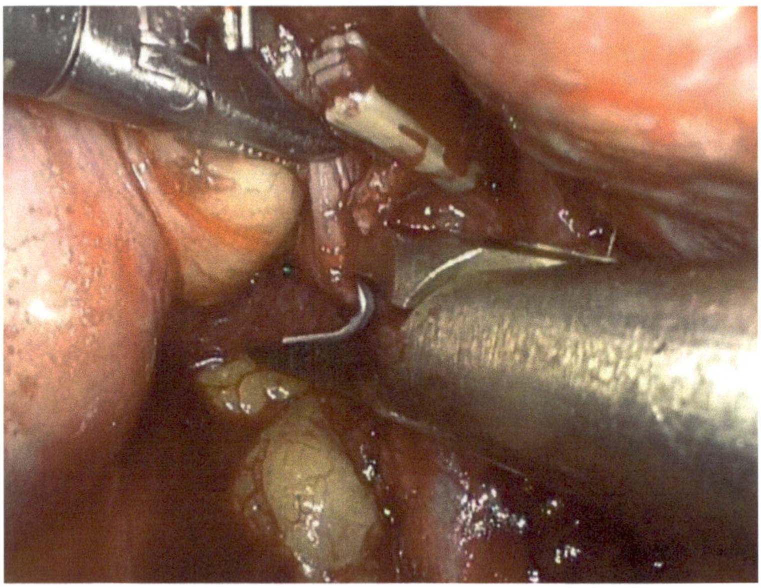

Fig. 8.51 The cystic duct (CD) is clamped with titanic clips after being dissected

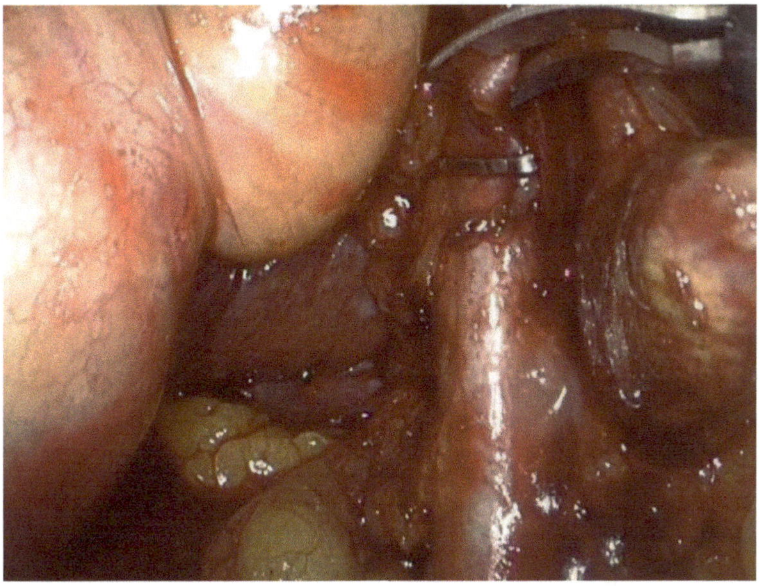

Fig. 8.52 The cystic duct is divided after being clamped with titanic clips

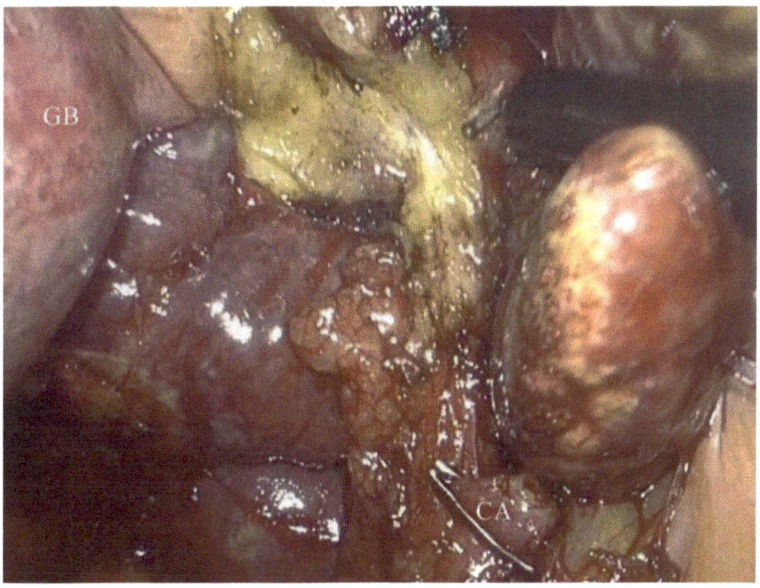

Fig. 8.53 The gallbladder (*GB*) is resected

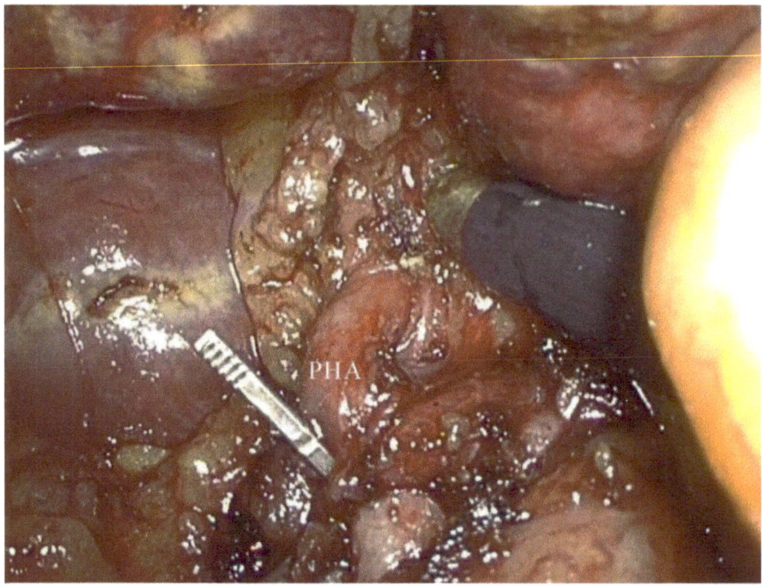

Fig. 8.54 The hepatic arteries are dissected with LPMOD

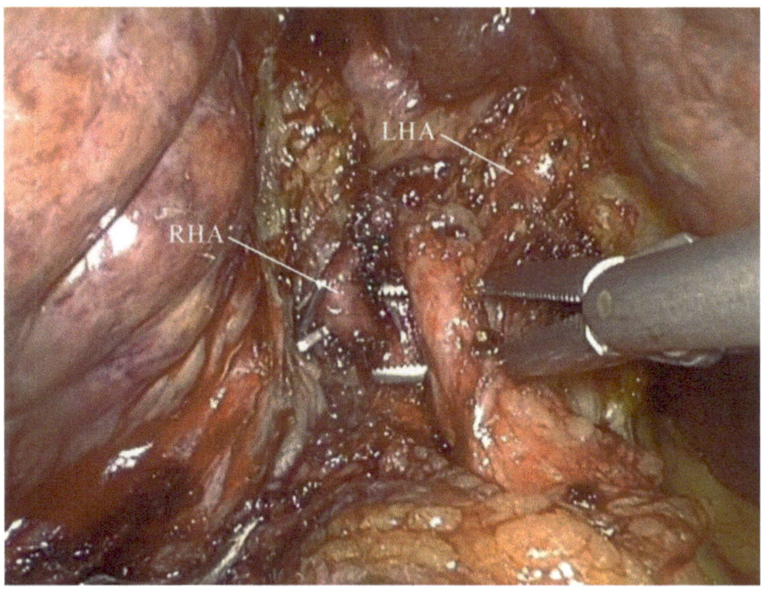

Fig. 8.55 The proper hepatic artery (PHA) is freed with the 90°-curved dissecting forceps

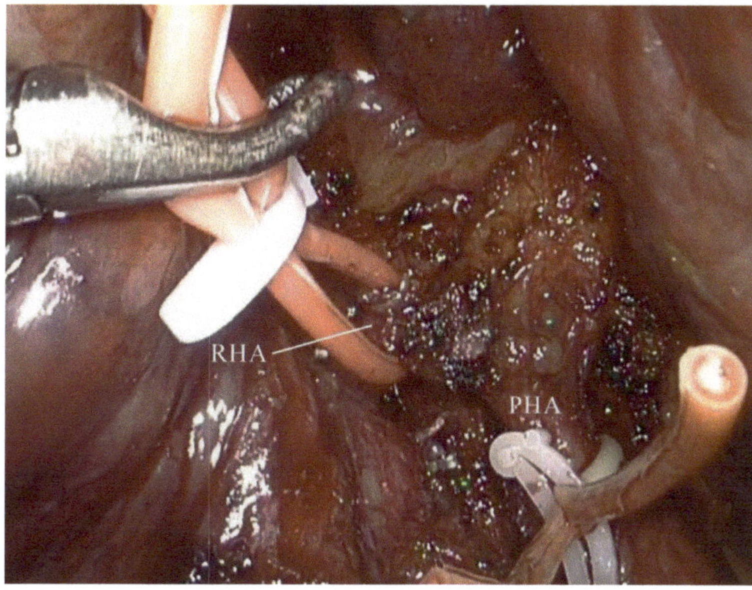

Fig. 8.56 Two elastic tapes are rounded the common hepatic artery (CHA) and the right hepatic artery (*RHA*) for the traction respectively

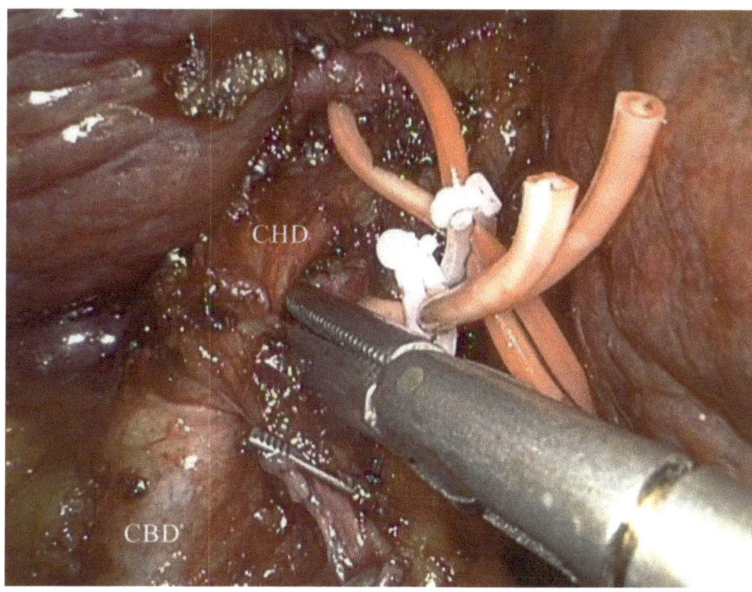

Fig. 8.57 The common hepatic duct (*CHD*) is freed with the 90°-curved dissecting forceps

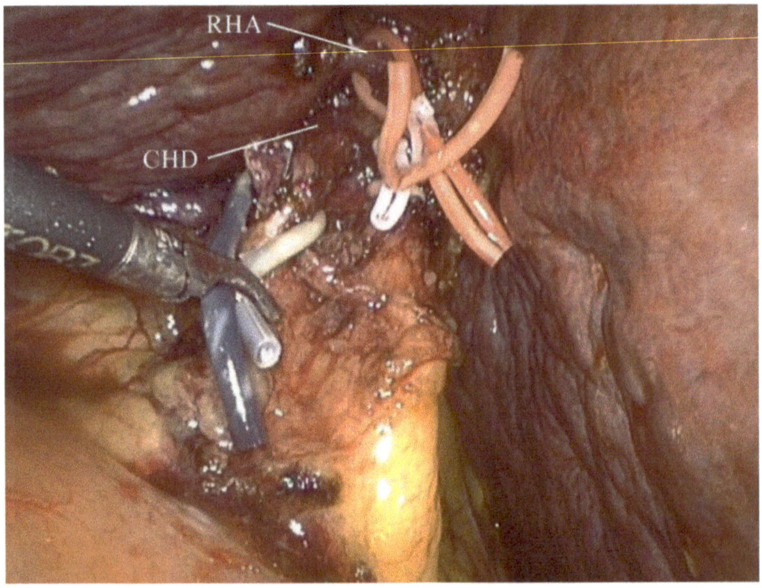

Fig. 8.58 Another elastic tape is rounded the CHD

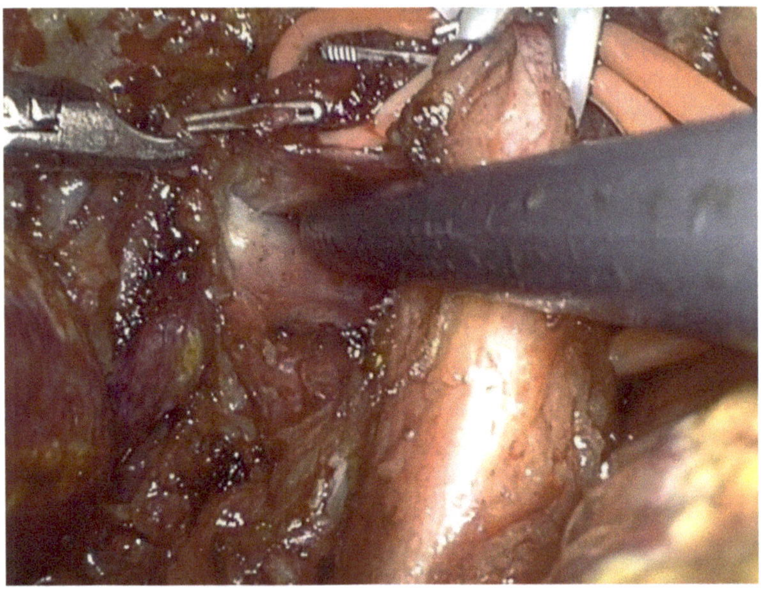

Fig. 8.59 The right branch of portal vein (RPV) is dissected with LPMOD

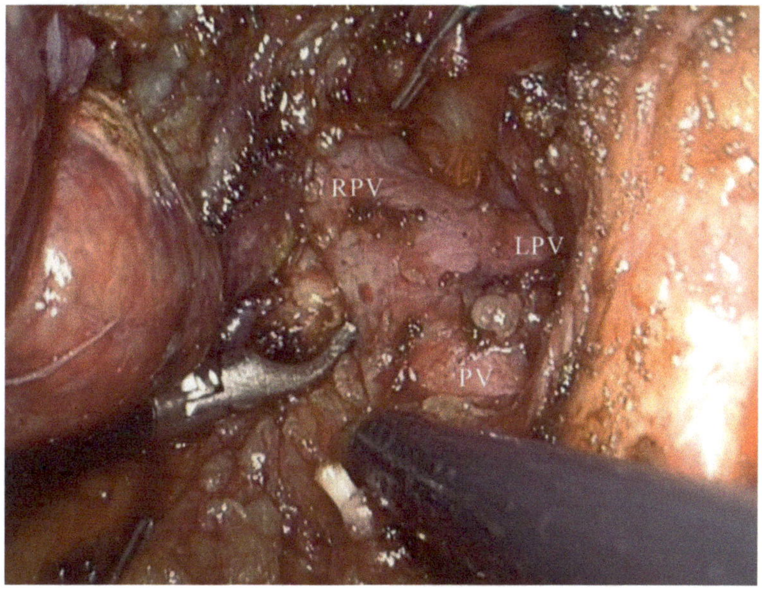

Fig. 8.60 The bifurcation of portal vein (BPV) is identified

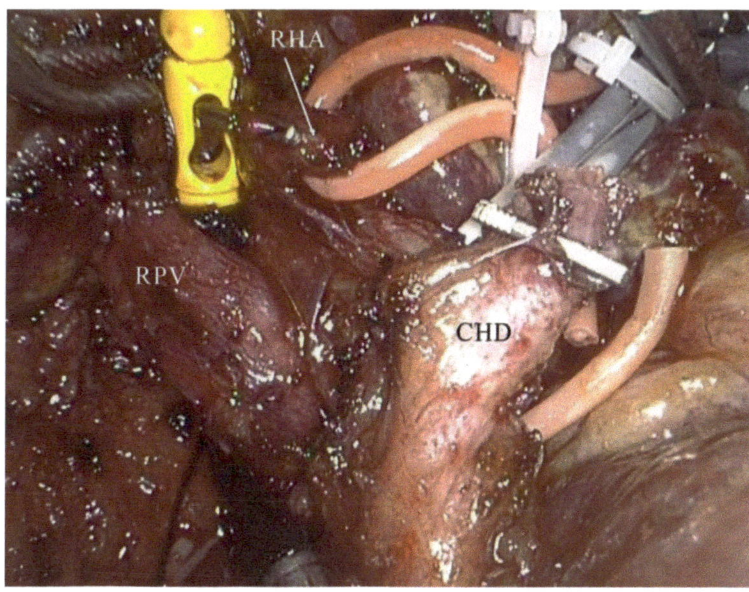

Fig. 8.61 The RPV is freed, and a suture is passed through the back of the RPV with the guidance of the "gold finger" liver retractor

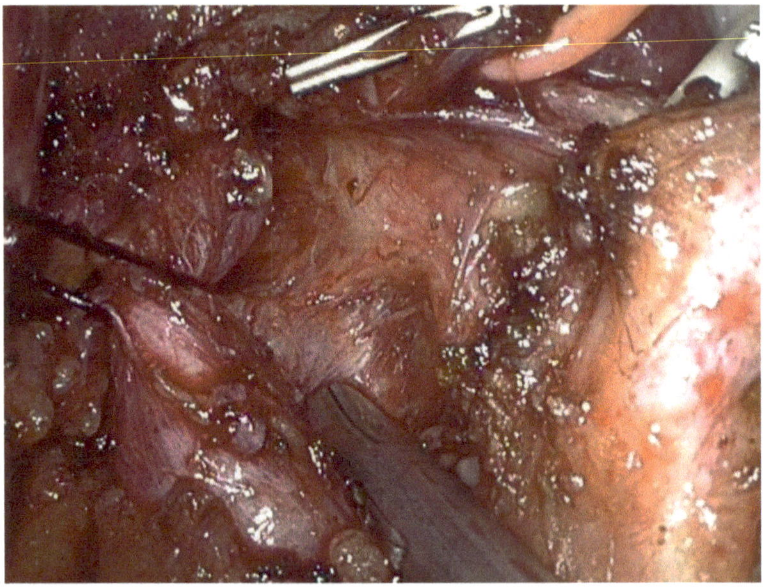

Fig. 8.62 The suture is rounded the RPV

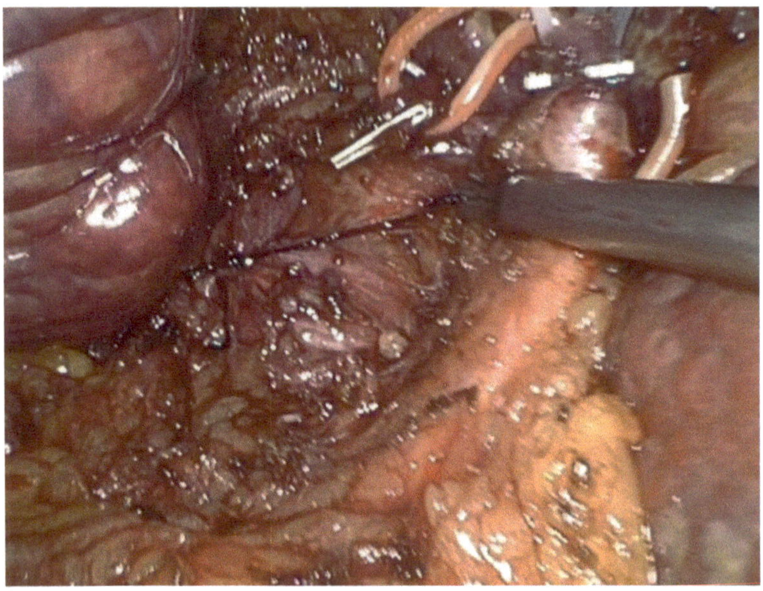

Fig. 8.63 The RPV is ligated with the suture

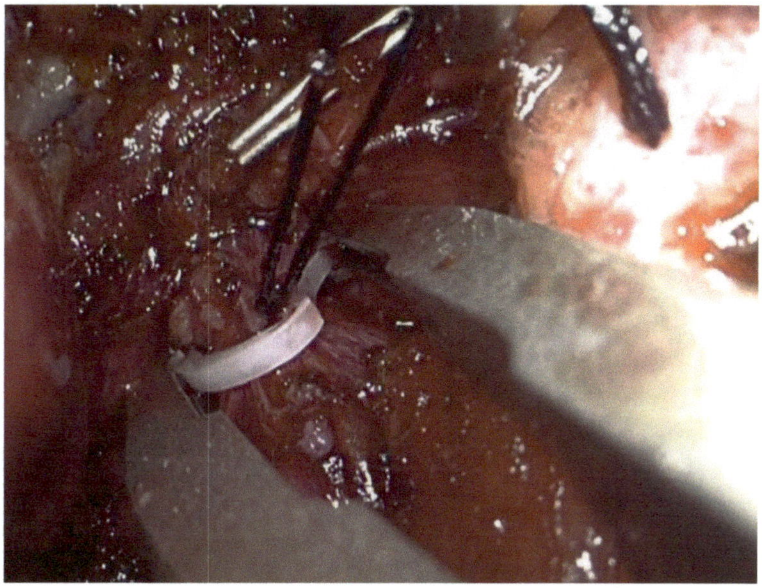

Fig. 8.64 A nonabsorbable polymer clip is applied on the RPV

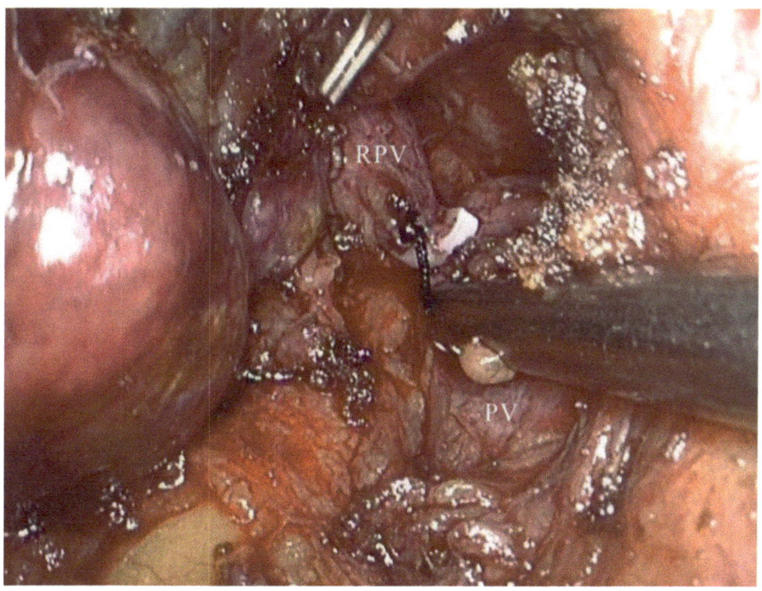

Fig. 8.65 The RPV is occluded by the ligation and the nonabsorbable clip

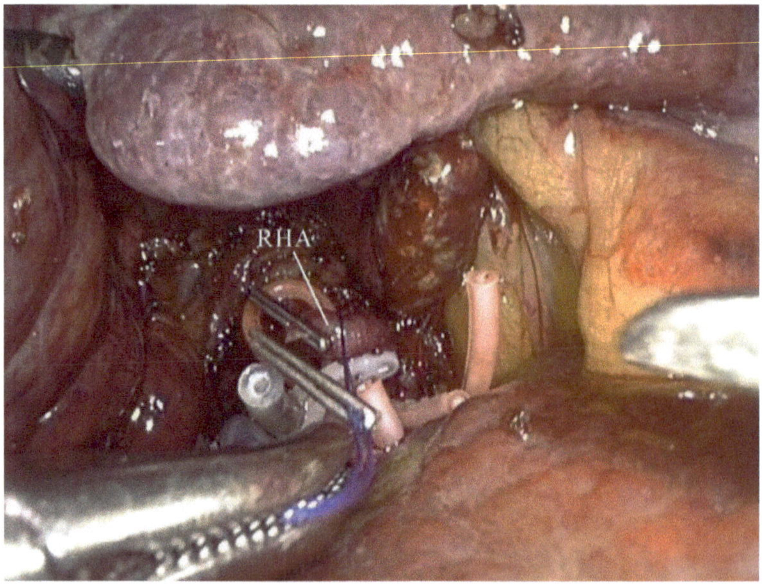

Fig. 8.66 A suture is placed around the RHA for the future management of the RHA in the second-stage operation

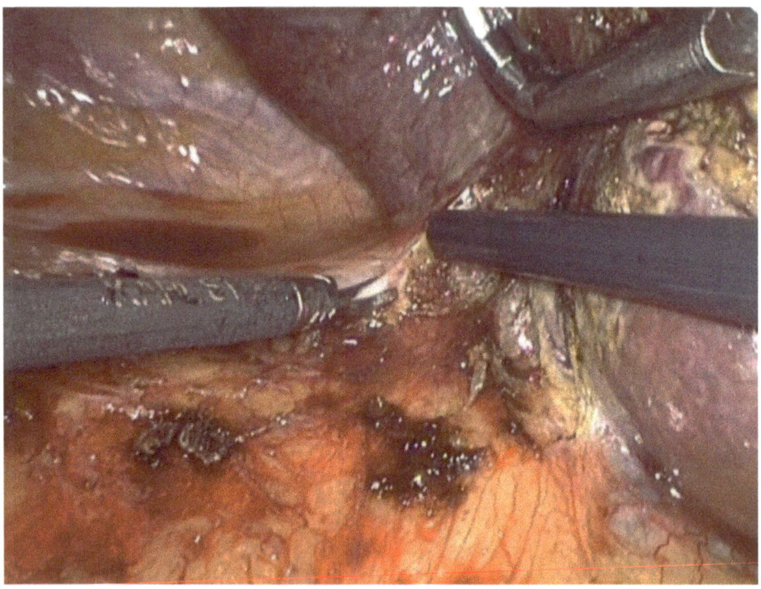

Fig. 8.67 The right lobe is mobilized to the left with a liver retractor, and the right side of inferior vena cava (IVC) is dissected with LPMOD

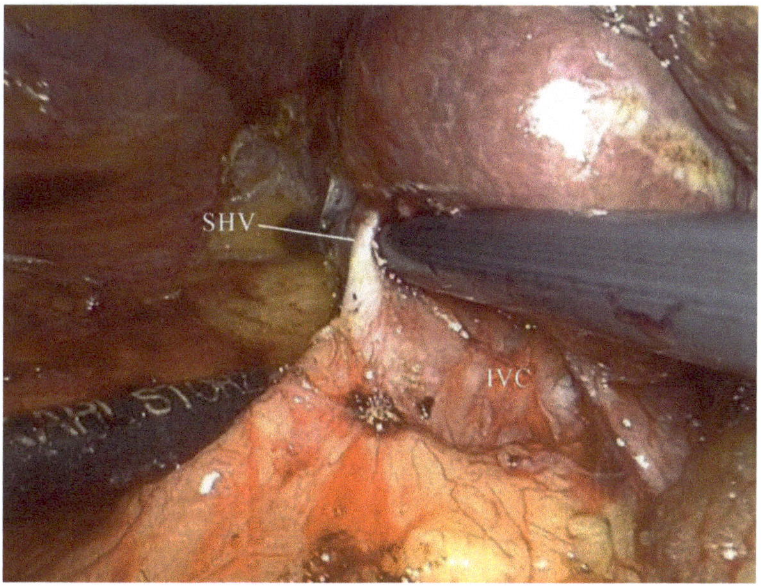

Fig. 8.68 A short hepatic vein (*SHV*) is dissected with LPMOD

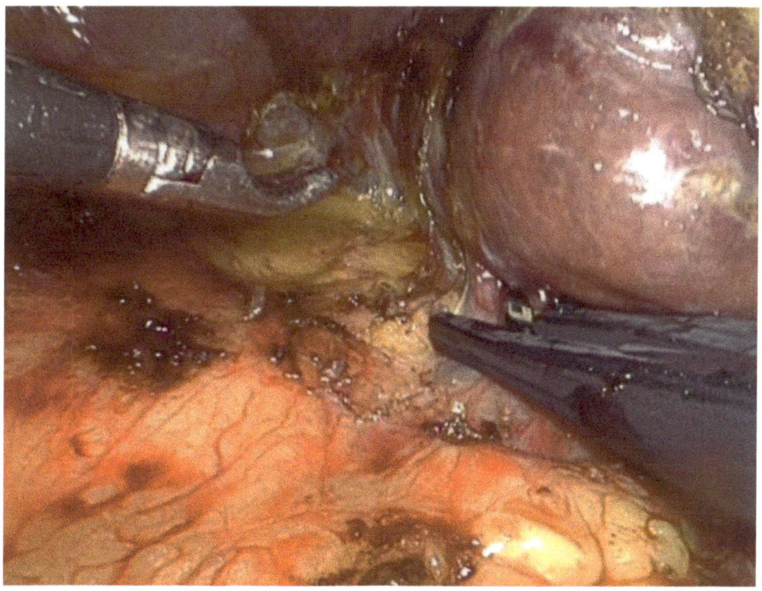

Fig. 8.69 The SHV is clamped with one absorbable clip

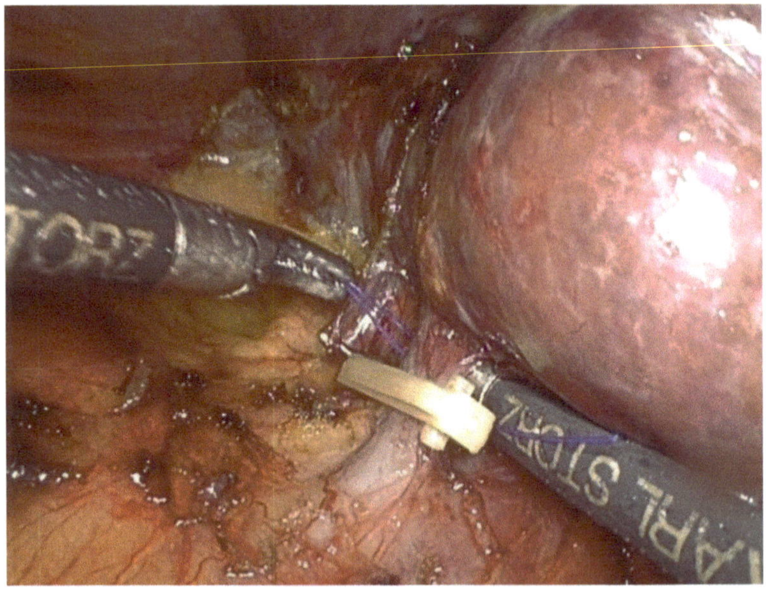

Fig. 8.70 A suture is passed through the back of the SHV with the guidance of the curved dissecting forceps

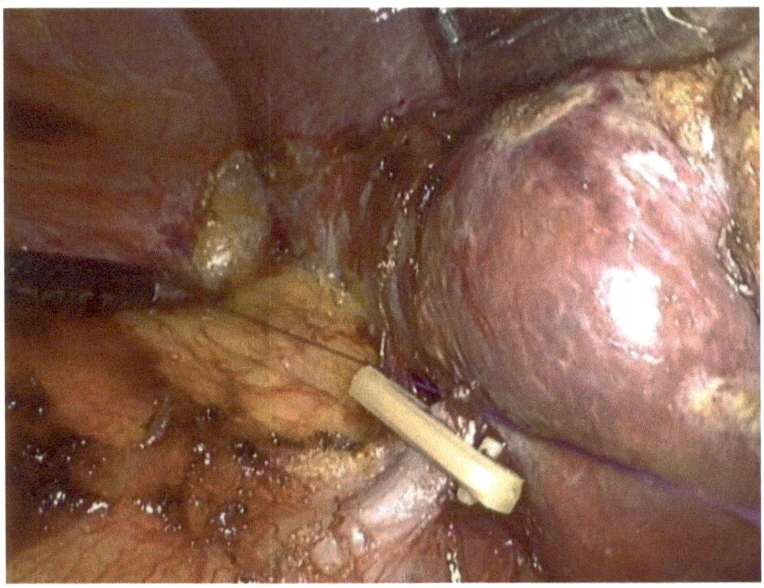

Fig. 8.71 The SHV is ligated with the suture

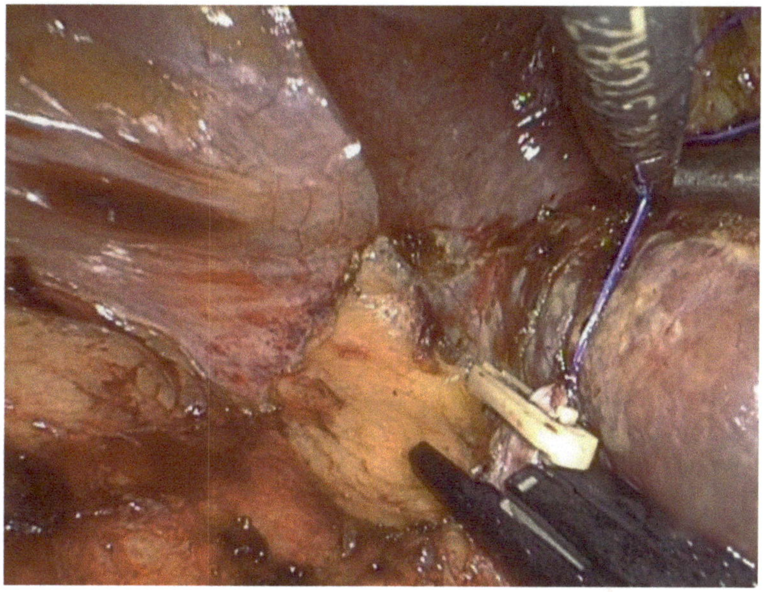

Fig. 8.72 The other absorbable clip is applied on the SHV

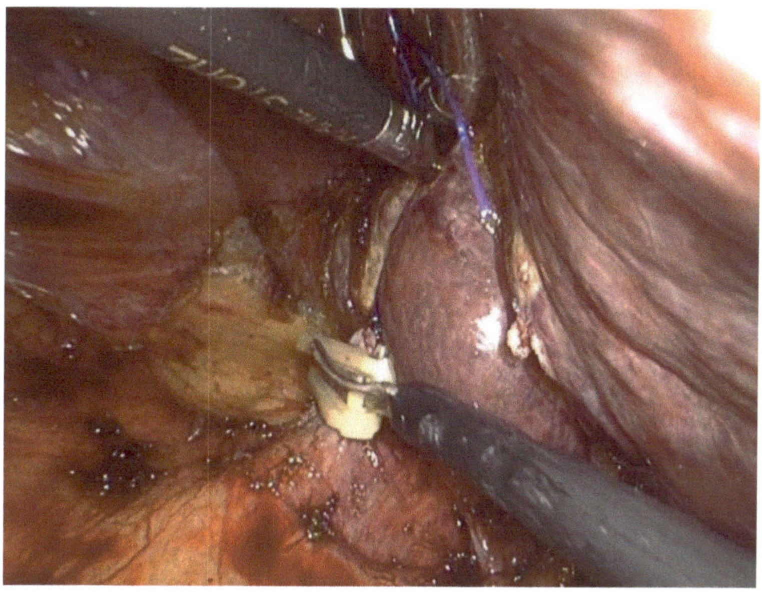

Fig. 8.73 The SHV is divided between the two clips

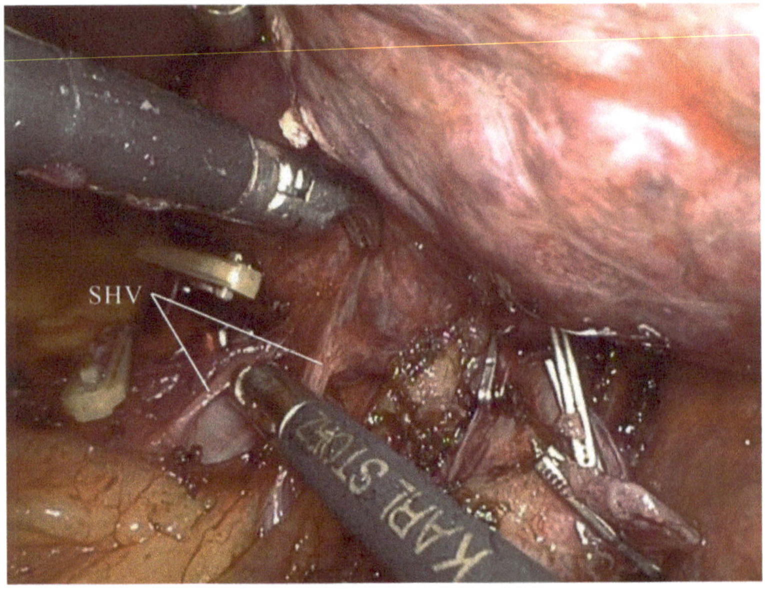

Fig. 8.74 SHVs are dissected

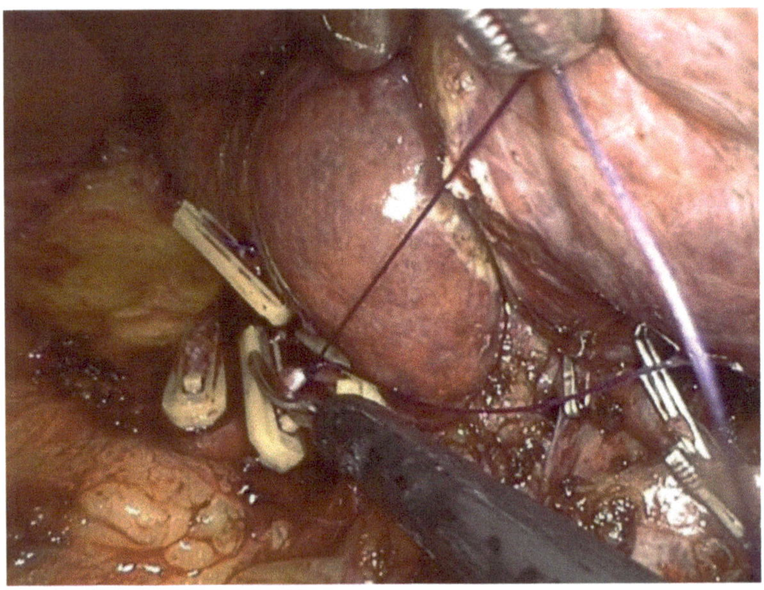

Fig. 8.75 A SHV is divided after being double clamped and ligated

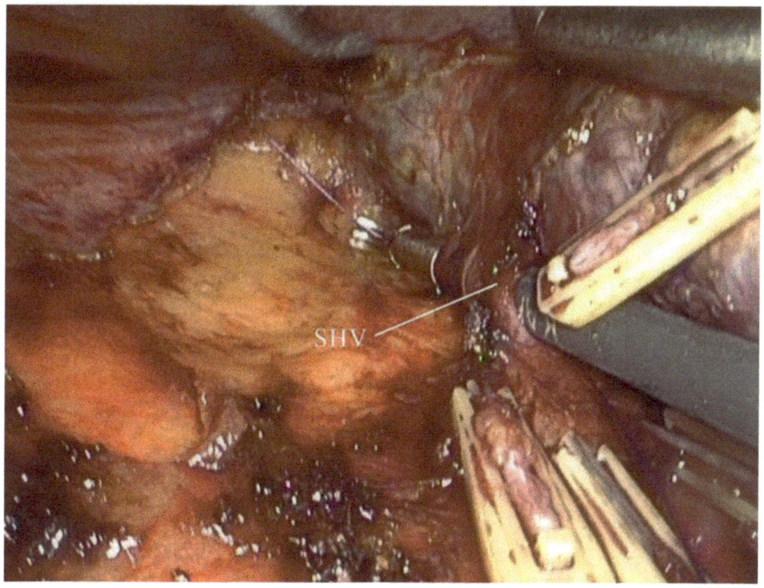

Fig. 8.76 Another SHV is dissected, and a suture is passed through the back of the vein with the guidance of the curved dissecting forceps

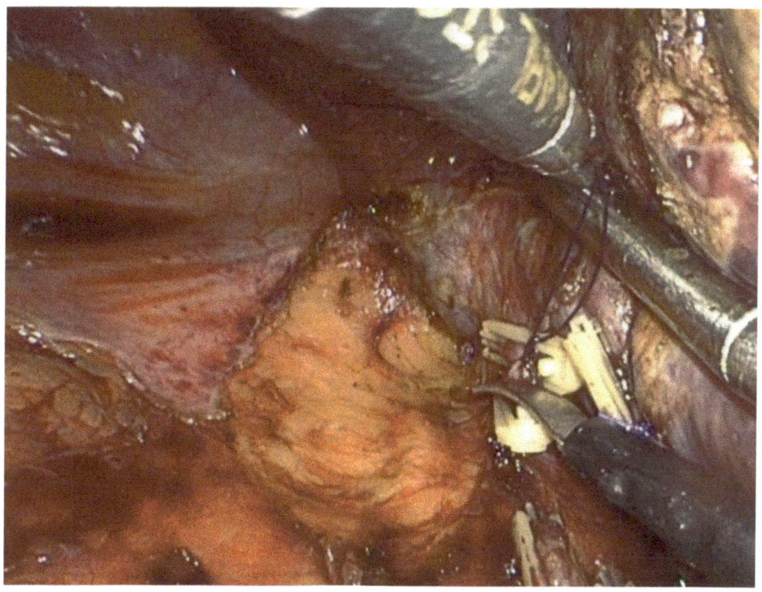

Fig. 8.77 The SHV is divided after being double clamped and ligated

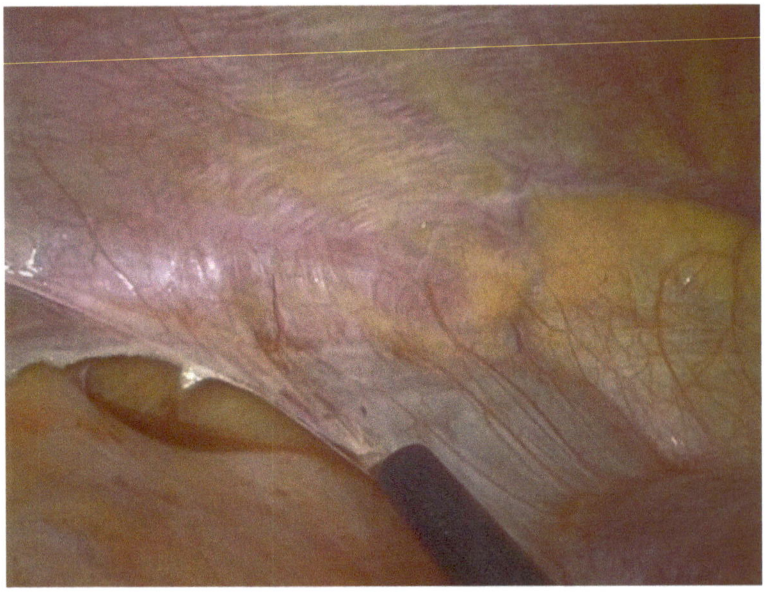

Fig. 8.78 The right lobe of the liver is pressed downward, and the right coronary ligament (RCL) is divided with LPMOD

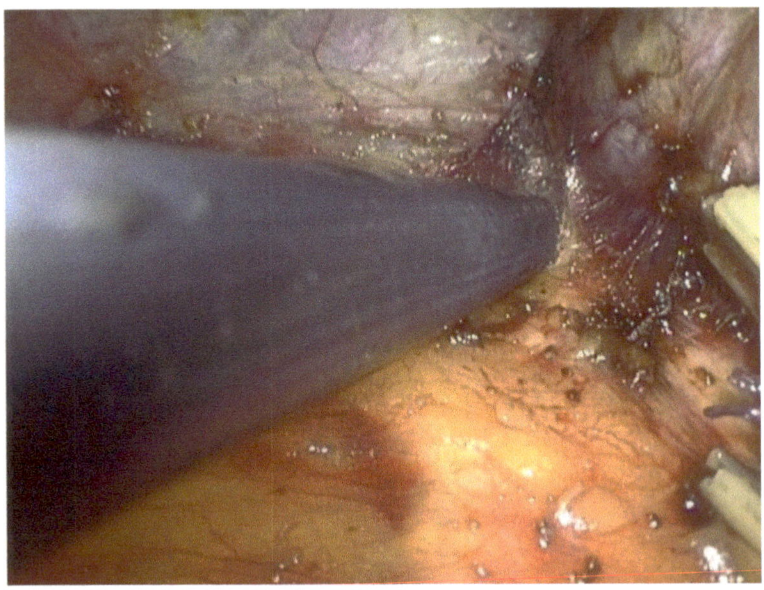

Fig. 8.79 The right lobe is mobilized to the left, and the right hepatic vein (RHV) is dissected with LPMOD

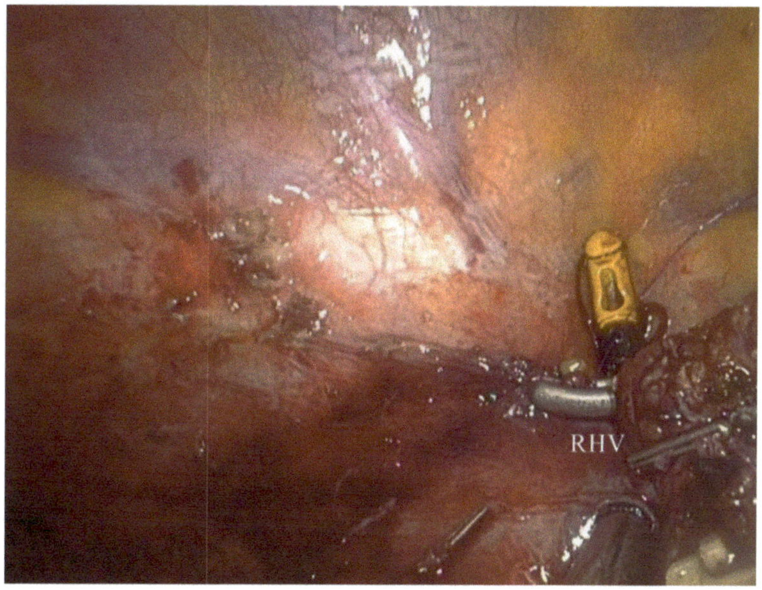

Fig. 8.80 The RHV is freed, and a suture is passed through the back of the RHV with the guidance of the "gold finger" liver retractor

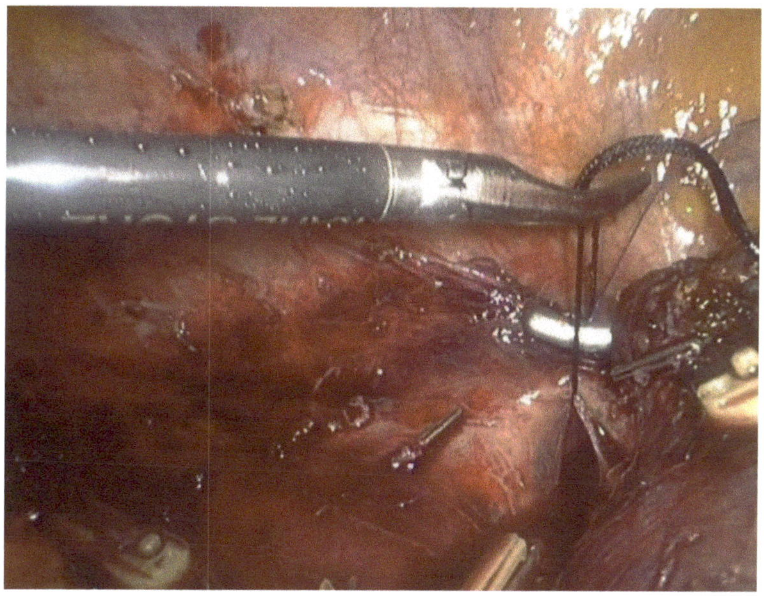

Fig. 8.81 The suture is rounded the RHV

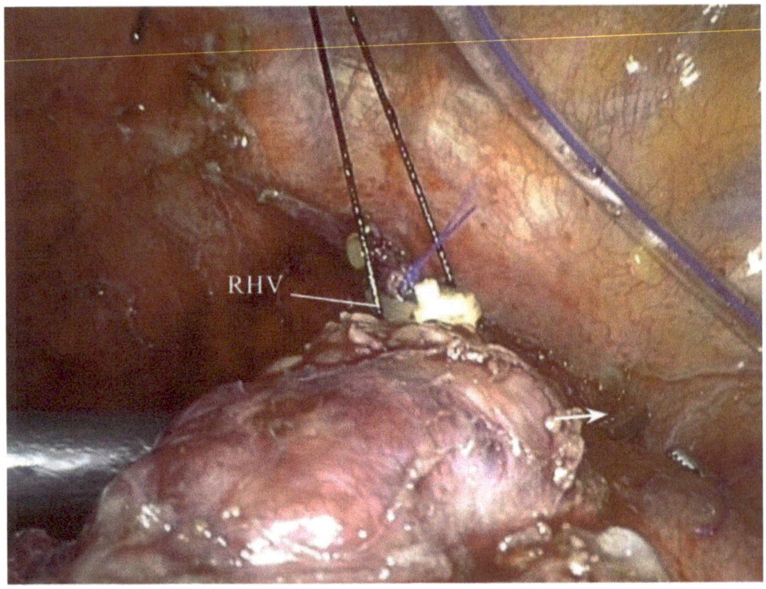

Fig. 8.82 The tip of the curved dissecting forceps (*arrow*) is passed through the back of the RHV, and the round-the-liver ligature, a nasogastric tube with a guide wire inside, is to be passed the back of the RHV with the guidance of the curved dissecting forceps

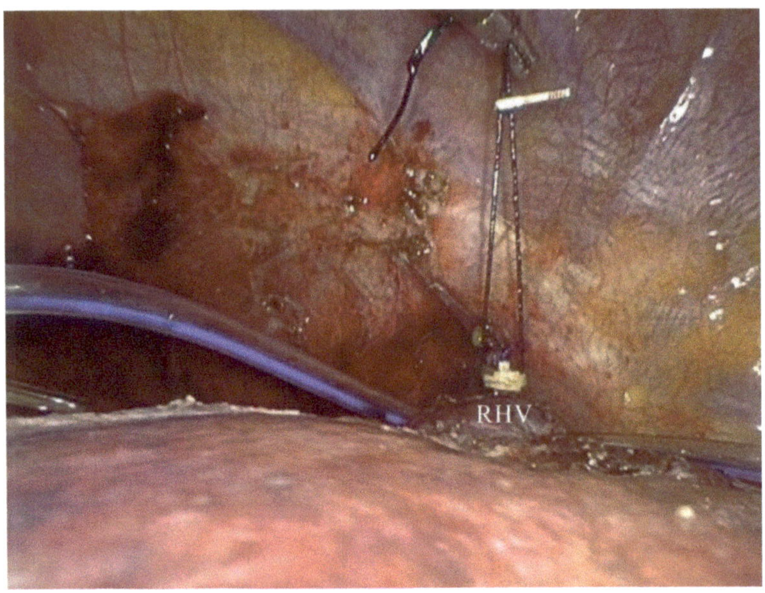

Fig. 8.83 The round-the-liver ligature has passed through the back of the RHV with the guidance of the curved dissecting forceps

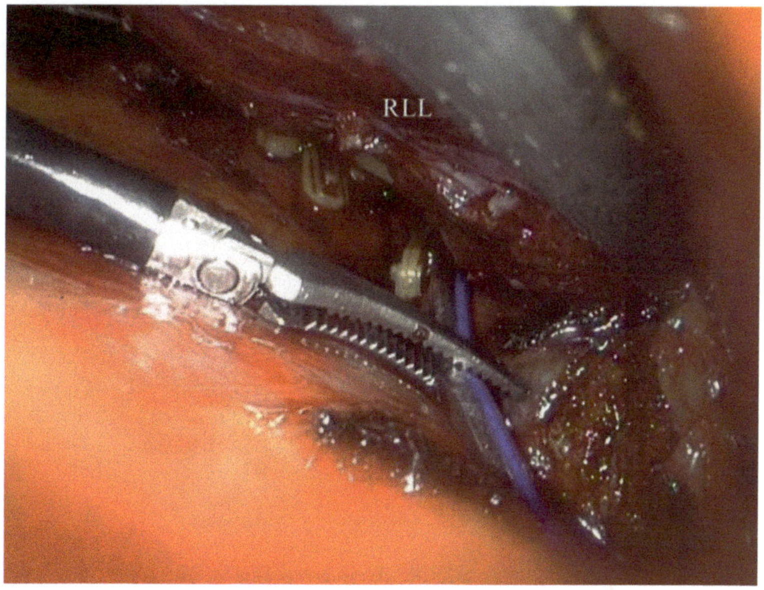

Fig. 8.84 The round-the-liver ligature is mobilized to pass through the below-the-right-lobe space

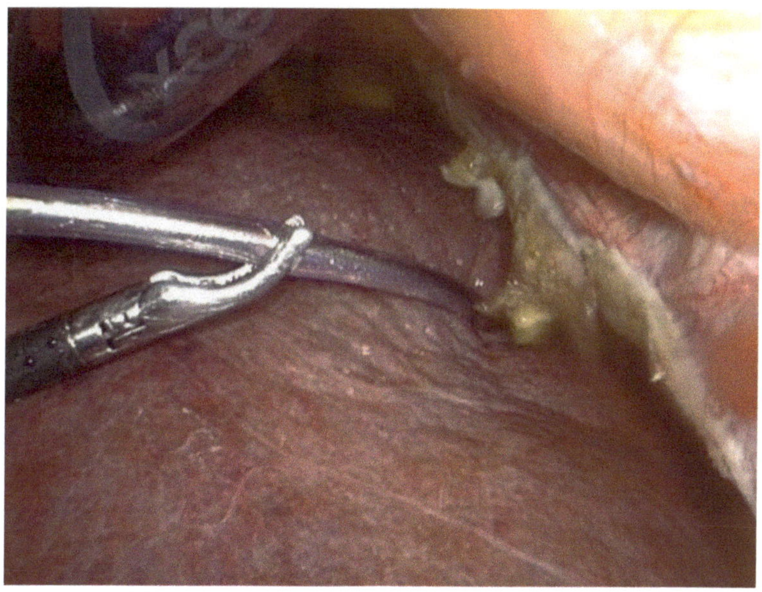

Fig. 8.85 The round-the-liver ligature is mobilized to round the liver

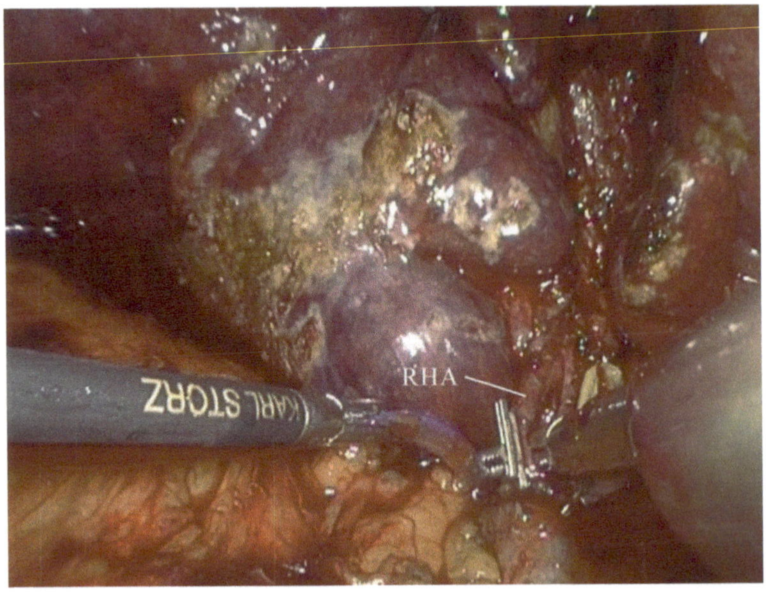

Fig. 8.86 The round-the-liver ligature is passed through the back of the RHA with the guidance of the curved dissecting forceps

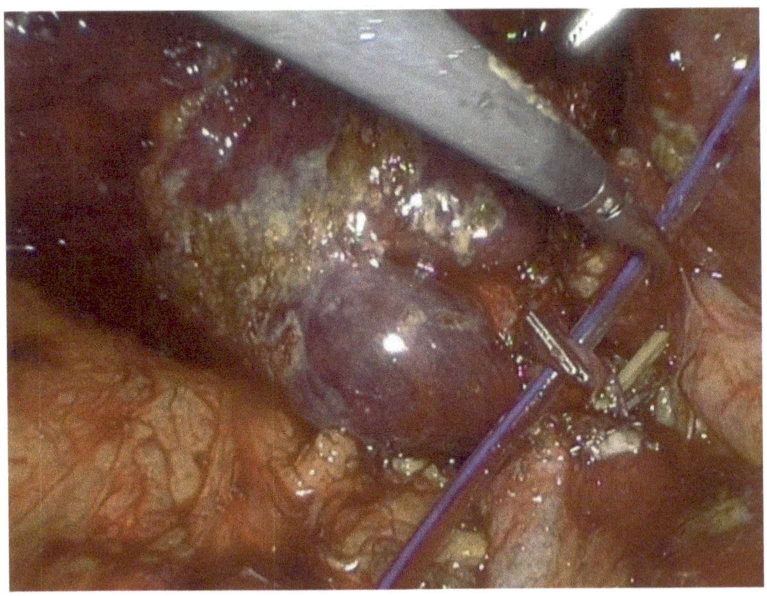

Fig. 8.87 The round-the-liver ligature has passed through the back of the RHA

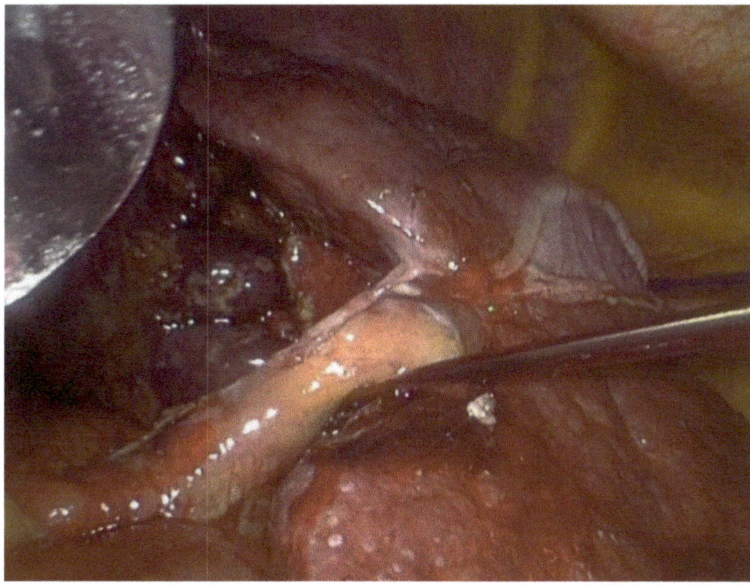

Fig. 8.88 The round-the-liver ligature is rounded the liver, and both ends of the ligature are extracted outside the abdominal cavity through the manipulation port

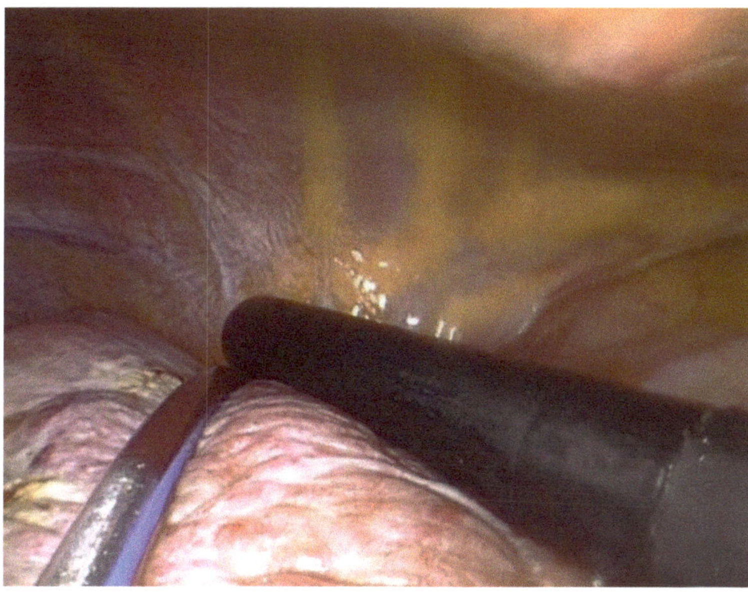

Fig. 8.89 Laparoscopic ultrasound is performed to guide the location of the round-the-liver ligature

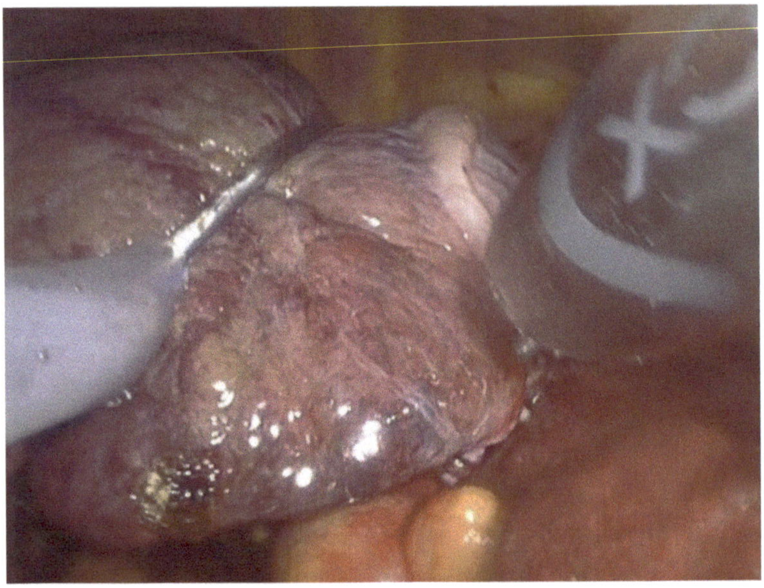

Fig. 8.90 A thoracic tube is inserted through the 12-mm trocar, and both ends of the ligature are passed through a thoracic tube. The ligation is executed by closing and fixing the ligature by using the manner which is usually used in totally vascular occlusion in open liver surgeries

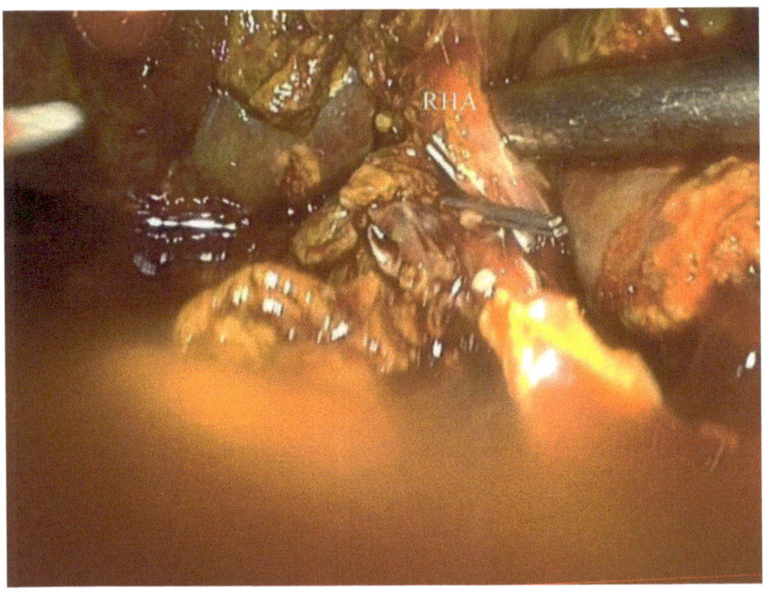

Fig. 8.91 The right hepatic artery is visualized

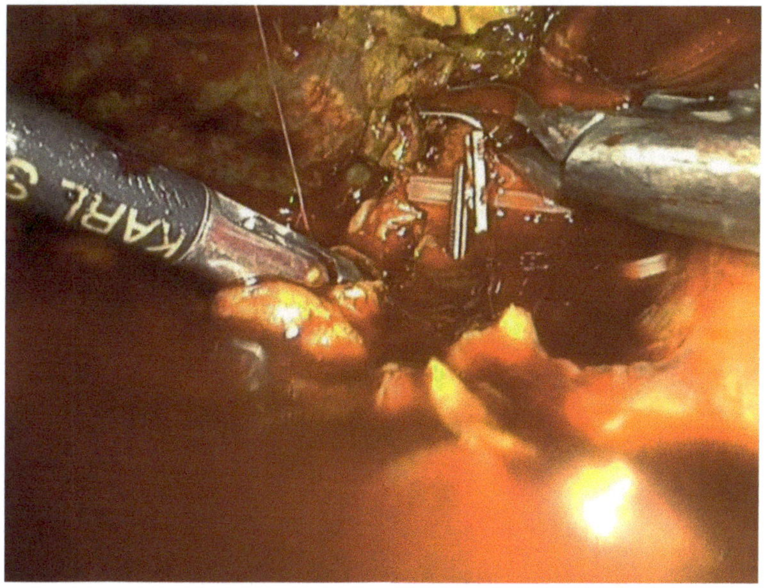

Fig. 8.92 The right hepatic artery is clamped with an absorbable clip and a titanic clip

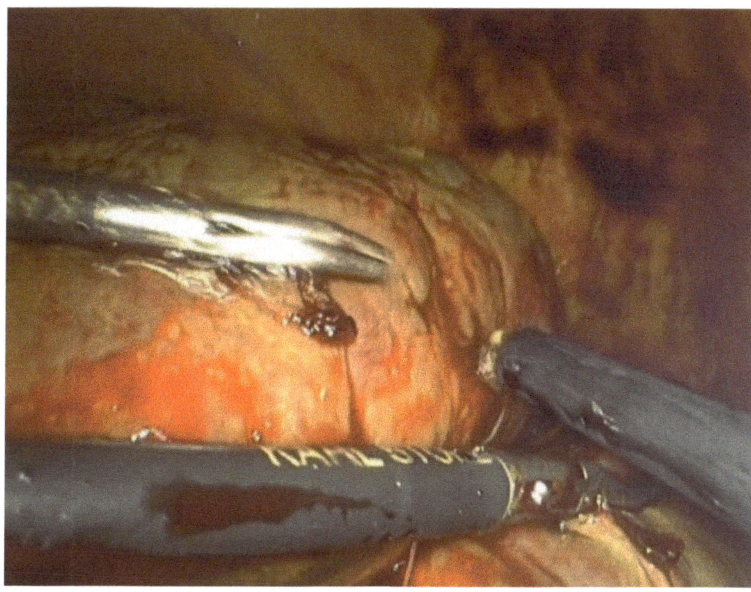

Fig. 8.93 The right lobe is mobilized by pulling the ligature, and the liver parenchyma is transected with LPMOD along the ligature

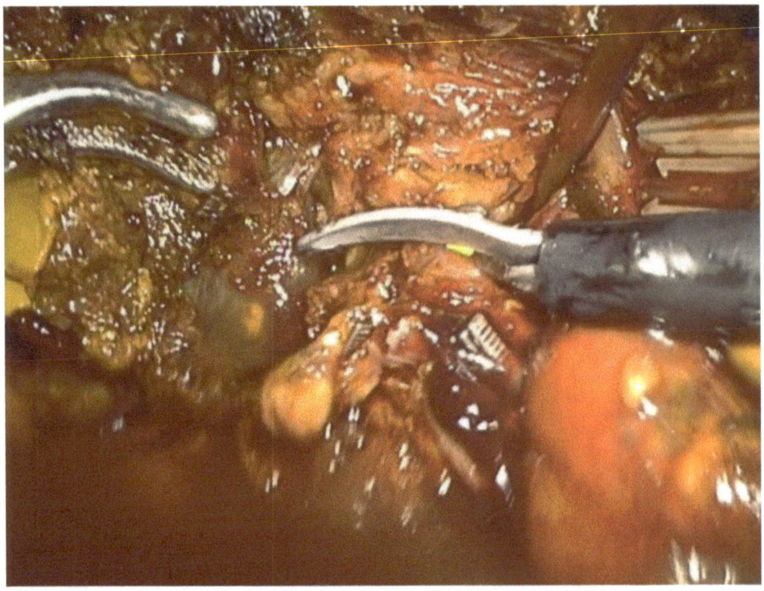

Fig. 8.94 The right hepatic artery is divided

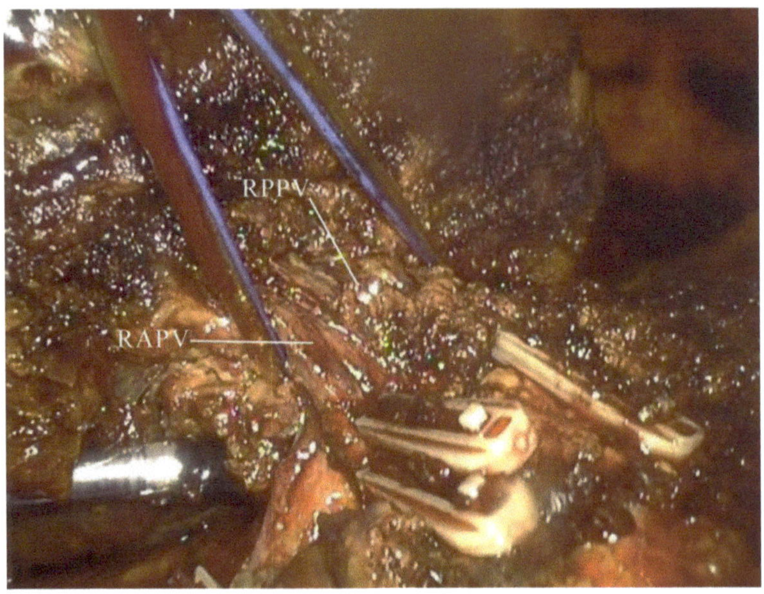

Fig. 8.95 The right anterior branch of portal vein (*RAPV*) and the right posterior branch of portal vein (*RPPV*) are visualized in the transection of the liver parenchyma

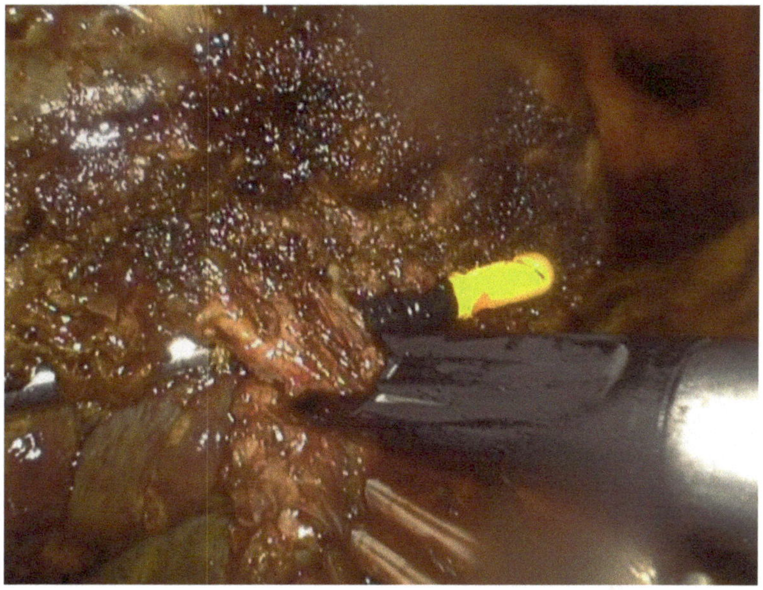

Fig. 8.96 The RAPV is clamped with the absorbable clips

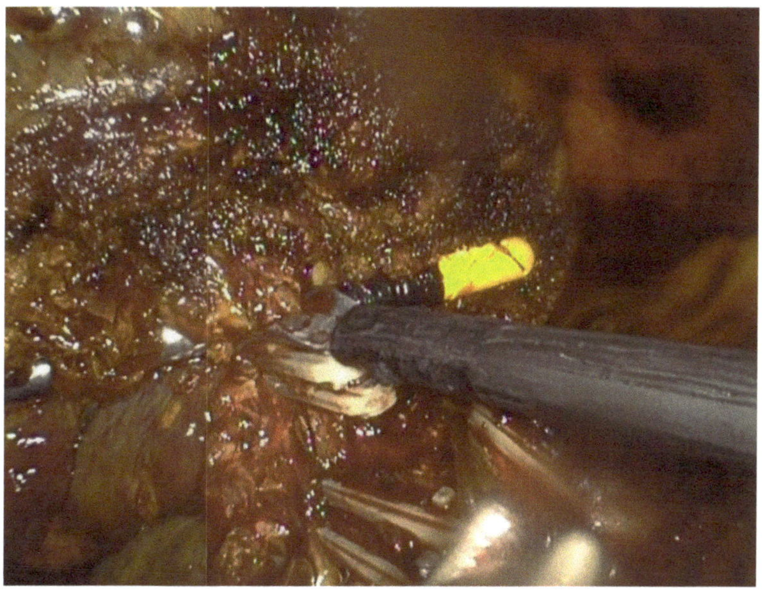

Fig. 8.97 The RAPV is divided

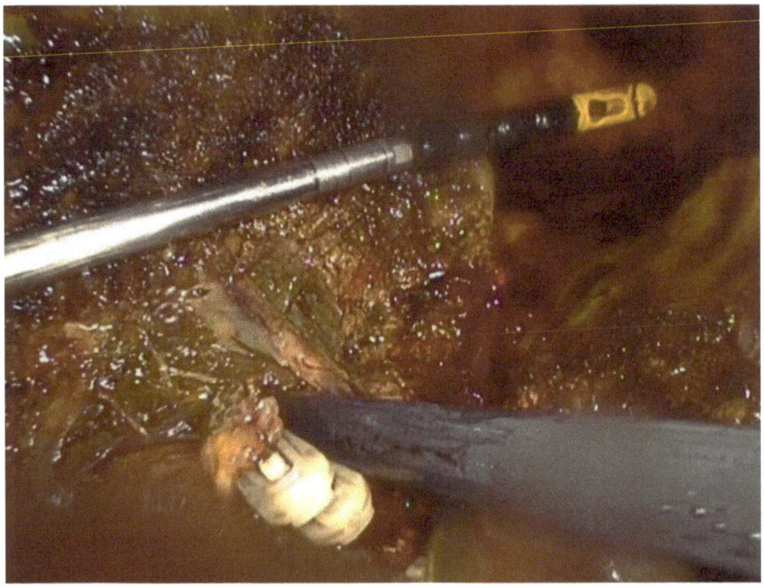

Fig. 8.98 The RPPV is dissected

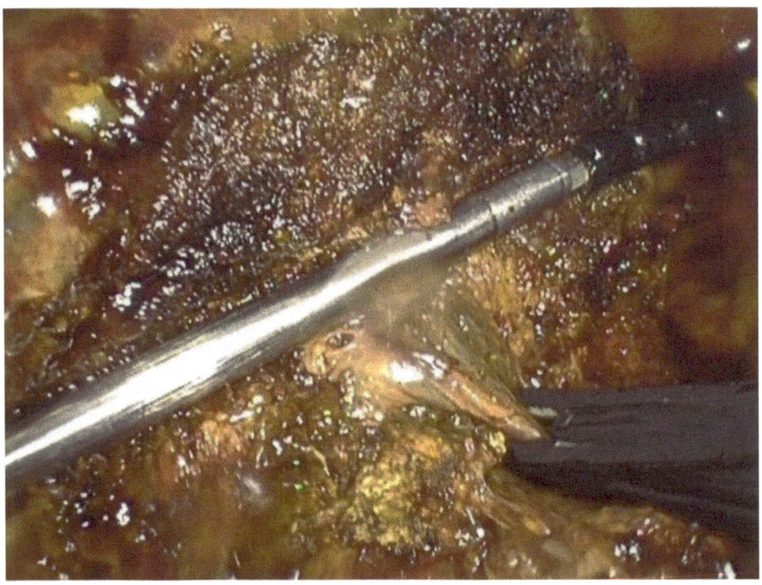

Fig. 8.99 The RPPV is clamped with an absorbable clip

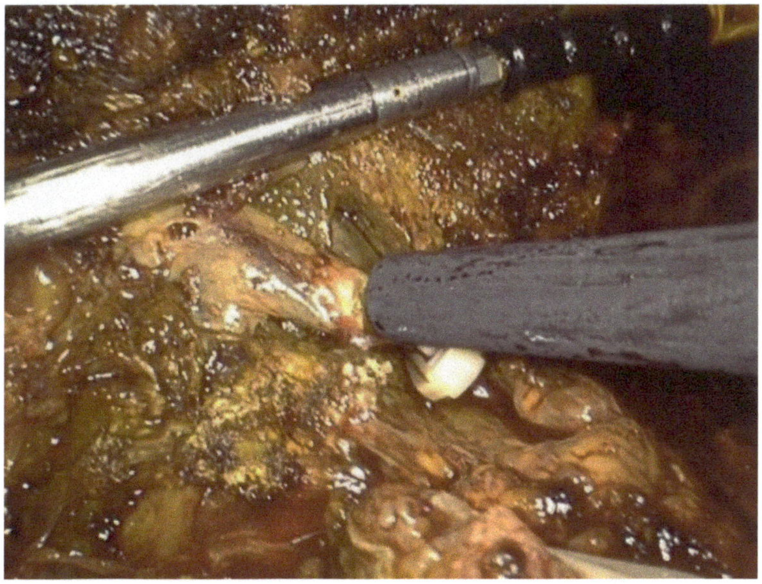

Fig. 8.100 The RPPV is divided

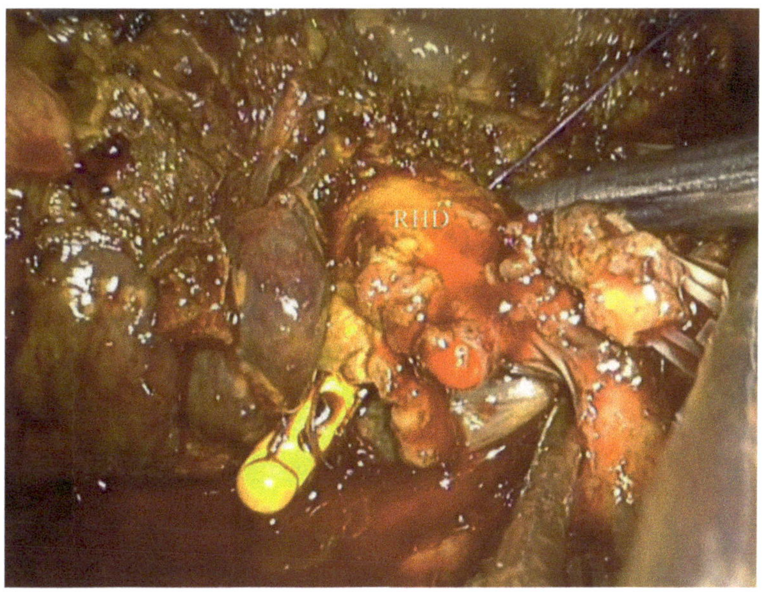

Fig. 8.101 The RHD is dissected, and a suture is passed through the back of the RHD with the guidance of the "gold finger" liver retractor

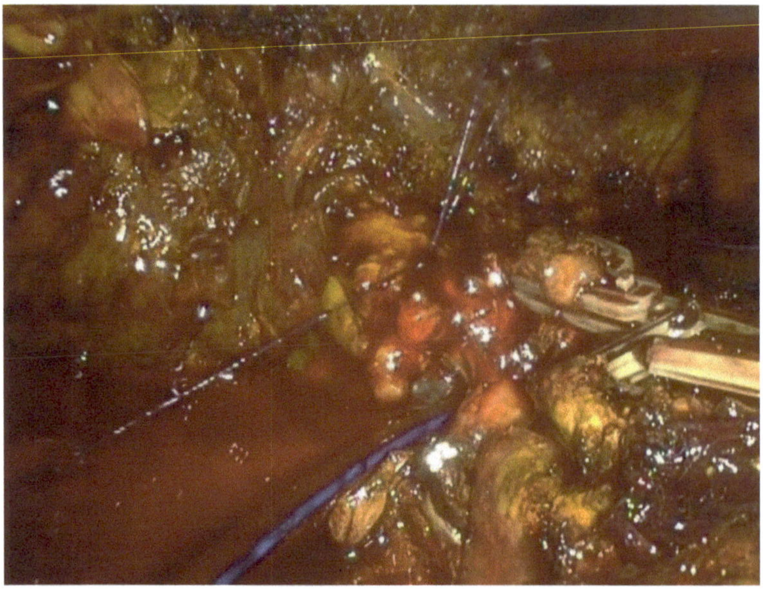

Fig. 8.102 The RHD is ligated with the suture

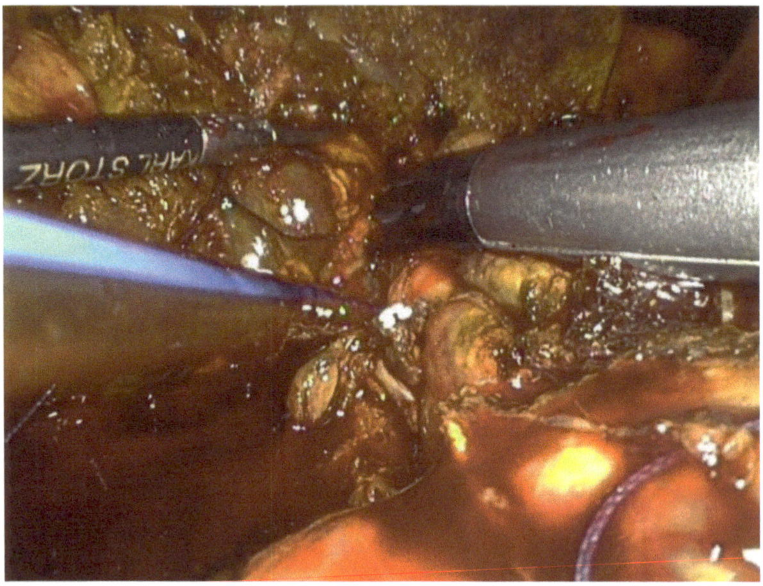

Fig. 8.103 The RHD is clamped with an absorbable clip

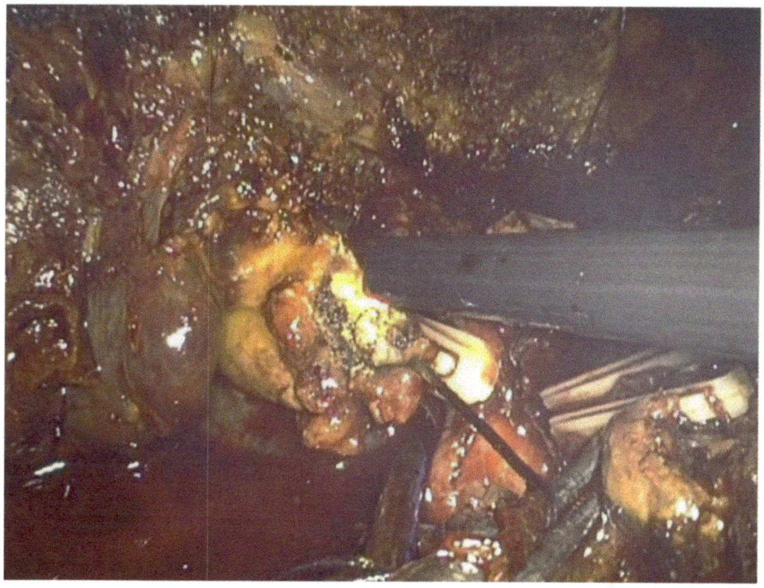

Fig. 8.104 The RHD is divided with LPMOD

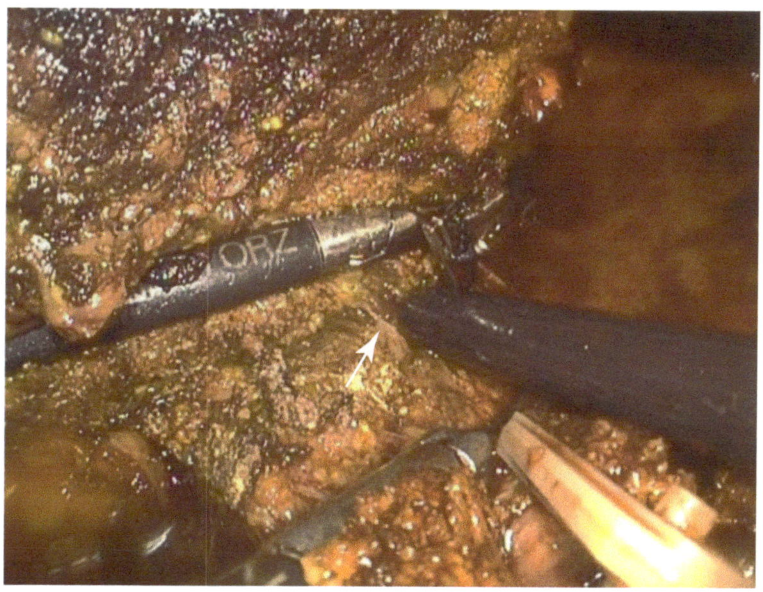

Fig. 8.105 A branch of the middle hepatic vein (MHV) is dissected with LPMOD

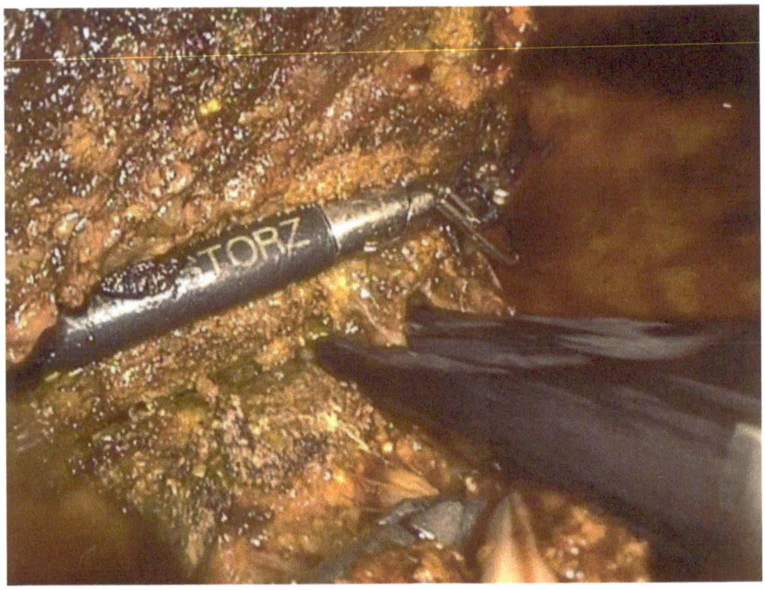

Fig. 8.106 The branch of the middle hepatic vein is clamped

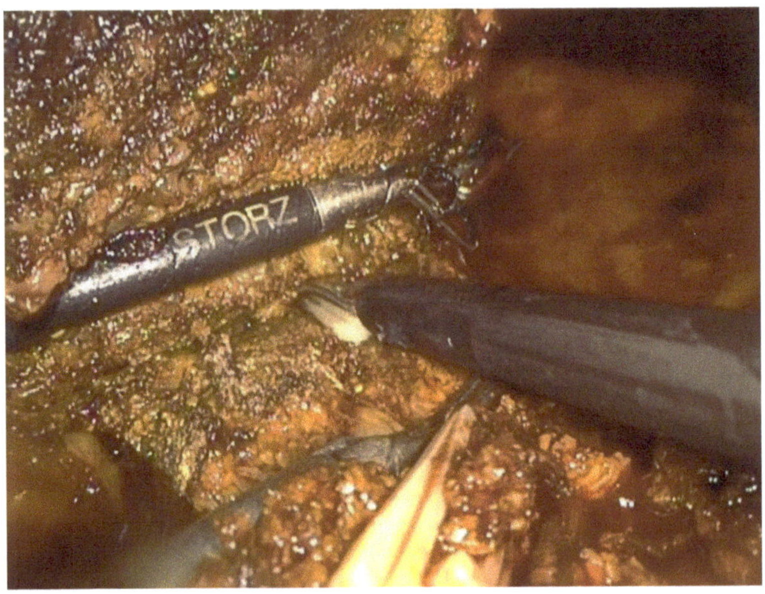

Fig. 8.107 The branch of the middle hepatic vein is divided

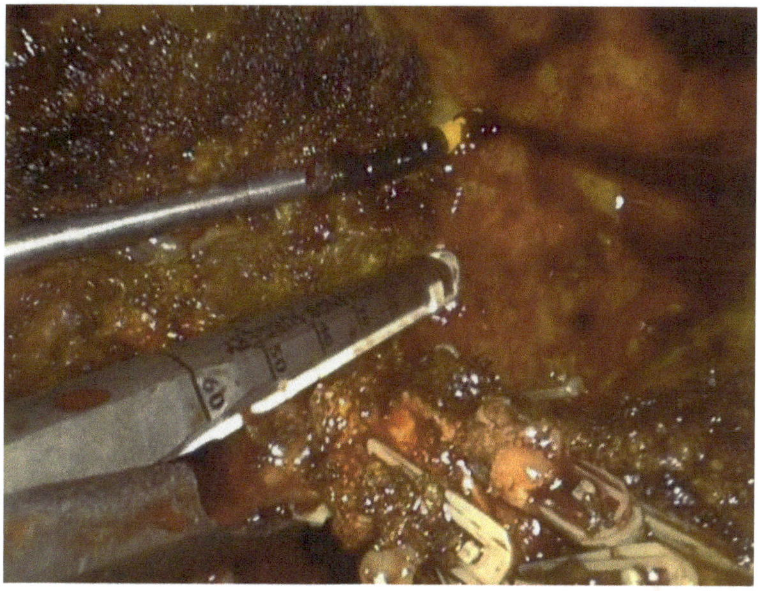

Fig. 8.108 The remaining liver parenchyma is transected with a laparoscopic linear stapler

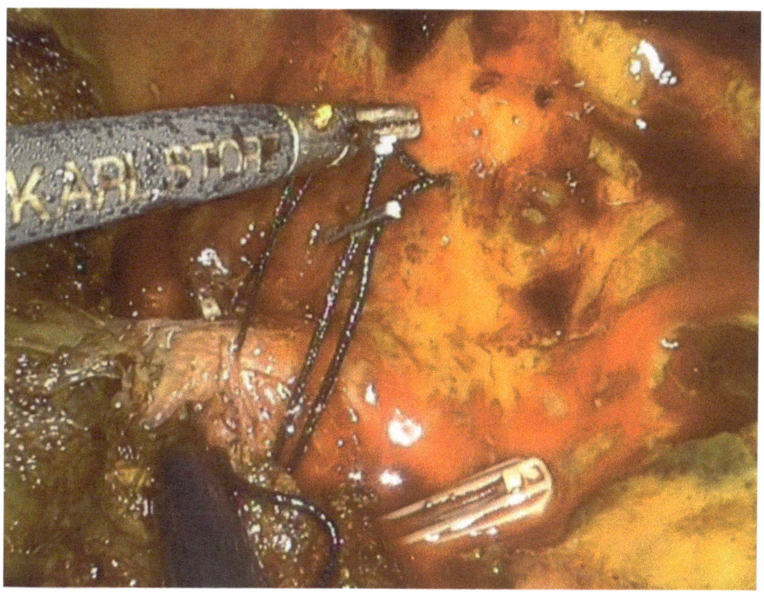

Fig. 8.109 The right hepatic vein is visualized after the liver parenchyma was transected

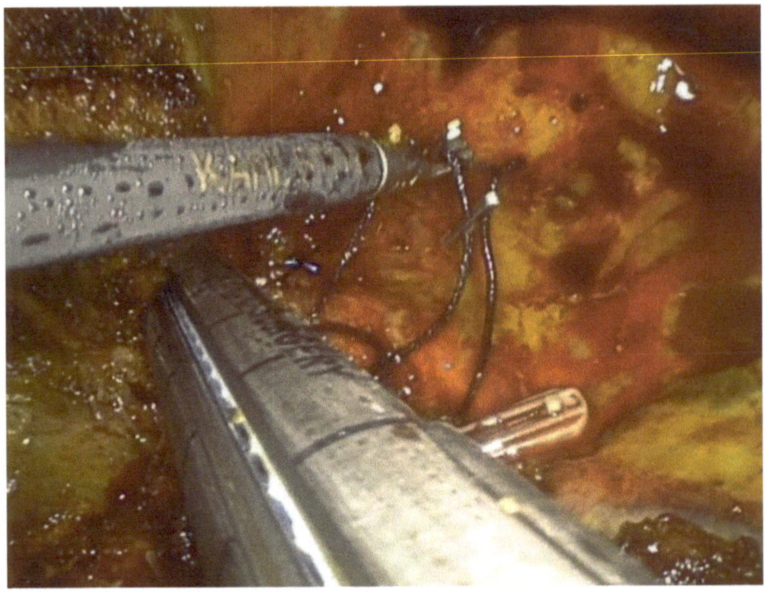

Fig. 8.110 The right hepatic vein is transected with the other laparoscopic linear stapler

References

de Santibañes E, Clavien PA. Playing Play-Doh to prevent postoperative liver failure: the "ALPPS" approach. Ann Surg. 2012;255:415–7.

Hayashi S, Baba Y, Ueno K, et al. Acceleration of primary liver tumor growth rate in embolized hepatic lobe after portal vein embolization. Acta Radiol. 2007;48:721–7.

Kokudo N, Shindoh J. How can we safely climb the ALPPS? Updates Surg. 2013;65:175–7.

Kokudo N, Tada K, Seki M, et al. Proliferative activity of intrahepatic colorectal metastases after preoperative hemihepatic portal vein embolization. Hepatology. 2001;34:267–72.

Machado MA, Makdissi FF, Surjan RC. Totally laparoscopic ALPPS is feasible and may be worthwhile. Ann Surg. 2012;256:e13.

Robles Campos R, Parrilla Paricio P, López Conesa A, et al. A new surgical technique for extended right hepatectomy: tourniquet in the umbilical fissure and right portal vein occlusion (ALTPS). Cir Esp. 2013;91:633–7.

Schnitzbauer AA, Lang SA, Goessmann H, et al. Right portal vein ligation combined with in situ splitting induces rapid left lateral liver lobe hypertrophy enabling 2-staged extended right hepatic resection in small-for-size settings. Ann Surg. 2012;255:405–14.

9 Laparoscopic Radical Resection of Gallbladder Cancer

Gallbladder (GB) cancer is an aggressive malignancy, and the prognosis for most patients is poor. The median overall survival time is 10 months (Duffy et al. 2008). Patients with gallbladder cancer confined to the mucosa or submucosa (T1a) are usually diagnosed by the postoperative pathological examination, and a simple cholecystectomy is adequate for them. A radical resection of the localized gallbladder cancer, including cholecystectomy, partial hepatectomy, and skeletonization of hepatoduodenal ligament (HDL), could gain a better result in patients with gallbladder cancer invading into (T1b) or beyond (stages II–IVa) the gallbladder muscularis. Laparoscopic surgery is adopted for treating gallbladder cancer, but port-site recurrence and intra-abdominal dissemination are concerns of surgeons (Kais et al. 2014; Lee et al. 2011). The rupture of gallbladder should be avoided to prevent intra-abdominal dissemination, and the specimen should be properly retrieved from the abdominal cavity. In our institute, the plastic Endobag is routinely used to capsule the specimen in the extraction of the specimen out of the abdominal cavity to prevent port-site recurrence.

9.1 Indications and Contraindications

Indications include gallbladder cancer invading into or beyond the gallbladder muscularis and liver function of Child A to B classification. Contraindications include malignant tumor involving porta hepatis or with intra-abdominal dissemination.

Electronic supplementary material The online version of this chapter at (doi: 10.1007/978-94-017-9840-2_9) contains supplementary material, which is available to authorized users.

X. Cai, *Laparoscopic Hepatectomy: Atlas and Techniques*,
DOI 10.1007/978-94-017-9840-2_9,

9.2 Patient Position and Trocars' Position

Patients are placed in the supine position under general anesthesia. Three surgeons are needed in the operation. The senior surgeon stands on the left side of the patient, one assistant surgeon stands on the right side of the senior surgeon manipulating the aspiration device, and the other assistant surgeon stands on the other side of the patient. Four entries are made. A supraumbilical 10-mm trocar is inserted as the observation port. A 12-mm trocar below the left costal margin is inserted as the main manipulation port. And two 5-mm trocars are inserted at the right flank area as assistant manipulation ports (Fig. 9.1).

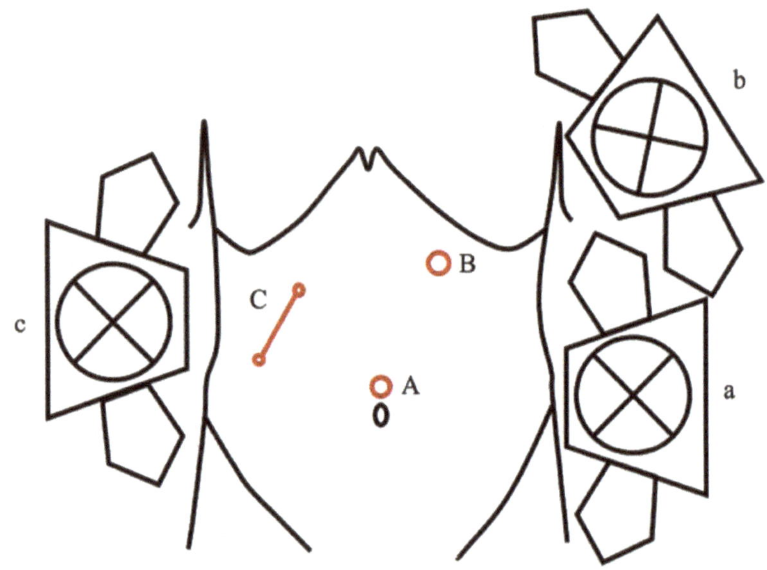

Fig. 9.1 Trocars' position and surgeons' position. (*A*) Observation port; (*B*) Main manipulation port; (*C*) Two assistant ports and the incision for removing specimen; (**a**) The senior surgeon stands on the left side of the patient; (**b**) One assistant surgeon stands on the right side of the senior surgeon controlling the aspiration device; (**c**) The other assistant surgeon stands on the right side of the patient

9.3 Laparoscopic Radical Resection of Gallbladder Cancer

See Figs. 9.2, 9.3, 9.4, 9.5, 9.6, 9.7, 9.8, 9.9, 9.10, 9.11, 9.12, 9.13, 9.14, 9.15, 9.16, 9.17, 9.18, 9.19, 9.20, 9.21, 9.22, 9.23, 9.24, 9.25, 9.26, 9.27, 9.28, 9.29, 9.30, 9.31, 9.32, 9.33, 9.34, and Video 9.1.

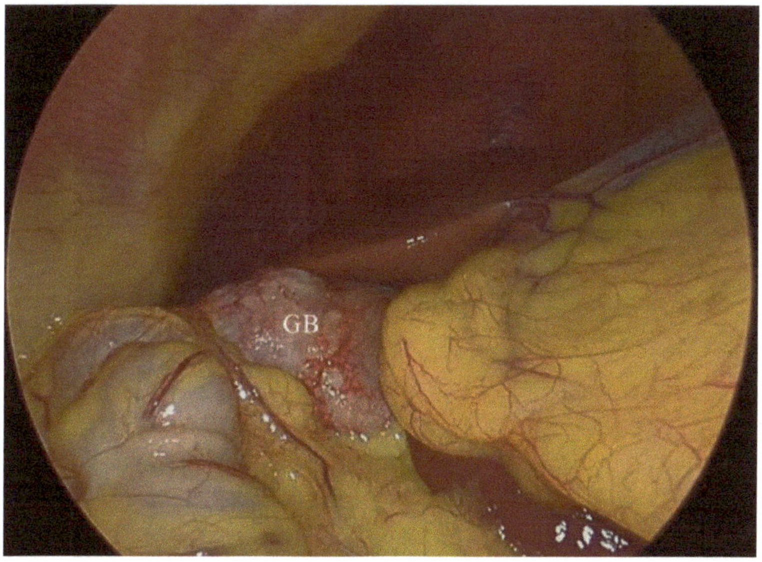

Fig. 9.2 A tumor is visualized in the GB, but no intra-abdominal dissemination is visualized

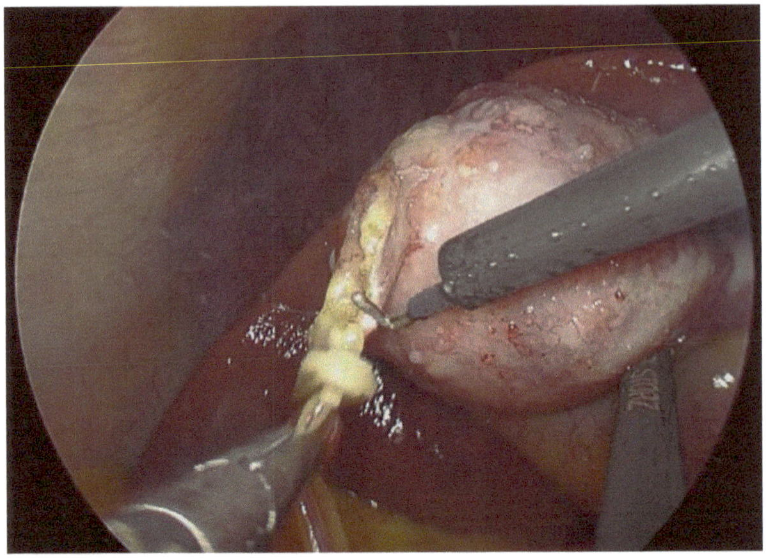

Fig. 9.3 Adhesion between the GB and the omentum majus is divided

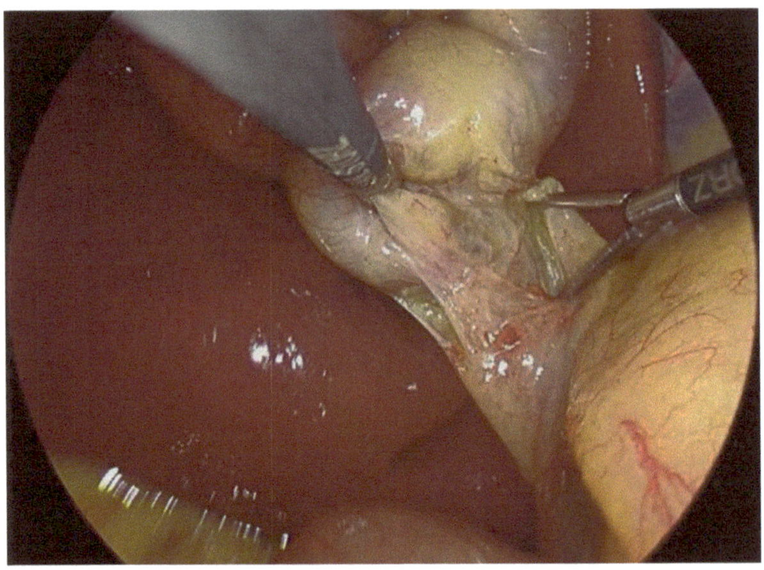

Fig. 9.4 The Calot's triangle is dissected

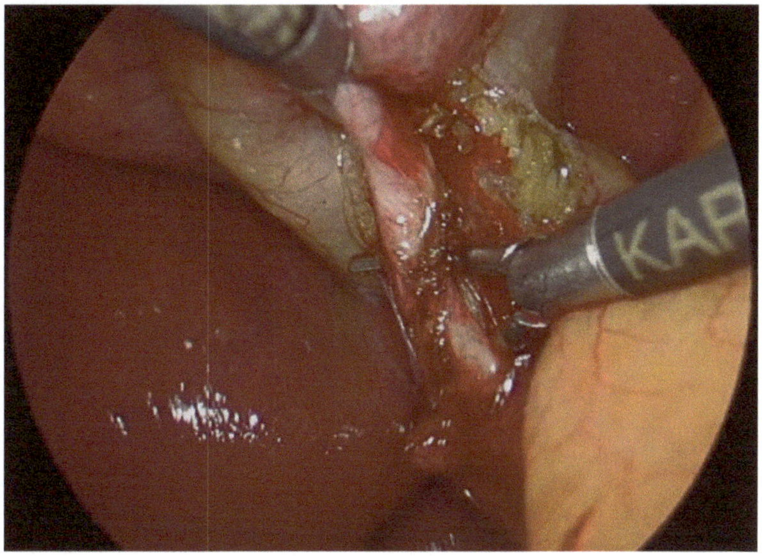

Fig. 9.5 The cystic duct (CD) is freed with a dissection forceps

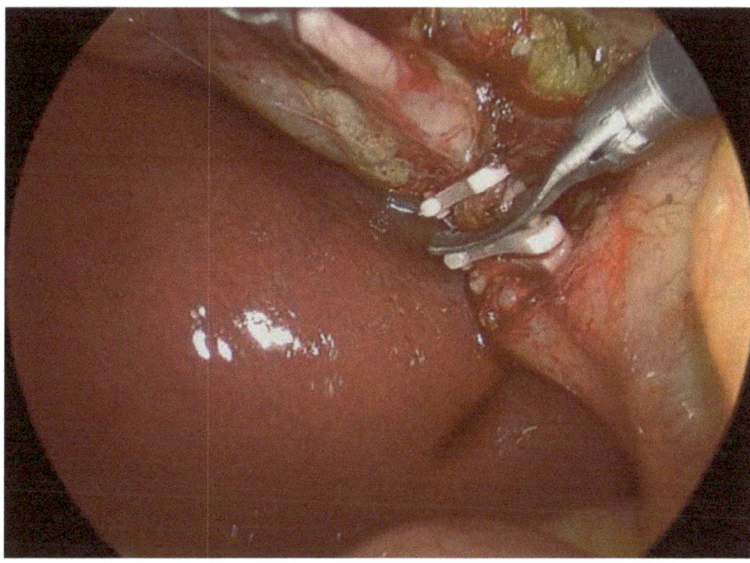

Fig. 9.6 The cystic duct is divided

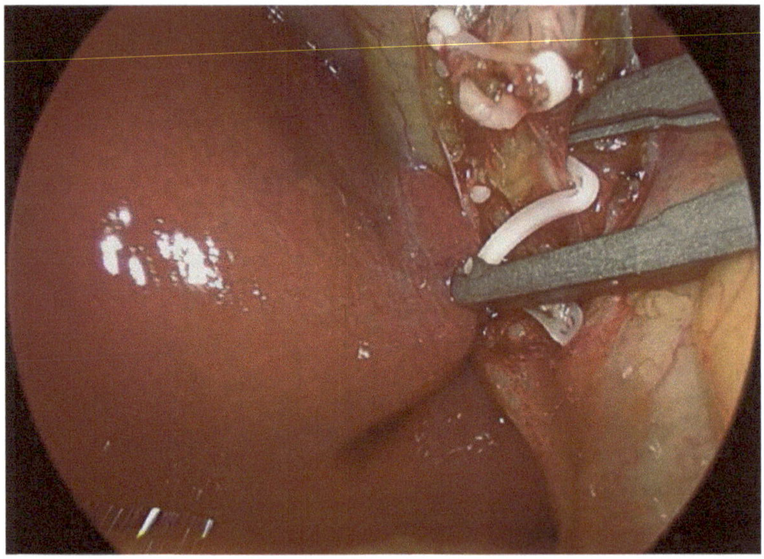

Fig. 9.7 The cystic artery is freed and is clipped

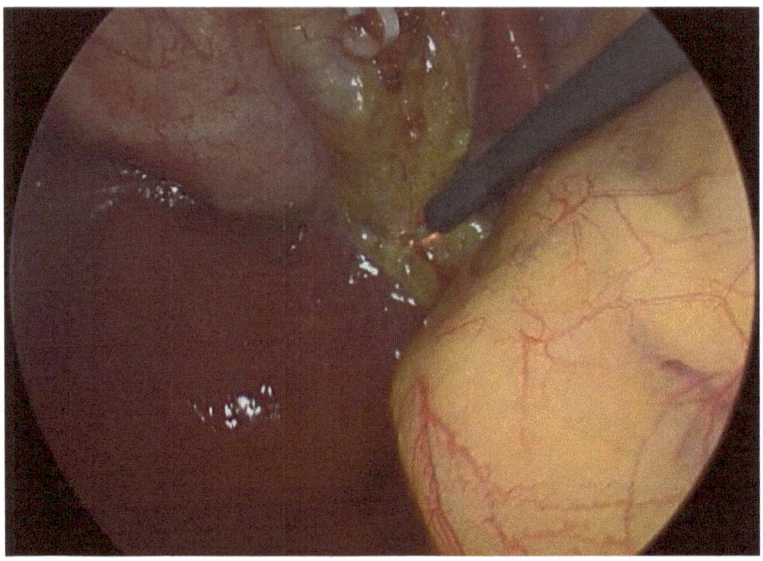

Fig. 9.8 The gallbladder is freed from the hepato-duodenal ligament after the cystic duct, and the cystic arteries (CA) were divided

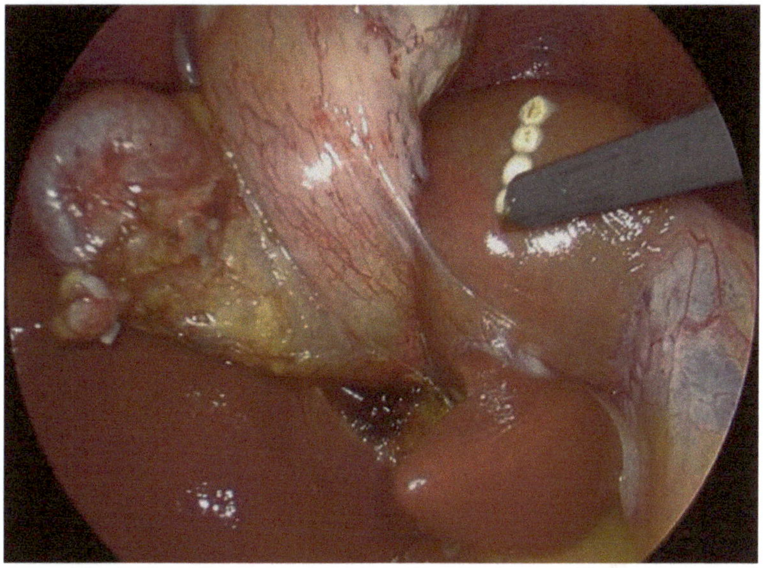

Fig. 9.9 The liver is mobilized upward by the traction of the neck of the gallbladder, and the transection line is marked on the liver surface about 2 cm to the tumor

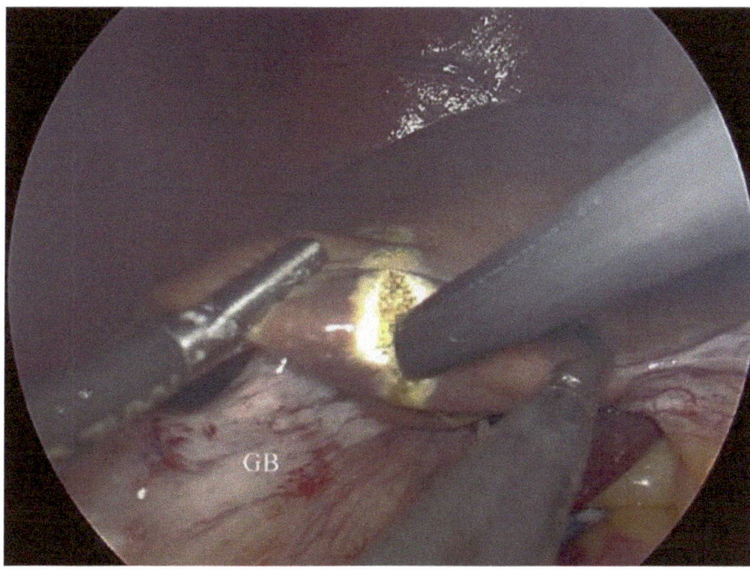

Fig. 9.10 The liver capsule is cut along the transection line with LPMOD

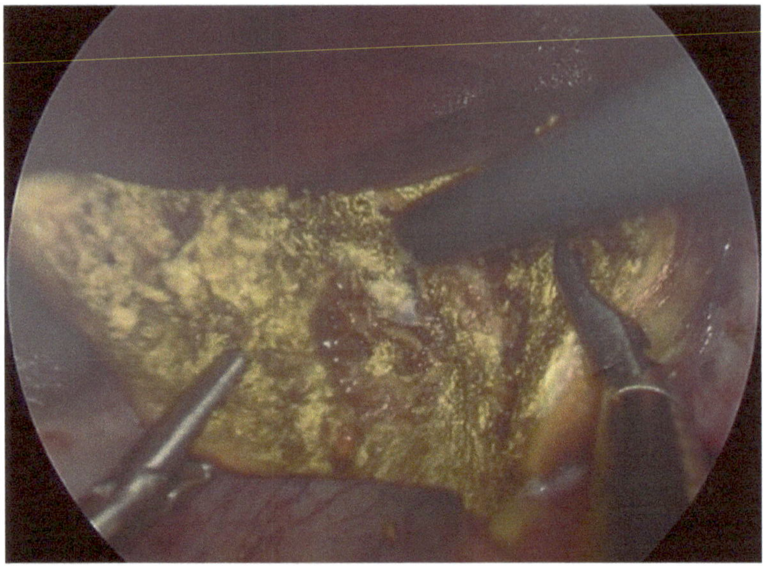

Fig. 9.11 Liver parenchyma is transected, and a small vessel is visualized in the transection

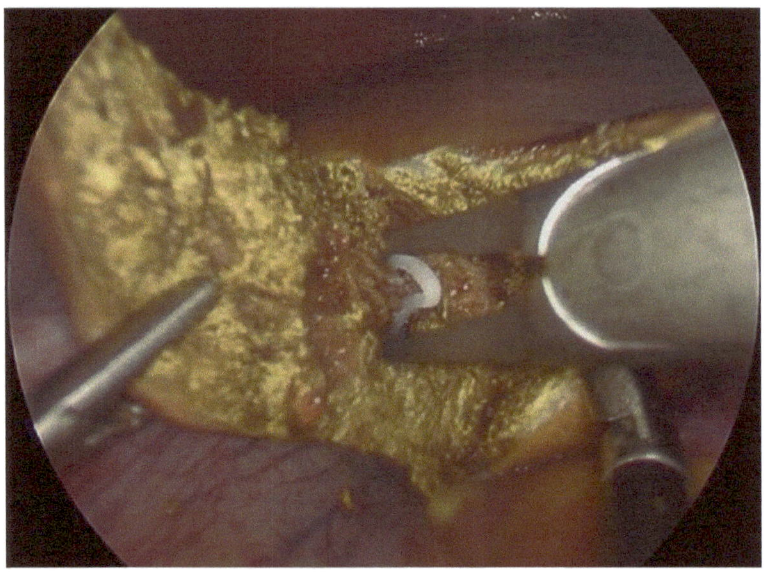

Fig. 9.12 The vessel is dissected and is clipped with a nonabsorbable polymer clip

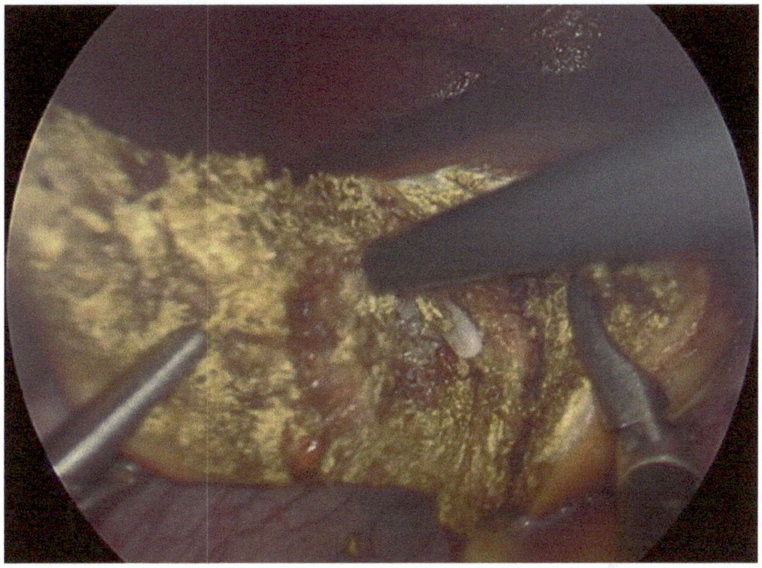

Fig. 9.13 The vessel is transected with LPMOD after being clipped

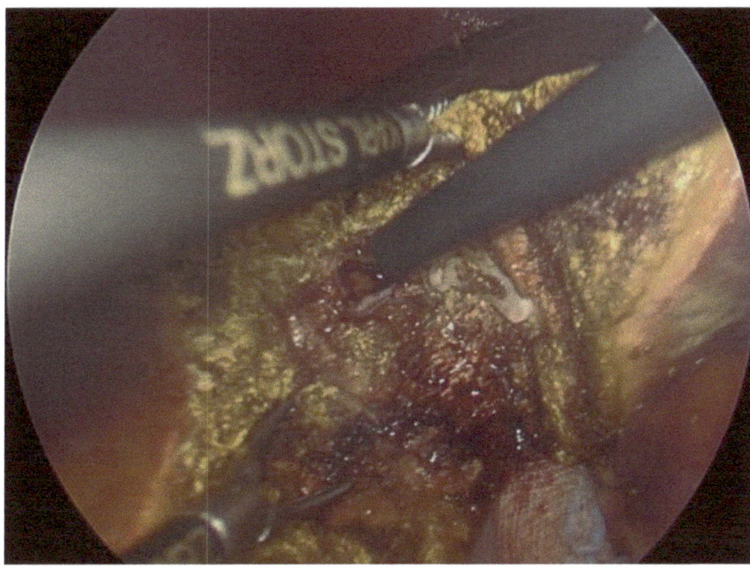

Fig. 9.14 Another vessel is visualized in the liver transection

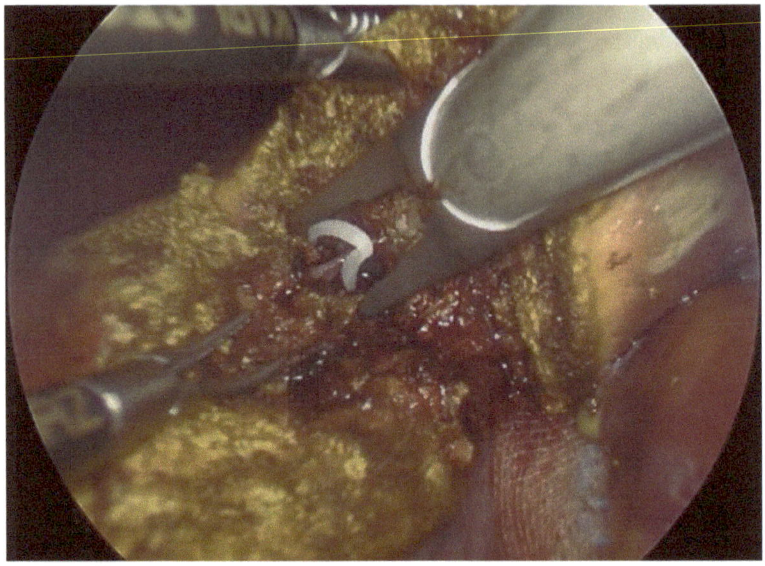

Fig. 9.15 The vessel is dissected and is clipped with a nonabsorbable polymer clip

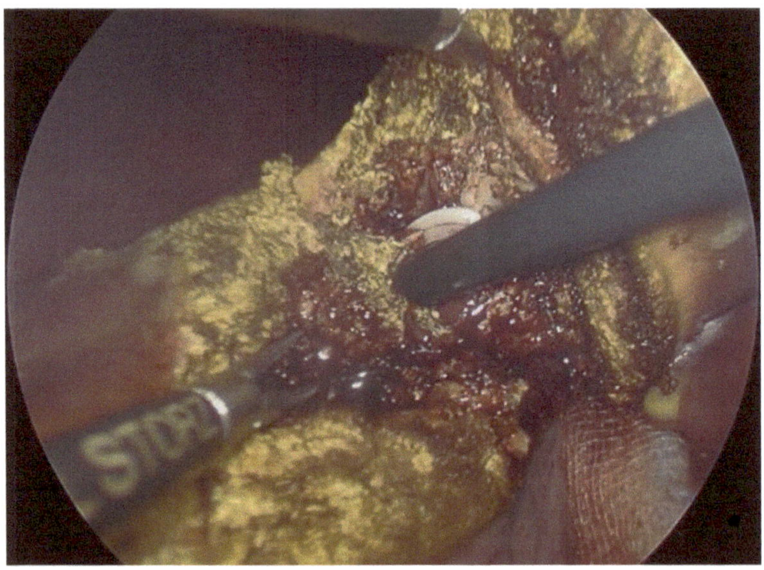

Fig. 9.16 The vessel is transected with LPMOD

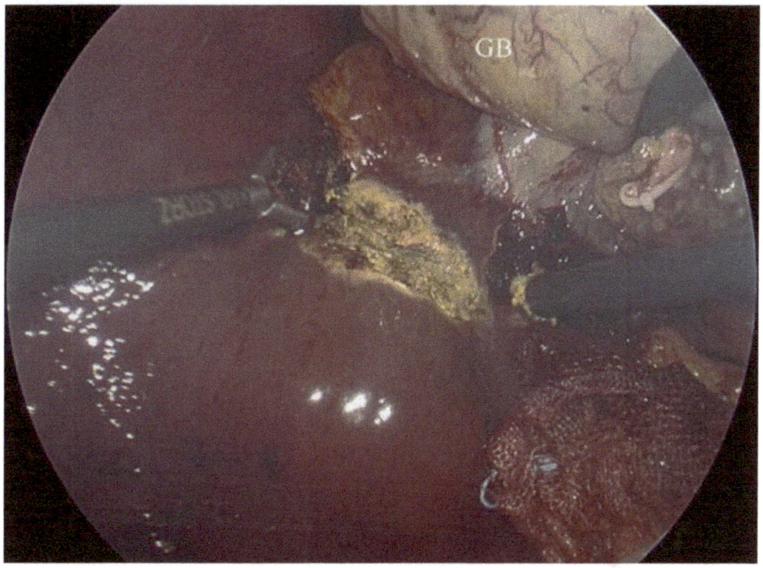

Fig. 9.17 The inferior margin of the liver is mobilized upward, and the liver parenchyma is continued to be transected with LPMOD

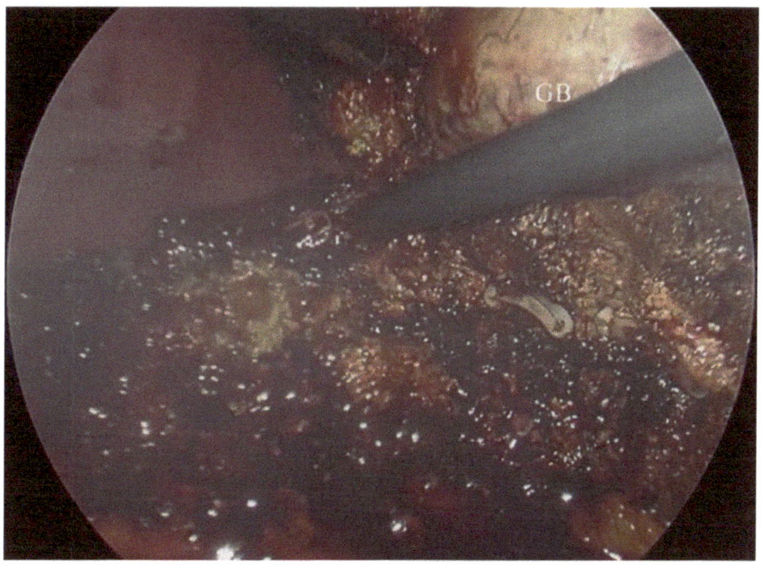

Fig. 9.18 The GB and the adjacent liver parenchyma is lifted, and the liver parenchyma is transected with LPMOD until the tumor is radically resected

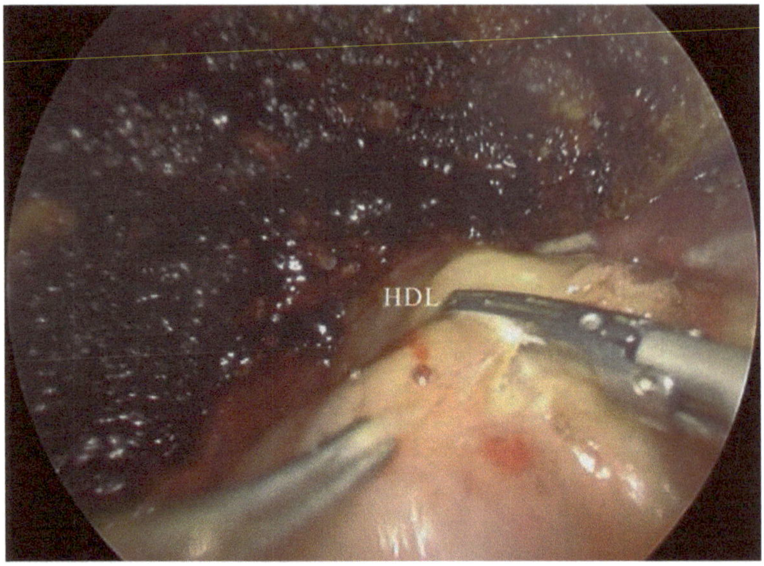

Fig. 9.19 The capsule of the HDL is cut open near the pancreas with a laparoscopic ultrasonic scalpel

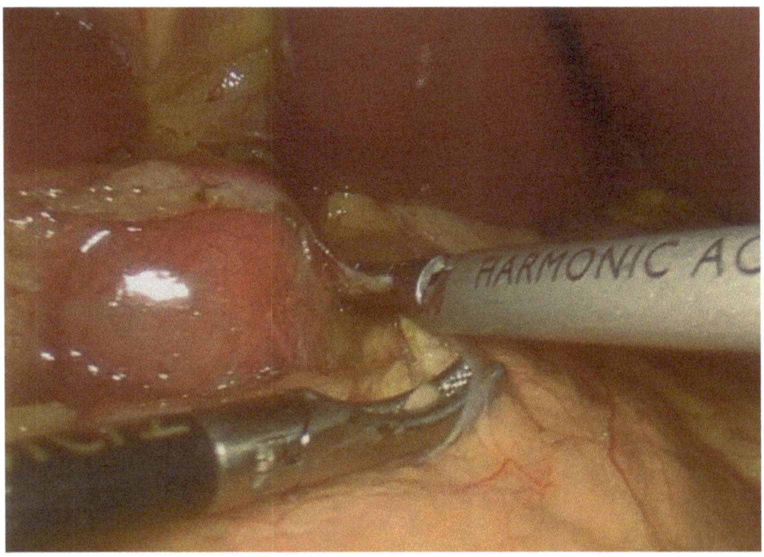

Fig. 9.20 The lesser omentum near the HDL was divided with the laparoscopic ultrasonic scalpel

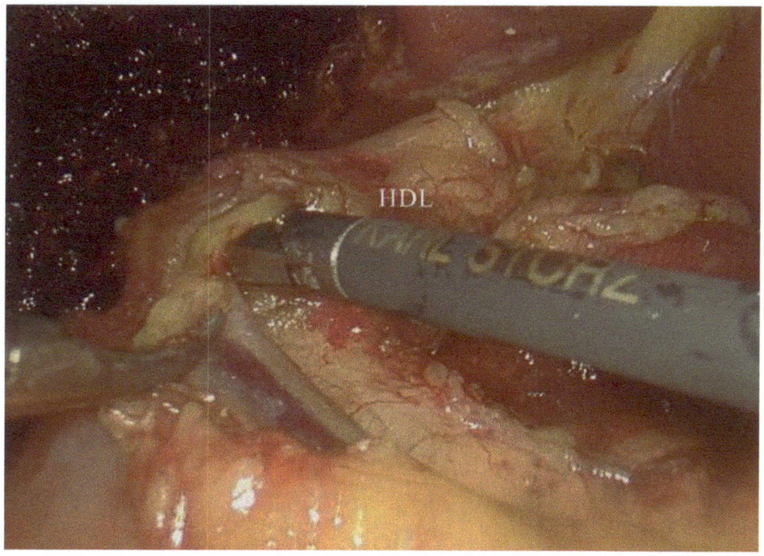

Fig. 9.21 A piece of tissue was freed from the HDL

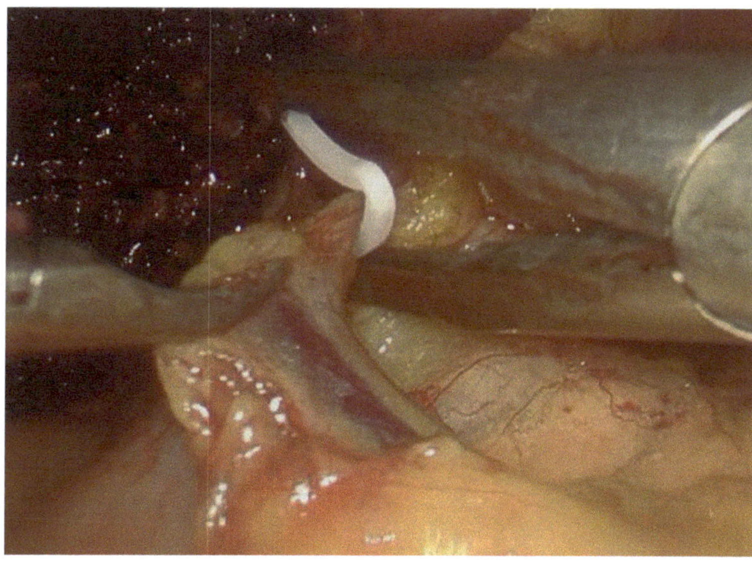

Fig. 9.22 The tissue is clipped en bloc with a nonabsorbable polymer clip

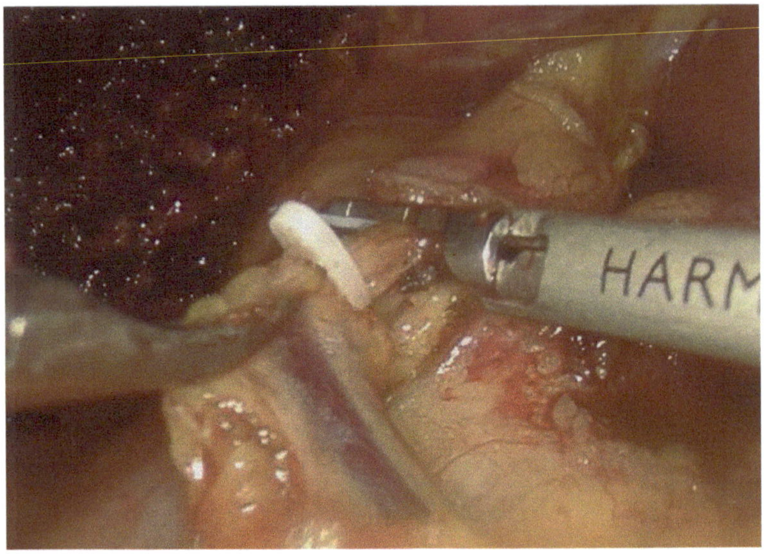

Fig. 9.23 The tissue is divided with the laparoscopic ultrasonic scalpel

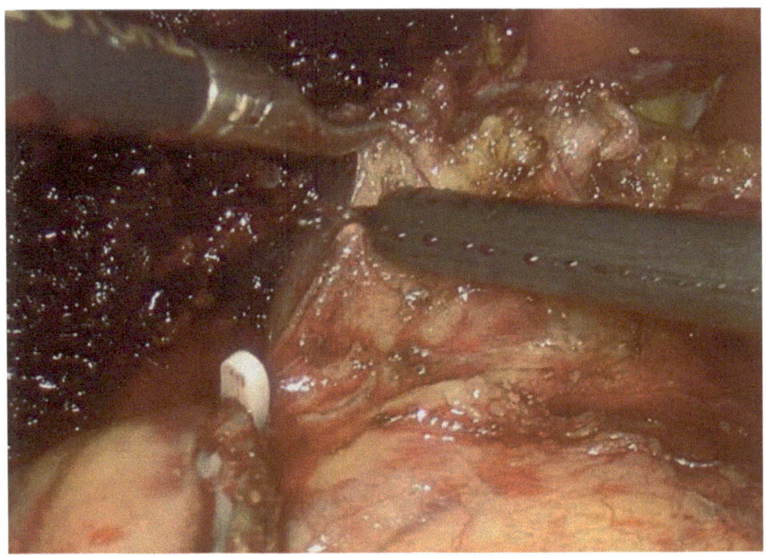

Fig. 9.24 The HDL is skeletonized from the pancreas to the porta hepatis (PH)

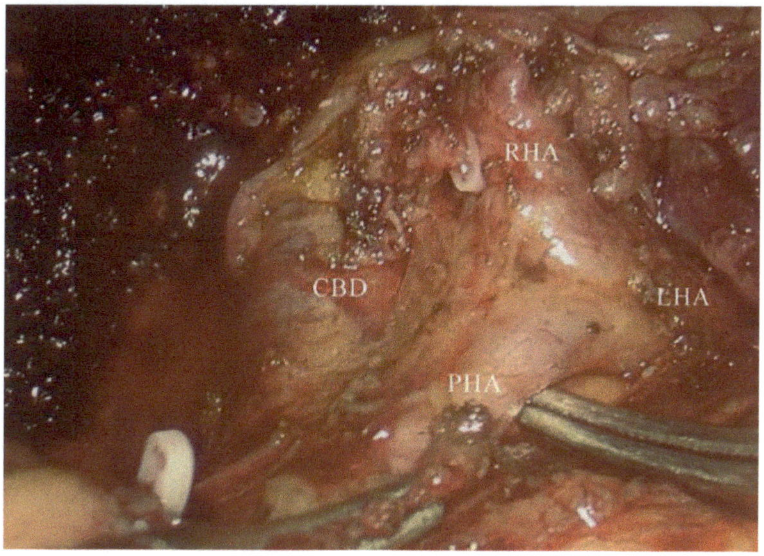

Fig. 9.25 After meticulous dissection, the common bile duct (*CBD*), the proper hepatic artery (*PHA*), the left hepatic artery (LHA), and the right hepatic artery (*RHA*) are visualized

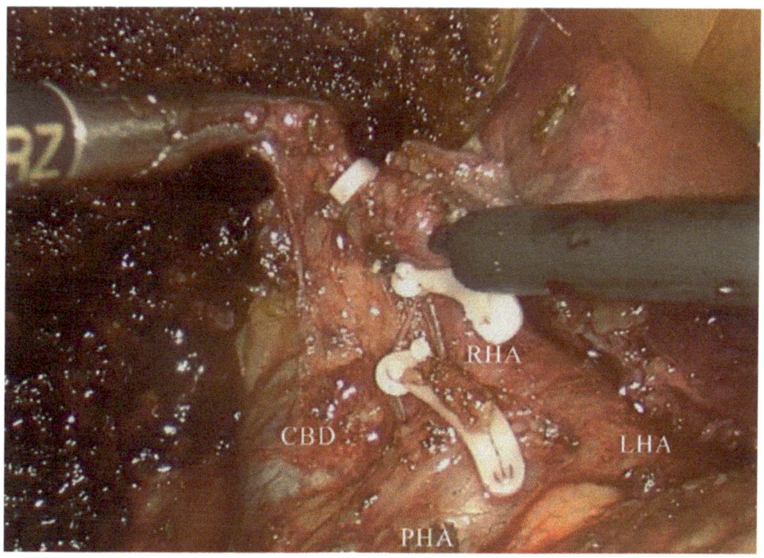

Fig. 9.26 The RHA was dissected

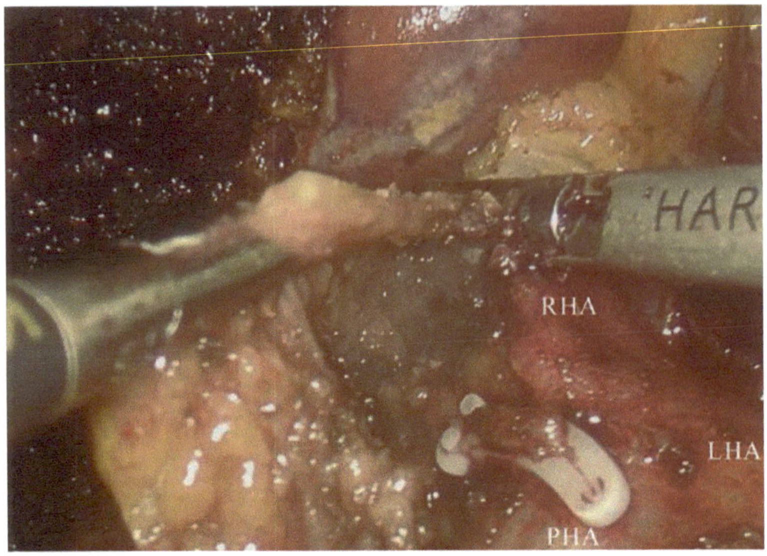

Fig. 9.27 The structures near the porta hepatis are dissected, and tissues are excised with the laparoscopic ultrasonic scalpel

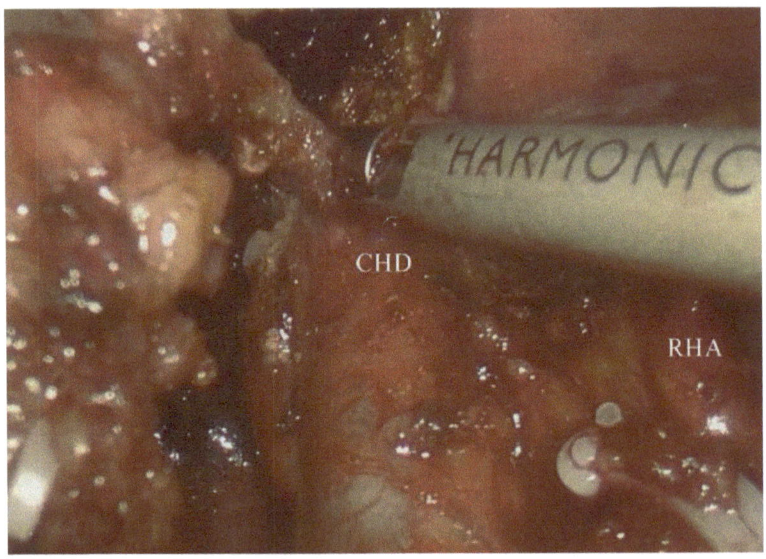

Fig. 9.28 The common hepatic duct (*CHD*) is dissected

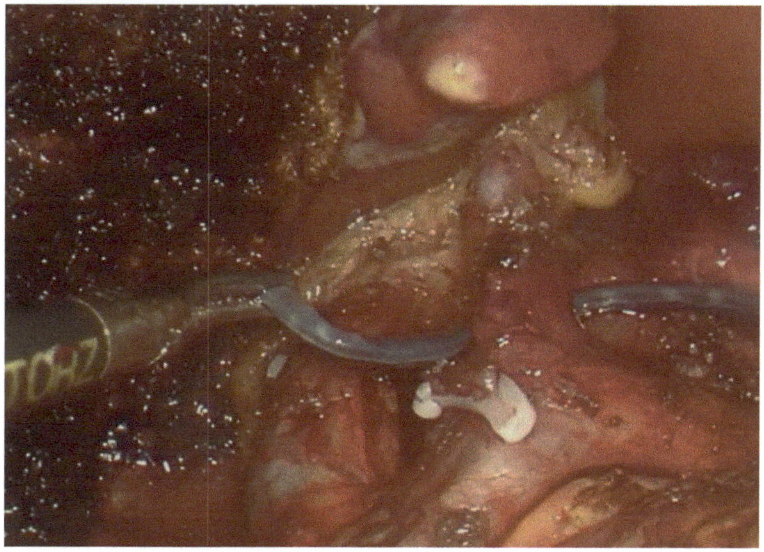

Fig. 9.29 The RHA is freed, and an elastic tape rounded it for traction

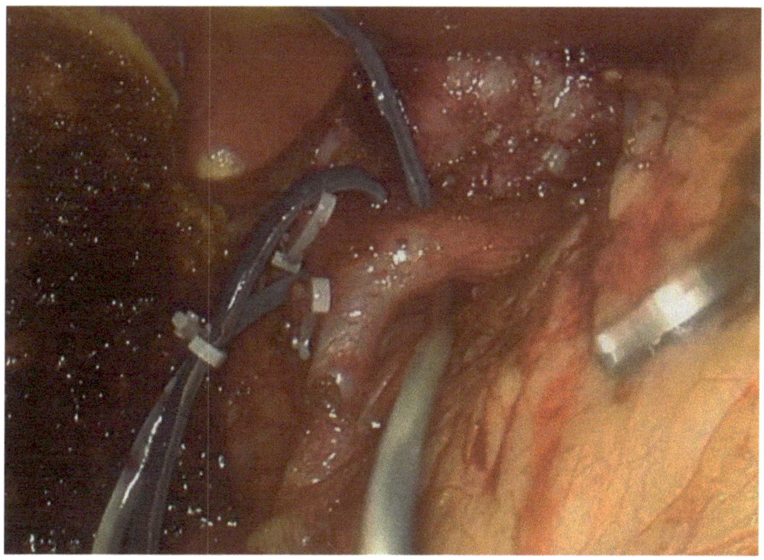

Fig. 9.30 The LHA is freed, and an elastic tape rounded it for traction

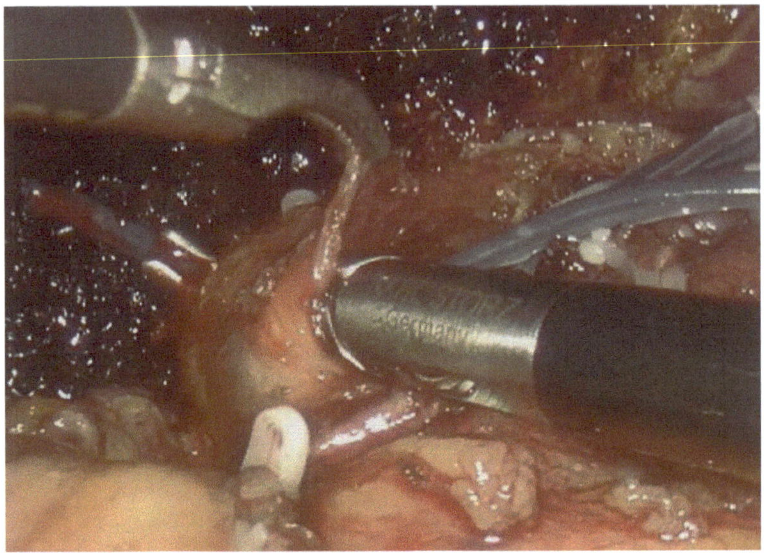

Fig. 9.31 The CBD is freed, and an elastic tape rounded it for traction

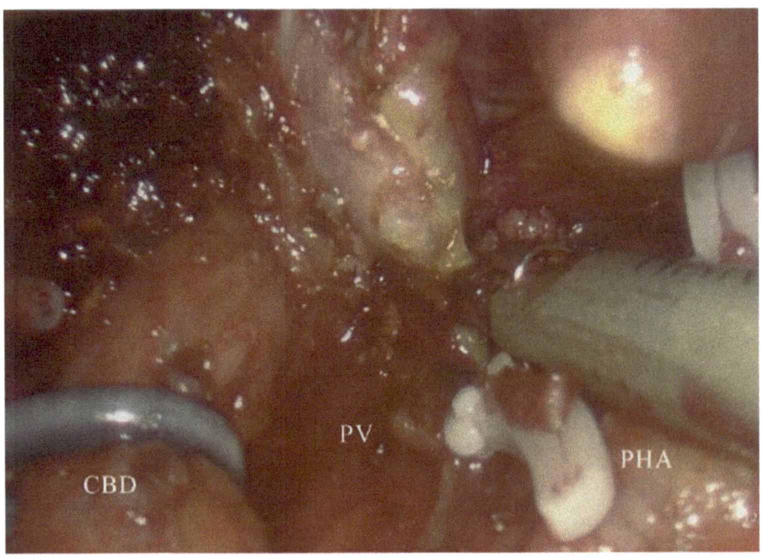

Fig. 9.32 The CBD and the RHA were mobilized, and a lymph node is exposed and is excised with the laparoscopic ultrasonic scalpel

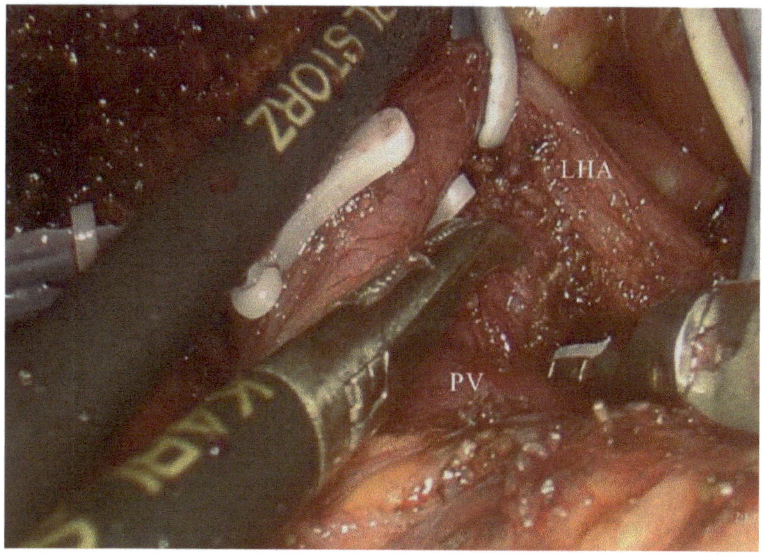

Fig. 9.33 The LHA is mobilized upward, and a lymph node is exposed and is excised with the laparoscopic ultrasonic scalpel

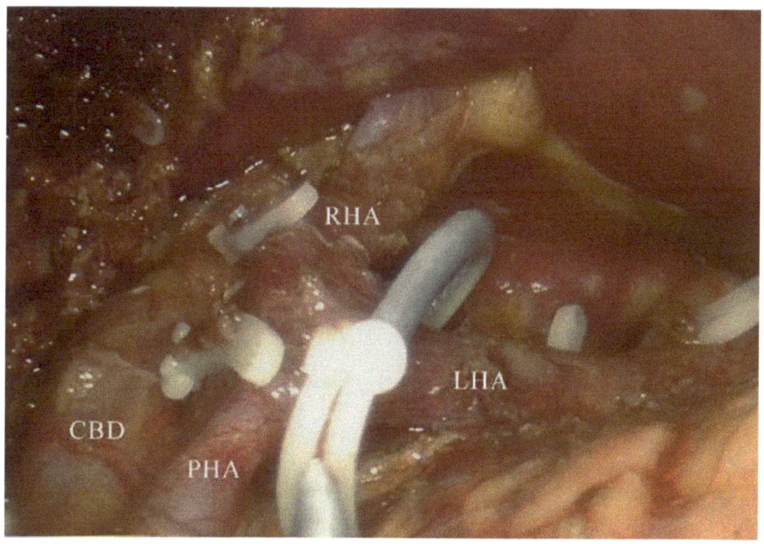

Fig. 9.34 After meticulous dissection, structures in the HDL are skeletonized

References

Duffy A, Capanu M, Abou-Alfa GK, et al. Gallbladder cancer (GBC): 10-year experience at Memorial Sloan-Kettering Cancer Centre (MSKCC). J Surg Oncol. 2008;98:485–9.

Kais H, Hershkovitz Y, Sandbank J, et al. Port site metastases in squamous cell carcinoma of the gallbladder. Isr Med Assoc J. 2014;16:177–9.

Lee JM, Kim BW, Kim WH, et al. Clinical implication of bile spillage in patients undergoing laparoscopic cholecystectomy for gallbladder cancer. Am Surg. 2011;77:697–701.

10 Other Techniques for Laparoscopic Hepatectomy

The laparoscopic approach allows patients a rapid return to daily activity and has been adopted almost worldwide. Laparoscopic hepatectomy has developed for two decades, but it is still a developing procedure and is performed only in a few institutes in the world. The liver has rich blood supply, and most intraoperative bleeding could not be effectively managed in a laparoscopic condition which is the major reason hindering the development of laparoscopic liver resection. A technique which could avoid intraoperative bleeding or could significantly decrease the occurrence rate of intraoperative bleeding was highly demanded by surgeons. Until now, the majority of techniques available for laparoscopic liver resection initiated from open procedures. Major changes include the minimization and elongation of instruments to fit laparoscopic manipulation, the modification of surgical procedures, and finally establishing special techniques.

Any technique for laparoscopic liver resection could not leave a special instrument for liver transection. That is to say, an instrument may represent a technique. Apart from LPMOD, there are other instruments used in laparoscopic liver resection, and some techniques are developed based on these special instruments. In this chapter, other techniques and instruments for laparoscopic liver resection will be introduced.

10.1 Laparoscopic Liver Transection with an Ultrasonic Dissector

Patients are usually placed in the lithotomy position. Three surgeons are needed in the operation. The main surgeon stands between the patient's legs and two assistants stand on each side. Four ports are made. The observation port is placed under or above the umbilicus, and the major manipulation port is usually placed subxiphoid. Firstly, some perihepatic ligaments are divided with the ultrasonic dissector according to the resection extent. Then a transection line is marked on the liver surface, and the liver parenchyma is transected with an ultrasonic dissector along the transection line. Because of the absence of large vessels and hepatic ducts, the superficial liver tissue can be transected directly without dissection which nearly no bleeding or bile leakage occurring (Fig. 10.1). In the transection of deeper liver parenchyma, the ultrasonic dissector should be moved in a "painting" motion (Aldrighetti et al. 2008) along the transection groove for the purpose of detecting large vessels and hepatic ducts without any injury. After vessels or hepatic ducts were detected, they are dissected and freed with the ultrasonic dissector for laparoscopic dissecting forceps and are disposed of depending on their size. Normally, vessels less than 4 mm in diameter could be coagulated and divided with the ultrasonic dissector, and the vessels larger than 4 mm should be clipped or transected with a laparoscopic linear stapler.

X. Cai, *Laparoscopic Hepatectomy: Atlas and Techniques*,
DOI 10.1007/978-94-017-9840-2_10,

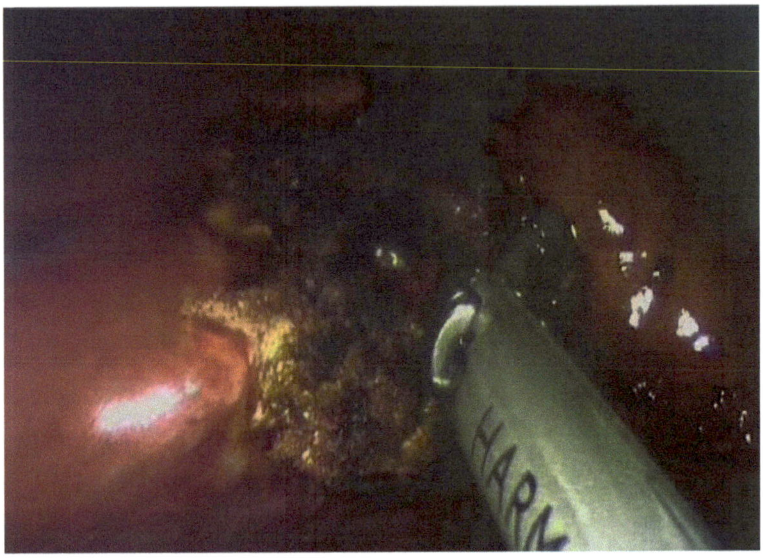

Fig. 10.1 Superficial liver parenchyma is transected with a laparoscopic ultrasonic dissector

10.2 Laparoscopic Liver Transection with the Cavitron Ultrasonic Surgical Aspirator (CUSA)

The CUSA is an instrument for dissecting the liver parenchyma. It is a powerful ultrasonic aspirator and dissector and is widely used in surgeries. CUSA has the effect on low-strength tissue and high-strength tissue, and the effect depends on the amount of high-strength intercellular bonds in tissue. It could dissect the liver parenchyma without injuring vessels and bile ducts. The procedure of laparoscopic liver resection with CUSA is similar to the ultrasonic dissector. It has the function of ultrasonic aspiration and irrigation. The action of fragmentation, aspiration, and irrigation could occur simultaneously which allows the surgeon to remove the liver parenchyma with meticulous dissection and accurate transection. CUSA enables the dissection around any structure that needs to be preserved exposing the Glisson capsule, hepatic veins, and vessels across the transection plane for further ligation or clipping (Honda et al. 2013).

10.3 Laparoscopic Liver Resection Using a Bipolar Vessel-Sealing Device: LigaSure

The LigaSure device uses physical compression, computer-controlled radiofrequency energy, and a brief cool-down period to produce the fusion of collagen and elastin of the vessel walls to achieve a translucent seal (Slakey 2008). Vessels less than 7 mm in diameter could be sealed with the LigaSure. Large vessels or hepatic ducts are usually managed with linear stapler. The procedure is also similar to the ultrasonic dissector in which the dissection motion was used. Ultrasound is usually used to locate major vessels.

10.4 Laparoscopic Liver Transection with Linear Staplers

Patients are placed in the supine position or lithotomy position. Usually, three surgeons are used and four ports are made. The major surgeon stands on the patient's left side or stands between the patient's legs. Firstly, some perihepatic ligaments are divided with an ultrasonic dissector, bipolar cutter, or other energy devices. Then the transection line is marked on the liver's surface with the guidance of ultrasound or according to anatomical marks on the liver's surface. The liver capsule is divided with diathermy. In hemihepatectomies, the hepatic pedicle could be dissected and divided en bloc with a linear stapler before the liver transection. In the liver transection, vessels and hepatic dusts are located by ultrasound, then the liver parenchyma is fractured stepwise with a vascular clamp, and tunnels are created in the liver parenchyma free of major vessels and hepatic ducts. Jaws of a laparoscopic linear stapler are inserted into tunnels. The laparoscopic linear stapler is fired. The liver parenchyma, vessels, and hepatic ducts between the jaws are divided. This procedure is repeated until the transection is completed. After completing the transection, coagulation is applied to stop minor bleeding or bile oozing on the raw surface.

The laparoscopic linear stapler is useful for the transection of major portal branches and hepatic veins during laparoscopic major hepatectomy (Fig. 10.2). After the linear stapler is applied, staples could hinder the further hemostasis of the raw surface with electrocautery (Gumbs et al. 2008). Combined use of laparoscopic linear stapler and other dissecting devices and energy devices might improve the efficiency of liver transection.

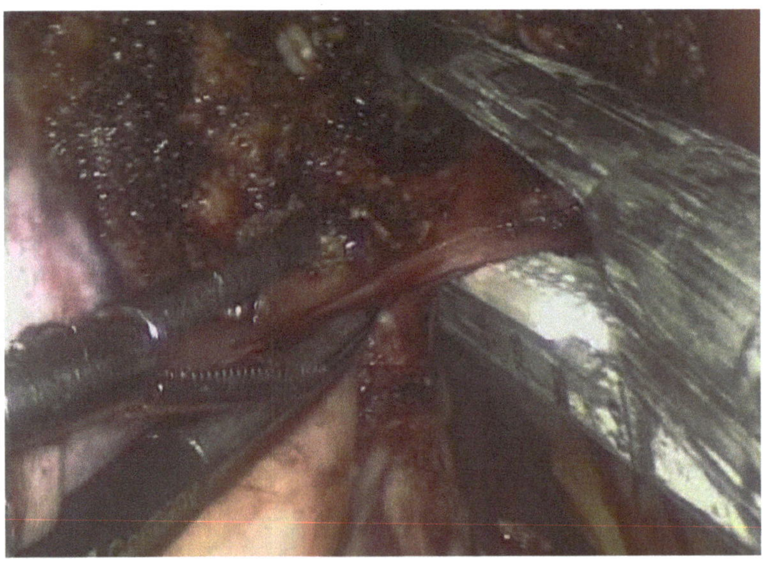

Fig. 10.2 The left hepatic pedicle is transected with a laparoscopic linear stapler

10.5 Laparoscopic Liver Transection with the Habib 4× Device

The Habib 4× consists of a 2×2 array of metallic needles arranged in a rectangle and uses bipolar radiofrequency energy to coagulate the liver parenchyma and vessels and bile ducts. Patients are usually placed in the supine position. Two surgeons are needed in the operation. The major surgeon stands on the patient's left side. Four ports are made. The observation port is placed under or above the umbilicus, and the major manipulation port is usually placed subxiphoidly. Some perihepatic ligaments are divided with energy devices. The lesion, major vessels, and bile ducts are located with ultrasound, and the transection line is marked on the liver surface with the guidance of ultrasound or according to anatomical marks on the liver surface. The Habib 4× is then inserted into the liver parenchyma free of major vessels and bile ducts and is activated to cause coagulative necrosis along the transection line (Fig. 10.3). The coagulated parenchyma is transected with a laparoscopic scissors after the radiofrequency coagulation was completed (Fig. 10.4). This procedure is repeated until the liver parenchyma is transected. Major vessels are dissected with dissection devices and are ligated or clipped followed by cutting (Zacharoulis et al. 2013).

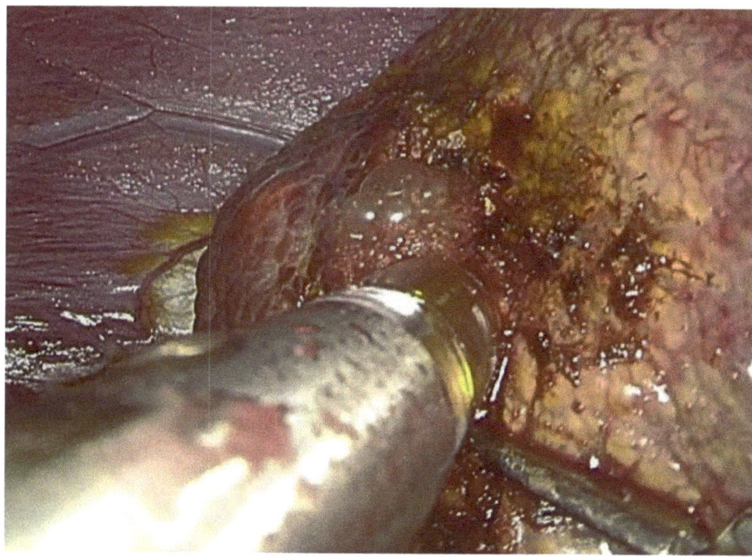

Fig. 10.3 Liver parenchyma is coagulated with the Habib 4×

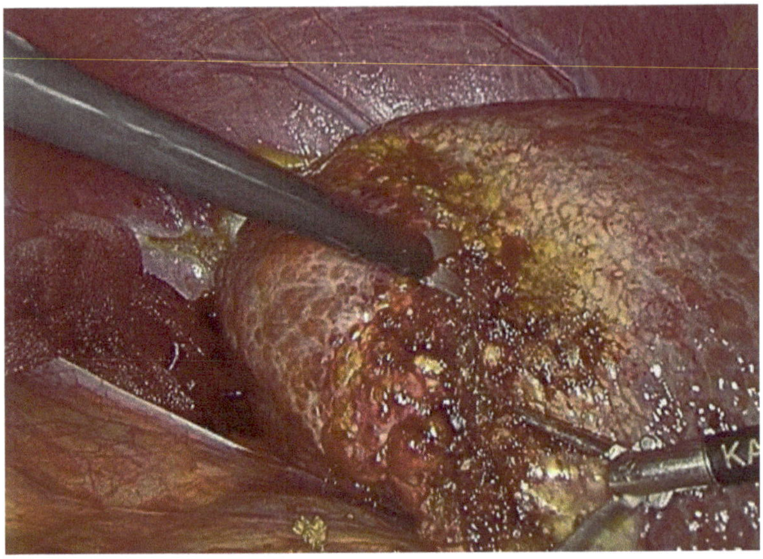

Fig. 10.4 The coagulated liver parenchyma is cut with a laparoscopic scissors

References

Aldrighetti L, Pulitanò C, Arru M, et al. Ultrasonic-mediated laparoscopic liver transection. Am J Surg. 2008;195:270–2.

Gumbs AA, Gayet B, Gagner M. Laparoscopic liver resection: when to use the laparoscopic stapler device. HPB (Oxford). 2008;10:296–303.

Honda G, Kurata M, Okuda Y, et al. Totally laparoscopic hepatectomy exposing the major vessels. J Hepatobiliary Pancreat Sci. 2013;20:435–40.

Slakey DP. Laparoscopic liver resection using a bipolar vessel-sealing device: LigaSure. HPB (Oxford). 2008;10:253–5.

Zacharoulis D, Sioka E, Tzovaras G, et al. Laparoscopic left lateral sectionectomy with the use of Habib 4x: technical aspects. J Laparoendosc Adv Surg Tech A. 2013;23:549–52.

Index

X. Cai, *Laparoscopic Hepatectomy: Atlas and Techniques*,
DOI 10.1007/978-94-017-9840-2,

FSC
www.fsc.org
MIX
Papier | Fördert gute Waldnutzung
FSC® C083411

Kolibri 360 GmbH
Ferdinand-Jühlke-Straße 7
99095 Erfurt, Deutschland
produktsicherheit@kolibri360.de